Computed Tomography of the Thorax

COMPUTED TOMOGRAPHY
of the
THORAX

David P. Naidich, M.D.
Assistant Professor
Department of Radiology
Bellevue Hospital
New York University Medical Center
New York, New York

Elias A. Zerhouni, M.D.
Associate Professor
Department of Radiology
De Paul Hospital
Eastern Virginia Medical School
Norfolk, Virginia

Stanley S. Siegelman, M.D.
Professor of Radiology
Director of Division of Diagnostic Radiology
Russell H. Morgan Department of
Radiology and Radiologic Science
The Johns Hopkins Medical Institutions
Baltimore, Maryland

Contributing Author
Rogelio Moncada, M.D.
Professor of Radiology
Foster G. McGaw Hospital
Loyola University of Chicago
Maywood, Illinois

Raven Press ▪ New York

Raven Press, 1140 Avenue of the Americas, New York, New York 10036

Made in the United States of America

The material contained in this volume was submitted as previously unpublished material, except in the instances in which credit has been given to the source from which some of the material was derived.

Great care has been taken to maintain the accuracy of the information contained in the volume. However, Raven Press cannot be held responsible for errors or for any consequences arising from the use of the information contained herein.

Library of Congress Cataloging in Publication Data

Naidich, David P.
    Computed tomography of the thorax.

    Includes bibliographical references and index.
    1. Chest—Radiography.   2. Tomography.   3. Chest—
Diseases—Diagnosis.   I. Zerhouni, Elias A.
II. Siegelman, Stanley S., 1932–   III. Title.
[DNLM: 1. Thoracic radiography.   2. Tomography, X-Ray
computed.   WF 975 N155c]
RC941.N27   1984   617′.5407572   82-42898
ISBN 0-89004-982-3

To Jocelyn and Zachary, and to my father, Harry, for his devoted contribution to the teaching of radiology

D.P.N.

To my wife, Nadia, and our children; to the memory of my father, Mohamed; and to the memory of my uncle, Djilali Rahmouni, formerly Professor of Radiology, University of Algiers, Algeria

E.A.Z.

To the memory of Charles Siegelman

S.S.S.

Preface

Diagnostic imaging has undergone a profound and astonishingly rapid transformation over the last decade, paralleling the rapid evolution of modern computer science. The first CT unit, conceived and developed by Godfrey Hounsfield, underwent initial clinical testing at theAtkinson Morley Hospital, Wimbledon, England, in 1971. This early scanner employed two sodium iodide crystals and produced an image based on an 80 × 80 matrix. The scan time of four and one half minutes effectively limited the machine to examination of intracranial pathology.

Within three years, Ledley developed a CT unit capable of imaging the body. In 1974 and 1975, whole body scanner prototypes were installed first at the Cleveland Clinic, and then at the Mallinckrodt Institute of Radiology, and the Mayo Clinic. Initial reports from these institutions were enthusiastic about the role of CT in the evaluation of the pancreas, liver, and retroperitoneum but pessimistic about the value of CT in the thorax.

Further improvements in instrumentation were necessary in order to assess the clinical role of thoracic CT. The pace of technological innovation was such that by 1977, scanners capable of scan times shorter than breath-holding had been developed. Additional improvements, including more detectors to increase resolution and finer collimation allowing a reduction in slice thickness to minimize partial volume averaging, soon became standard. As a result, initial pessimism about the role of CT in the thorax quickly gave way to considerable enthusiasm. This first became apparent as reports of the value of CT in analyzing mediastinal disease were published. Thereafter, an ever expanding range of uses for thoracic CT has evolved and continues to evolve.

In December 1977, a CT scanner was installed at the Johns Hopkins Hospital. At that time, Drs. Naidich and Zerhouni were residents under the tutelage of Dr. Siegelman, under whose auspices the three authors of this volume enthusiastically began a series of studies concerning the utility of thoracic CT in a wide range of clinical settings. In July 1980, Dr. Naidich joined the staff at New York University Medical Center, and in January 1981, Dr. Zerhouni moved to the East Virginia Medical Center. Despite this separation, the team continued their collaborative endeavours, and in 1982 and 1983, presented instruction courses in chest CT at the annual meeting of the American Roentgen Ray Society. From these presentations, the need for a volume representing the current status of thoracic CT became apparent.

This textbook has been organized primarily around the major anatomic subunits of the thorax. These include: the mediastinum, the airways, the hila, the pulmonary parenchyma, the pleura and chest wall, the pericardium, and the diaphragm. Additional chapters have been added specifically on the role of CT in evaluating lobar collapse and the pulmonary nodule, as these represent discrete topics best addressed apart. This organizational scheme represents the authors' views that CT is primarily an anatomic imaging modality. Specifically excluded from consideration is the use of CT in evaluating the heart. It is only appropriate to consider cardiac CT in comparison to other cardiac imaging modalities, including angiography, echocardiography, and nuclear cardiology. It is the authors' feeling that this is outside the intended scope of the present volume as initially conceived.

Thoracic CT has become an integral part of the daily practice of radiology. With the ever increasing number of diagnostic modalities, the task of deciding which diagnostic test is the most appropriate for a given clinical problem has become a significant part of medical practice. The authors believe that an adequate understanding of clinical issues is necessary for practicing radiologists to best help the referring physician. Consequently, throughout the text, a strong emphasis has been placed on discussing CT as it relates to clinical issues, especially as compared to other routine imaging modalities.

It is to be anticipated that further technologic advances in diagnostic imaging will further complicate the role of radiologists. It is hoped that this text will prove valuable in assisting this process.

D. P. Naidich
E. A. Zerhouni
S. S. Siegelman

Contents

---

* This chapter was written by Rogelio Moncada, M.D., Professor of Radiology, Foster G. McGaw Hospital, Loyola University of Chicago, Maywood, Illinois.

Acknowledgments

The preparation of this manuscript was aided by a large number of devoted friends at three separate institutions.

From New York University Medical Center, we wish to thank our technologists, Irene Cleary, Barbara Coakley, Bruce Foster, Ladislav Kamenar, Larry Mark, Robert Rabinowitsch, Rudi Rosa, John Sabellico, Roy Thompson, Thomas Tortorici, Raymond Tuthill, and Carolyn Tyson for their tireless cooperation in performing studies and constant re-loading and re-imaging of cases. Special thanks are owed to Herbert O'Brien and Daniel Rivera, supervisors extraordinaire. We also wish to express our thanks to Martha Helmers, whose photographic expertise has added considerably to the quality of this text.

From the Eastern Virginia Medical School, DePaul Hospital, we wish to express our appreciation to our technologists, Michele Newbold, Maureen Shirey, and Duane Stone for performing the studies. Rebecca Jennette, and, in particular, Nicky Liberty deserve credit for the countless deadlines they managed to keep in the preparation of manuscripts. John Keith, Thomas Xenakis, Robert Robinson, and Rachel Scott prepared the illustrations.

From the Johns Hopkins Medical Institutions, our gratitude to Pat McMillan for her patience in helping to co-ordinate this work, and to Henri Hessels for his photographic talents.

We would also like to acknowledge the valuable input of a large number of our colleagues: Nagi F. Khouri, M.D., Donald Hulnick, M.D., Mohamed Boukadoum, M.D., M. Ali Siddiky, M.D., Domingo Tan, M.D., and Lee Lampton, M.D., for the multiple forms of support they have provided during the preparation of this text. In particular, we would like to express our gratitude to Frederick P. Stitik, M.D., Chairman of the Department of Radiology, DePaul Hospital, Virginia, and Dorothy I. McCauley, Director of Thoracic Radiology, New York University Medical Center, for their advice, editing, constant support and endless patience in the preparation of each phase of this work.

Finally, special mention must be made of two Raven Press editors, namely, Anne Patterson, without whose inspiration this text would never have been written; and above all, Mary Rogers whose dedication, forebearance, and talents were a constant source of inspiration.

Chapter 1

Principles and Techniques of Chest Computed Tomography

The contribution of computed tomography (CT) to diagnostic imaging is based on two unique properties: (a) the capability of CT to differentiate much smaller differences in radiographic density than can conventional techniques by a factor of ten and (b) the method's transaxial imaging capability (1, 2).

Computed tomography was first applied to the head and abdomen, where improvement in contrast resolution was most needed because of inherently poor natural radiographic contrast in these areas. It was only after the development and wide distribution of CT machines with scan times shorter than breath holding times that thoracic CT began to be evaluated effectively. The naturally high contrast of thoracic structures provided by the aerated lungs has always made conventional techniques extremely effective in the evaluation of pulmonary pathology. The superior contrast resolution of CT is a less critical asset in the thorax, except when investigating the mediastinum or the CT density of pulmonary nodules.

The cross-sectional depiction of anatomy achieved by CT provides an additional dimension to conventional radiology and helps to clarify or detect suspected pathology in regions where overlapping structures prevent a full two-dimensional evaluation. This is particularly true in the subpleural, peridiaphragmatic, and perimediastinal areas (2–9).

Computed tomography is not a screening procedure. In the majority of cases, CT is called on for the further investigation or clarification of pathology already detected by conventional chest radiography. Abnormal mediastinal or hilar contours, complex pleural disease, and staging of carcinoma are a few examples (4). In a minority of cases, CT is primarily used to detect suspected but not demonstrated pathology. Specific instances are patients with normal chest X-ray films, but (a) abnormal sputum cytology and hence a possible bronchogenic cancer; (b) myasthenia gravis and thus a possible thymoma; (c) a primary malignancy with a propensity for pulmonary metastasis such as melanoma or osteosarcoma; and (d) clinical evidence of a parathyroid adenoma, but a negative neck exploration (10,11).

The problem-solving function of CT and the boundless variations of pathologic presentations make it necessary to tailor each CT examination to the particular diagnostic task. To that effect, the on-line intervention of the radiologist is required at all stages of the examination to (a) review the available radiological and clinical data to determine which components of the thoracic anatomy need to be clarified, (b) define the best strategy of examination for the case, and (c) modify the course of the study in light of evolving findings. The advent of image reconstruction times on the order of seconds has eased these tasks by permitting on-line reviewing of the CT examination before the patient is removed from the CT gantry.

Modern scanners have reached a stable and mature stage in their development. An array of once desirable functions has now become standard (12). The operations of a CT scanner are complex and highly automated, but several technical parameters remain operator-dependent.

Given the variety of clinical presentations and the expanding indications for thoracic CT, no single technique is optimal (13). The cardinal principle of "maximum diagnostic value for minimum risk and cost" is best served by understanding the correlation between the physics of CT and the various forms of pathology investigated.

Throughout this chapter, these correlations are stressed as we discuss the concepts underlying the choice of the most appropriate slice thickness and spacing, exposure factors, scan time, circle of reconstruction, image display, positioning, and method of contrast enhancement. Our goal is to integrate these factors into a coherent technical approach to thoracic CT.

SLICE THICKNESS

The CT image is the two-dimensional representation of a three-dimensional slice of space. The third dimension, or thickness of the cross section, is not displayed but does directly affect the quality of the image in the other two dimensions (1,14). All structures within a unit volume of space, or voxel, of the cross section are averaged and represented by a single CT number for the unit surface of the image, or pixel. For example, if a 5-mm spherical object in the lung is registered in a slice 10 mm thick, the attenuation values for each pixel displaying the object will be averaged with the attenuation values of 5 mm of adjacent lung parenchyma. The thicker the slice is, the more averaging of adjacent structures occurs, with a resultant loss of spatial resolution in the CT image. This phenomenon is termed partial volume averaging. To correct for this effect, CT scanners offer a choice of slice thicknesses, varying from 1 to 10 mm. Slice-thickness variance is achieved by placing collimators in front of the X-ray-generating tube to reduce beam width. However, narrowing the beam width decreases the number of sampling photons and increases image noise unless higher exposures are used. The constant trade-off between partial volume averaging and image noise is the most important technical consideration in slice-thickness selection. The correlation of this trade-off with the range of density in the body part examined or subject contrast, the orientation of the investigated anatomy relative to the scan plane,

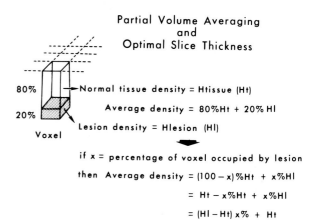

FIG. 1. The mathematics of partial volume effect. The basic equation governing CT density changes with different slice thicknesses and tissues is simple: the change in CT density of a voxel of normal tissue partially occupied by a lesion depends on the gradient of CT density between the lesion (Hl) and surrounding tissue (Ht) or (Hl − Ht) multiplied by the percentage (x) of the slice occupied by the lesion. Let us assume that the illustrated example is applied to the lungs: Ht measures −750 HU and a mass measuring +50 HU occupies 20% of the slice. The CT number change created by the mass will be equal to [50 − (−750)] × 20% = 160 HU. This lesion will be visualized, since current scanners can detect changes of 10 to 20 HU. In short, the larger is the density gradient between pathologic and normal tissues, the wider the CT slice can be.

and the size of the abnormalities to be demonstrated determines optimal slice thickness.

Partial Volume Averaging, Subject Contrast, and Optimal Slice Thickness

The detection of a lesion by CT depends on the density gradient between the lesion and the surrounding normal tissue. The larger is the density difference, the less pathologic tissue needs to be included in the slice to create a significant difference in CT number between lesion and normal tissue (Fig. 1).

In the low-density lung parenchyma, a large slice thickness is very advantageous because most pulmonary pathologic processes are of much higher density than normal lung. If only a small portion of such an abnormality is included in the slice, averaging of densities will be sufficient to make the abnormality visible. In the lung, nodules at the limit of resolution of a scanner (approximately 1 mm) can be seen with a 10-mm thick section (Figs. 2 and 4). Conversely, in the liver, for example, a lesion needs to be as large as the slice thickness to be detectable (Fig. 2).

There is another significant advantage in using large sections for the lungs: structures such as ves-

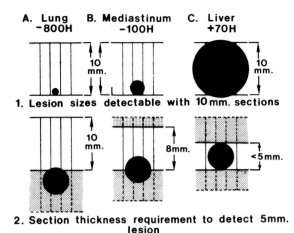

A. Lung **B. Mediastinum** **C. Liver**
-800H **-100H** **+70H**

1. Lesion sizes detectable with 10 mm. sections

2. Section thickness requirement to detect 5mm. lesion

FIG. 2. Correlations among slice thickness, tissue density, and lesion size. **1 (top):** Minimum size of lesions of average soft tissue density (50 HU) detectable with 10-mm section in (A) lung, of density of −800 HU—1 mm; (B) mediastinum with normal amount of fat, of density of −100 HU—3 mm; (C) liver of density of +70 HU—10 mm. **2 (bottom):** Maximum thickness of contiguous slices to detect a 5-mm lesion of density +50 HU in (A) lung—10 mm or more if available on scanner; (B) mediastinum—8 mm (with only half of the lesion in the slice, the density change will be 45 HU as per the equation in Fig. 1, and the lesion will be easily detected; if less than half of the lesion is included in a slice, the contiguous slice will contain more than half of the lesion, which will be detected); (C) liver—5 mm or less. The radiologist's choice of slice thickness should be determined by the density of the tissues investigated, as well as the size of the abnormality to be demonstrated.

sels that run obliquely to the plane of the scan are better appreciated using thick sections, which makes their differentiation from pathology easier (Figs. 3 and 4). In the mediastinum, when enough contrasting fat is present, 10-mm sections allow detection of lesions as small as 3 mm.

The radiologist should always estimate the minimum size of the lesions he or she wishes to demonstrate before determining slice thickness. Reliable detection of a 5-mm lesion of soft-tissue density can be achieved with a 10-mm section in the lungs, 8-mm section in a mediastinum with normal amounts of fat, and a section of 5 mm or less if the amount of fat is reduced (Fig. 2).

For structures of relatively equal density, optimal slice thickness will also depend on the orientation of these structures relative to the scan plane. Unless enough contrasting fat is present, thinner sections are required for adjacent structures oriented obliquely to the scan plane (Fig. 5). This is especially important with the hila and nearby large vessels.

Noise and Optimum Slice Thickness

Noise in CT is perceived by the human eye as a graininess in the image. Each step of the CT process introduces noise into the image (15). Noise degrades resolution and is in great part dependent on the dose of radiation used to generate the image. This is known as the "dose–noise-resolution trade-off" (16–21). The number of photons reaching any recording medium will vary from point to point solely on the basis of statistical variation. Noise increases when the total number of photons used to generate the image decreases because the relative variation at each point is increased. An analogy is useful in comprehending this phenomenon. A light rain will sprinkle the soil, giving it a spotty or "noisy" appearance. If the rain lasts long enough or

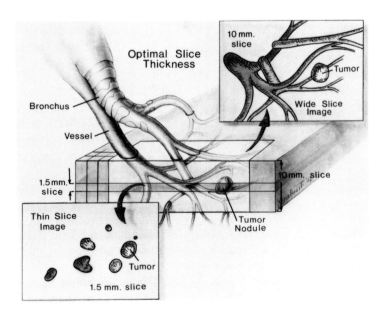

FIG. 3. Specific advantage of wide slices in lung. Tubular structures such as vessels running obliquely to the scan plane are included over a longer distance in a 10-mm slice than in a 1.5-mm slice. Vessels will be seen over much of their course in a wide slice image (upper right, inset) because they are of higher density than the surrounding lung. Bronchi will be recognized in their thicker parts only because they are not as different from the lung in density. Conversely, in a thin slice image (lower left, inset), vessels and bronchi appear round rather than tubular. A tumor nodule, as illustrated, is easier to recognize with thicker sections.

4a,b

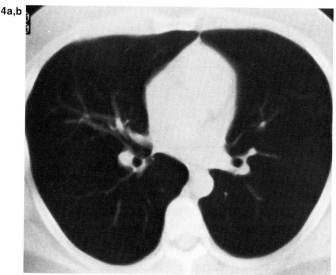
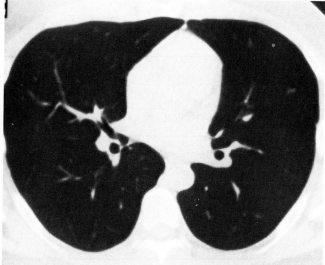

4c

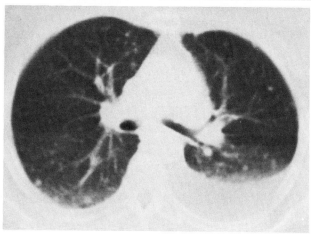

FIG. 4. Advantage of thick sections in recognition of metastatic nodules. **a:** Normal patient, 10-mm section. Vessels and bronchi are recognized as such even though they do not occupy the whole slice thickness, because partial volume averaging makes them visible and reveals their tubular shape. **b:** Same patient as in (a) (same anatomic level), 1.5-mm section. Vessels are more difficult to recognize. Several nodular images representing vessels in cross section are seen. (Compare with (c).) **c:** 59-year-old female with autopsy-proven metastatic breast carcinoma, 10-mm section. Numerous small metastatic deposits are seen, along with clearly identifiable vessels. Except for the larger metastases, it would have been difficult to recognize the pathology in a thinner section.

becomes heavy enough, no areas will be left dry, and thus a smoother, less "noisy" appearance results. In cases in which we have to decrease slice thickness to better visualize pathology, we should keep in mind that the number of photons is proportionally reduced. The resultant image is noisier, leading to a loss of resolution (Fig. 6). The expected advantage of thin slices due to the reduction in partial volume averaging may be lost if noise is not checked by an adequate increase in exposure time ("long, light rain") or intensity ("short, heavy rain"). For practical purposes, scan time or milliamperage needs to be increased when thinner sections are used if image quality is to be preserved (21–24). The degree of dose correction with thin slices depends on the natural contrast of the object scanned. In the lungs, where contrast differences are much larger than noise variations, diagnostic value is not significantly decreased by noise. In the mediastinum or chest wall, the attainment of low noise

levels is more important, especially when fat is lacking (25).

SLICE SPACING

The chest radiograph is the guide to proper slice spacing. When the size of the abnormality is larger than the slice thickness, interspacing of slices by one slice width will be adequate. All too often, contiguous slices are obtained regardless of pathologic presentation, which unnecessarily increases patient exposure, examination time, and maintenance costs. Contiguous spacing should be selected (a) if the expected pathology could conceivably be smaller than the slice thickness (examples are searches for occult metastases or for occult primary carcinoma), (b) to better define areas of complex anatomy such as the hilum, and (c) in selected areas of significant pathology.

Scanner-generated digital images of the area to be

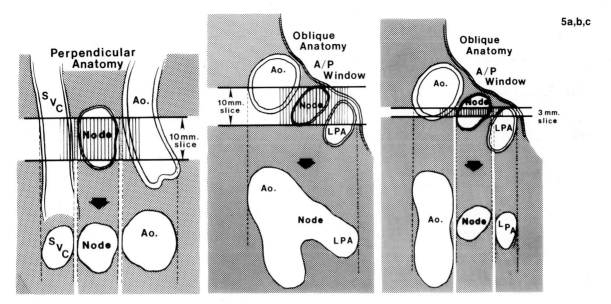

FIG. 5. Anatomic orientation and optimal slice thickness. **a:** Coronal representation (top) of space between superior vena cava (SVC) and ascending aorta (Ao). These structures are usually perpendicular to the scan plane. The node will be seen even with thick sections, provided a minimum amount of contrasting fat is present. Pixels containing only fat allow separation of SVC, Ao, and node in the resultant CT image (bottom). **b:** Coronal representation (top) of aorto-pulmonary window (A/P). The node between the arch of the aorta (Ao) and the left pulmonary artery (LPA) cannot be separated in the CT image (bottom) because the oblique orientation of the anatomy relative to the slice prevents having pixels containing fat only. **c:** When the slice width is reduced, the node becomes visible as a distinct structure. To select proper slice thickness, the radiologist should take into account the orientation as well as the contrast and size of the abnormality he wishes to investigate.

examined (scout view, scanogram, etc.) facilitate the programming of slice spacing. Such views obtained with the patient in scanning position decrease the number of unnecessary scans, and their use is encouraged.

EXPOSURE FACTORS

Proper exposure factors in CT are determined by the need for an adequate photon flux to the detectors (21,25). Optimally, the intensity and energy of the beam should fall within the most efficient part of the dynamic range of the detectors.

On most CT scanners, operating kilovoltages are limited to one or two values because detector performance and image reconstruction processes are heavily dependent on the spectral energy of the incident beam. The advantages of a higher or lower kilovolt potential in clinical experience have not yet been investigated fully. Manufacturers' recommendations should therefore be followed.

Milliamperage, scan time, and number of beam pulses per unit of time are the variables accessible to the radiologist. Photon flux is affected by the transmission characteristics of the object scanned. Large patients require more exposure than small or thin ones so that an adequate amount of information

is transmitted to the detectors. The thorax is not as dense as the head or abdomen, and lower exposure factors should generally be used.

It should be remembered that CT images are digitalized and easily manipulated by the viewer. Overexposure is therefore difficult to detect with CT, as opposed to standard radiography in which image quality cannot be artificially corrected. All too often, none of the necessary corrections for chest CT are implemented. The radiologist should make a point of verifying exposure factors in the thorax to ensure minimal patient exposure, as well as minimal tube heat loading.

On most scanners, good-quality CT scans of the thorax can be obtained at 150 to 250 mAs with 10-mm slice sections. Appropriately reduced exposure factors increase X-ray-generating tube life and decrease operational costs.

SCAN TIME

Short scan times are necessary in chest CT to reduce the effect of respiratory motion (26–28). Scanners that can acquire data in a reasonable breath holding period are now widely available.

Although short scan times improve image quality by reducing the deleterious effect of physiologic

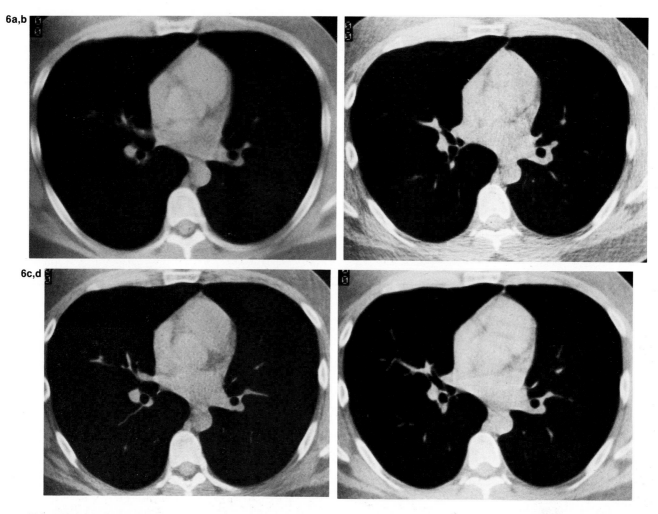

FIG. 6. Noise and slice thickness. **a:** 10-mm section at 160 mAs. **b:** 1.5-mm section at 80 mAs. **c:** 1.5-mm section at 160 mAs. **d:** 1.5-mm section at 384 mAs. All these sections are from the same patient. Noise is best appreciated in (b), at the lowest exposure. Heart and chest wall are the most affected because their natural contrast is lower than that of the lungs. (a) and (c) demonstrate the increase in noise when a thinner section is used without changing exposure levels. (d) shows restoration of image quality due to the larger number of photons used. With thin sections, spatial resolution is higher, as demonstrated by the sharper edges of anatomic structures in (c) and (d); however, noise can cancel this advantage, especially in lower-contrast structures such as the mediastinum, as shown in (b).

motion, it is important to remember that extremely short scan times (1 to 4 sec) are most often achieved by reducing the number of projections used to reconstruct the image. This is usually done by decreasing the angular rotation of the X-ray tube. Since the accuracy of the reconstructed image depends on the number of projections used, a certain loss of resolution occurs with shorter scan times. The reduction in the amount of data used to reconstruct the image is not fully correctable by using a higher photon flux, i.e., by increasing the beam intensity or milliamperage. Thus, we do not recommend the systematic use of the shortest scan time available on current scanners. Scan times shorter than 5 sec are not of significantly higher quality (26).

The great majority of patients can sustain breath holding periods of up to 10 sec if they are instructed properly before scanning. A few minutes of pre-scanning breathing instruction are very rewarding in terms of study quality. In our department, all patients are asked to rehearse the instructions they will have to follow during the examination. Very short scan times are selected only if it is apparent that longer breath holding may be a problem in a given patient.

In most centers, scanning of the thorax is performed at full lung capacity (end-inspiratory volume) (7). This is the most common way of suspending respiration. The instructions are simple: "Take a deep breath and hold it." Full inspiration also reduces the crowding of vascular structures.

However, the reproducibility of inspiratory breathing may be less reliable than breathing at resting lung volume (end-tidal volume). If we are concerned about the reproducibility of lung position, we prefer to scan the patient at resting lung volume. The instructions in this case are: "Breathe in . . . breathe out . . . relax and hold it." Lack of breathing reproducibility can sometimes create significant problems, such as the total miss of a known pulmonary nodule (29). Devices to control breathing have been developed, but have not yet been proven to be of definite clinical value (30).

CIRCLE OF RECONSTRUCTION

The CT image is the pictorial representation of a matrix of CT numbers (14). Matrices of 256 × 256, 320 × 320, and 512 × 512 rows and columns are the most frequently encountered. Each element of the matrix, or pixel, represents a small volume of space, or voxel. The matrix is the mathematical support of the computer calculations representing the space examined within the aperture of the scanner (1).

The portion of the space represented by an individual pixel will depend on the size of the circle examined, as indicated to the computer by the operator. This circle is called the circle of reconstruction or field of view. Current scanners offer a selection of different circle sizes in order to allow an optimal fit between the body part examined and the circle of reconstruction. This permits the full use of the computing capacity of the system.

Ideally, a pixel should be much smaller than the minimal distance resolvable by the scanner, currently varying between 0.6 and 1 mm. Current limits

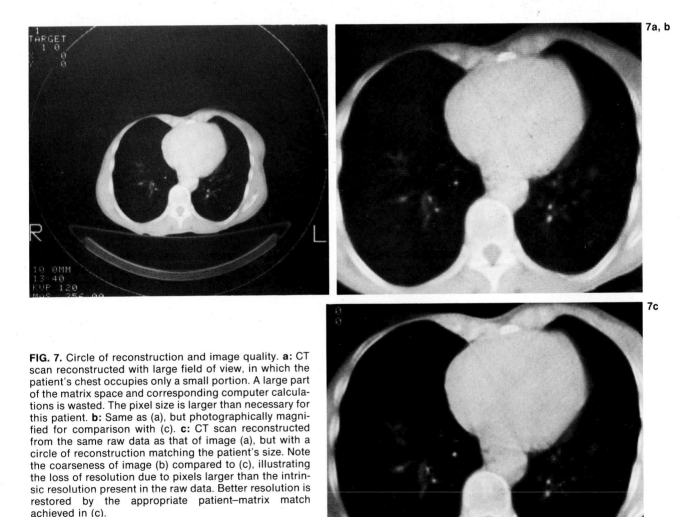

7a, b

7c

FIG. 7. Circle of reconstruction and image quality. **a:** CT scan reconstructed with large field of view, in which the patient's chest occupies only a small portion. A large part of the matrix space and corresponding computer calculations is wasted. The pixel size is larger than necessary for this patient. **b:** Same as (a), but photographically magnified for comparison with (c). **c:** CT scan reconstructed from the same raw data as that of image (a), but with a circle of reconstruction matching the patient's size. Note the coarseness of image (b) compared to (c), illustrating the loss of resolution due to pixels larger than the intrinsic resolution present in the raw data. Better resolution is restored by the appropriate patient–matrix match achieved in (c).

on computing capacity make very fine matrices impractical, since an increase in the number of pixels increases the amount of calculations necessary. With larger circles of reconstruction, pixel size can be larger than the 0.6- to 1-mm resolution of current scanners. For example, a patient measuring 42 cm in diameter and represented by a 320 × 320 matrix will be imaged with pixels measuring 1.3 × 1.3 mm. (This value is obtained by dividing the diameter of the circle of reconstruction, 420 mm, by the number of pixels in one row of the matrix, 320 in this case.)

To correct for this resolution loss, modern scanners offer the possibility of reconstructing, from the raw data, selected areas of the object scanned in order to reduce the pixel size to optimal values. This is sometimes called "zooming" or "targeting." It is often stated that this maneuver improves resolution, when, in fact, it only restores resolution otherwise lost with large circles of reconstruction. The spatial resolution of the scanner is essentially determined by the sampling frequency at the detectors and cannot be improved by computer manipula-

tions. However, resolution and image quality can certainly be degraded if the radiologist does not ensure that the smallest circle of reconstruction is selected to achieve a proper patient–matrix match. Too large a circle of reconstruction results in a waste of matrix space, a loss of resolution, and poor images (Fig. 7).

PATIENT POSITIONING

Scanning in positions other than the supine is most useful in patients with pleural or parenchymal fluid collections. In these patients, the question of whether additional positions could improve the diagnostic value of the ongoing examination should be constantly weighed as the study evolves. The effect of gravity may help in differentiating loculated from free effusion, and pulmonary edema from other causes of infiltrates (31). Displacement of fluids by the use of lateral decubitus or prone positioning can help define any underlying pathology (Fig. 8).

8a, b

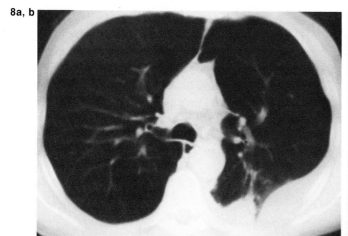 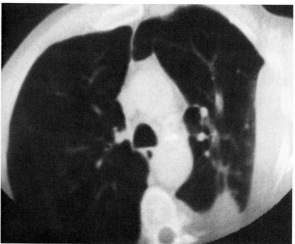

8c

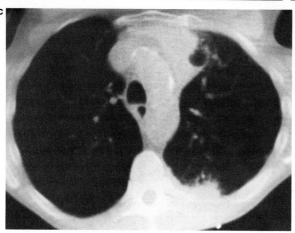

FIG. 8. Pleural effusions and gravity. Scans of a 67-year-old male with biopsy-proven adenocarcinoma (posterior segment, left upper lobe). **a:** Supine position: the tumor is located medially. Fluid with smooth margins is located laterally. In this position, it is difficult to separate mass from fluid. **b:** Left lateral decubitus (illustrated to correspond with (a)): the effusion has moved against left lateral chest wall. **c:** Prone position (illustrated to correspond with (a)): the effusion is now anteriorly located against the aorta. The tumor and its extent are better appreciated.

In the supine position, lung water may normally accumulate in the posterior dependent portions of the lung, rendering the vessels more prominent as well as increasing lung density. This water accumulation may lead one to suspect pulmonary nodules or infiltrates in those regions. The problem is best solved by placing the patient in a different position, usually prone, and repeating scans in the same area. Dependent lung water should shift to the anterior portions of the lungs.

In a few cooperative patients, the same problem can also be solved by scanning after deep inspiration, in which case lung density decreases and vessels appear less prominent, thereby allowing the radiologist to exclude infiltrates or nodules.

The pulsation of arterial vessels creates star-like artifacts, which are not present around nodules. This pulsation artifact, termed the "twinkling star sign," can sometimes help differentiate vessels from nodules, without having to resort to positional changes (32).

GANTRY ANGLE

Chest scanning is usually performed with the gantry in the vertical plane and the patient horizontal. Table tilt and gantry tilt capabilities are now widely available, and angles other than the vertical can be used for scanning. In a few selected cases, angled scanning can help sort out complex anatomy. In our experience, angle scanning has been helpful in the hilar regions, the aorto-pulmonary window, and the mediastinum near the base of the heart. In these cases, we attempt to obtain a scan angle almost perpendicular to the structures examined (Fig. 5). The question of whether angles other than the vertical would be most appropriate for thoracic CT has not been resolved. At this point, we suggest the use of angled scanning only as an adjunctive technique in difficult cases.

CONTRAST ENHANCEMENT

In most radiology departments, the CT section has become a major dispensing center for contrast agents. By definition, contrast agents are the means by which we can increase subject contrast to bring it within the detection range of a particular imaging system. The thorax is the body part with the highest natural contrast. Ribs and vessels are of markedly different density than the surrounding aerated lungs. Mediastinal structures are embedded in usually sufficient amounts of fat. In thoracic CT, therefore, the role of contrast agents is limited.

Knowledge of mediastinal and hilar anatomy is generally sufficient to determine whether a particular structure is abnormal. Contrast enhancement is necessary in the minority of cases in which mediastinal fat is lacking or a vascular abnormality is suspected, and is potentially useful in patients with complex pleuro-parenchymal pathology. (See Chapter 9.)

A brief review of the physiology of intravenous contrast distribution in the body is helpful in defining sensible strategies of contrast agent utilization.

First and foremost, a clear distinction should be made between contrast enhancement in the brain and contrast enhancement in the body. The vascular compartment of the brain is not permeable to intravascular contrast agents when the blood–brain barrier is intact (33). The depiction of the vascular compartment can therefore be easily achieved in the brain, provided enough iodine molecules are present in the vascular space for contrast against the normally iodine-free brain. In the body, however, the vascular compartment is freely permeable to contrast medium molecules (34–36). Rapid passage of contrast from the intravascular space into the extracellular, extravascular space occurs within seconds (36–38). Very shortly after injection (1 to 2 min), the majority of iodine molecules will be distributed in the extravascular space of tissue rather than in vessels (34,38) (Fig. 9). In the body, therefore, the differentiation of a lesion from its surrounding structures depends on several factors: (a) its vascularity, (b) the relative size of its extravascular space compared to normal tissue, (c) the permeability of its vascular space, which determines the rate of contrast agent exchange between intra- and extravascular compartments, (d) the amount of contrast agent injected, (e) the time elapsed following the end of contrast medium injection, and (f) renal excretion.

Understanding the dynamics of contrast medium distribution over time has major implications for the technique of contrast enhancement in the chest (39–41). For example, a bolus injection will provide sufficient vascular characterization only for the first few scans after injection, with progressively decreasing differentiation thereafter. Nonvascular structures such as nodes and masses can also progressively increase in density over time, depending on the amount of extravascular space and the permeability of the intravascular space (Fig. 9). On occasion, we have observed nonvascular masses becoming as dense as nearby vascular structures (Fig. 10). Serious error can result, since the determination of the vascular nature of an abnormality is

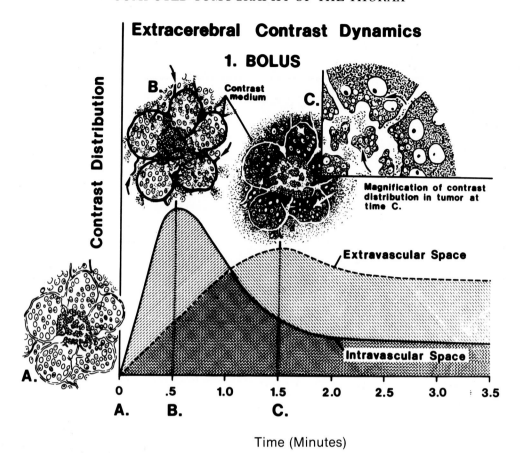

FIG. 9. Relationships of contrast distribution with time and CT appearance of lesions after bolus injection. A hypothetical tumor is graphically represented at three separate moments after a bolus injection. **A:** 0 sec. The hypothetical tumor, hypervascular with large and irregular vessels, is composed of small and tightly packed cells. Normal tissue, with fewer cells per unit of space and normal vessels, surrounds the tumor. Vessel walls are discontinuous, to indicate their normal permeability to contrast molecules. **B:** 30 sec. As indicated by the curves, most of the contrast is still intravascular at time (B). A small amount of contrast medium is already extravascular (small dots). The tumor appears denser than the surrounding normal tissue because it has a larger vascular bed. **C:** 90 sec. With the rapid redistribution known to occur in extracerebral tissues, most of the contrast medium is in the extravascular space at time (C). Because the tumor has tightly packed cells, its extravascular space is smaller than that in normal tissue (magnified view, inset). Relatively fewer contrast molecules are in the tumor, which therefore appears less dense. In the body, the best vascular differentiation occurs very early after bolus injection. The radiologist should keep in mind the complexity of contrast physiology when he or she reads CT images. CT contrast enhancement is fundamentally different from angiographic enhancement after the first few seconds following contrast administration.

usually made by comparing the density of a known vessel with that of the abnormality.

Continuous infusions of contrast medium have become more popular because a more constant intravascular contrast level can be maintained for the longer periods of time needed to complete scanning. The main drawbacks of this technique are the use of a higher total amount of contrast medium and the occurrence of a lower level of vascular enhancement than that in bolus injection methods.

The combination of a bolus injection of contrast medium followed by a rapid infusion can give more satisfactory results (Fig. 11). It is evident that with continuous methods of infusion contrast is administered at a time when no information is acquired, i.e., in the time interval between scans. Rapid se-

quential scanning can reduce the amount of contrast agent needed, especially if only a few scans in one given area are necessary. (See section on Dynamic Scanning following.)

An ideal method of contrast medium delivery for the mediastinum should provide a high level of vascular enhancement at the time of scanning, and only at that time (41). A working knowledge of the transit times of the intravenous bolus in the various vascular structures of the chest greatly helps in the timing of bolus injections and scans.

To define the range of transit times for thoracic vascular structures, we studied 35 consecutive patients referred for nuclear bone scanning, as follows: 20 mCi of technetium-99m methylene diphosphonate were diluted in 10 cc of normal saline

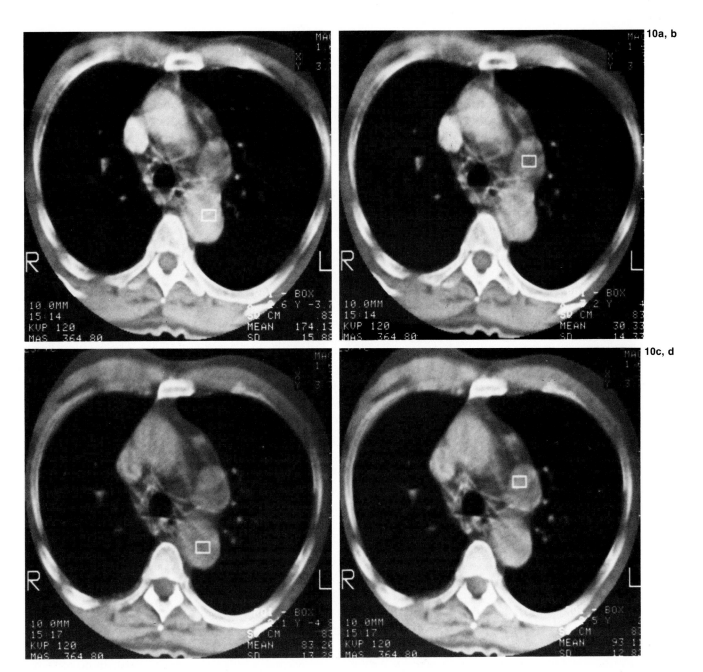

FIG. 10. a, b: Same section, at the level of the aortico-pulmonary window, immediately following a bolus of contrast agent (note time reference in the lower left corner—15:14). The descending aorta has a mean density of 174 HU; the well-defined mass in the aortico-pulmonary window has a mean density of 30 HU. **c, d:** Same section, at the same level as in (a) and (b), obtained 3 min later (note time reference in lower left corner—15:17). There has been a decrease in the density of contrast medium within the descending aorta, which now measures 83 HU [compare with (a)]. However, there has been a substantial increase in the density of the mass, which now measures 93 HU [compare with (b)]. The marked increase in density within this mass suggested the erroneous diagnosis of a saccular aneurysm of the undersurface of the aortic arch. This patient had known small cell carcinoma involving the left hilum. Following chemotherapy, a repeat scan showed total disappearance of the mass in the aortico-pulmonary window, confirming this mass to be mediastinal adenopathy. Density within masses is a function of the total dose of contrast agent, the vascularity of a lesion and the relative size of its extravascular space compared to normal tissue, the permeability of the capillaries within the mass, and the time elapsed from the end of the contrast medium injection. (Case courtesy of Dr. Norman Ettinger, New York University Medical Center, Manhattan VA Hospital.)

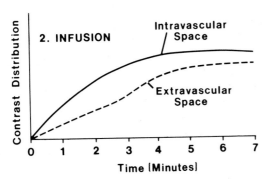

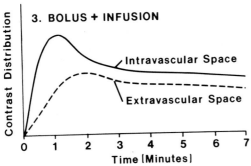

FIG. 11. Comparison of infusion of contrast medium versus bolus followed by infusion. Compare this figure with Fig. 9. Infusion maintains a slightly higher level of intravascular contrast medium for a longer period of time than does bolus injection. A combination of bolus followed by infusion provides a higher vascular differentiation initially. Larger amounts of contrast medium with lower differences in density between vessels and tissues are the most significant disadvantages of the technique.

TABLE 1. *Average thoracic transit times[a]*

	Bolus in (sec)	Bolus out (sec)
Superior vena cava	3.7 ± 1.5	9.0 ± 2.5
Pulmonary arteries	6.5 ± 2.5	10.0 ± 3.0
Ascending aorta	10.5 ± 3.0	17.8 ± 3.5
Descending aorta and neck vessels	12.3 ± 3.8	19.4 ± 3.8
Jugular vein	17.8 ± 5.0	27.0 ± 5.0
Inferior vena cava	16.0 ± 5.5	ND

[a] 2-sec i.v. bolus of 10 cc total volume in antecubital vein. Data were obtained by measuring transit times with a gamma camera set at one image per second from start of an injection of 20 mCi of technetium-99m methylene diphosphonate. The data of 35 consecutive patients of ages varying between 19 and 72 years were averaged. These average times should be taken into consideration when setting up dynamic scan programs or when obtaining individual scans of particular areas. Scans should start at the time of bolus arrival in the structures investigated. ND, not done.

solution and injected in an antecubital vein at the rate of 5 cc/sec. Gamma-camera images of the thorax in anteroposterior view were obtained at the rate of one image per second starting with the injection. Average times of bolus arrival and departure in the major vascular structures and standard deviations were calculated (Table 1). The ages of subjects ranged from 19 to 72 years. No attempt was made to define the cardiovascular status of the patients tested. The values in Table 1 represent a nonselected consecutive series.

The data on transit times are most useful when (a) a high level of enhancement is sought in more than one area of the thorax, (b) dynamic scanning cannot be used because it would require breath holding periods above the patient's capacity, and (c) selective enhancement of pulmonary arteries, veins, and/or aorta is needed.

In such cases, we use a technique of intermittent bolus injections. Instead of injecting a large bolus continuously, the dose of contrast medium is fractionated. Each scan is timed to ensure visualization of the investigated structures by taking into account the proper transit times (Table 1). No contrast agent is injected during the interscan times, when no information is acquired. Using this technique, high-quality studies can be achieved with reduced total amounts of contrast medium; a rate of injection of 4–5 cc/sec is usually adequate. Purely intravascular agents, without extravascular distribution, are in the early stages of development (42).

DYNAMIC SCANNING

Dynamic scanning can be defined simply as the ability to acquire several scans in a limited period of time. It has two major applications. The first is in the study of the vascularity of a lesion or structure at a single level during a contrast bolus transit (41). This application has been called "CT angiography" (42,43). The second use of dynamic scanning is in the acquisition of scans at different levels within a short period of time, either in an uncooperative patient to decrease sedation time or for study of the vascularity of a general area during an extended bolus injection of contrast medium. The latter has been called "dynamic incremental scanning" (44–47). In the thorax, dynamic scanning is best applied in the study of major vessels; aortic dissection is the prime example (48–50).

The number of scans obtainable with dynamic scanning is limited by the heat capacity of the X-ray tube, as well as the breath holding capacity of the patient. The shortest interval of time for the examination is limited to the scan time, plus the time needed between scans for table motion and/or information handling. To bridge the time gap between scans, certain machines have computer programs that can reconstruct several images, based on the data obtained from two successive scans at the same level, by using complementary sets of projections from both scans. To set optimal dynamic scan programs for the chest, the average time of arrival, peak, and end of the intravenously injected bolus should be taken into account (Table 1). If the number of scans needed cannot be obtained in either one breath holding period or one sequence because of exceeded tube heat capacity, we would recommend temporarily stopping the injection of contrast medium between scans to decrease total contrast medium dose. Automatic contrast agent injectors for CT applications may have a role in dynamic scanning (48).

INFORMATION DISPLAY

The full scale of CT numbers generated by the CT reconstruction process cannot be displayed in a single image because current electronic display systems utilize a limited number of gray shades, usually 16. The operator has to select the portion of the CT number range he or she wishes to display. This is done by using electronic windows and defining the width and level at which the window will be active. The range of CT numbers present in the thorax is the greatest of those for all body parts; it extends from the almost air density of the lungs to the high density of the bones. In thoracic CT, window widths of up to 2,000 Hounsfield units (HU) are therefore necessary and have become standard on recent scanners. Each thoracic CT examination should be viewed with at least two, and optimally three, sets of window settings: one for the lungs, one for the mediastinum and chest wall, and one for the bony structures whenever needed. The precise settings are often a matter of subjective preference, but guidelines can be used. The window width should be set at twice the CT number range of the organ examined. For example, in the lungs, if the lowest density is − 840 HU and the maximum density is + 60 HU (a pulmonary vessel, for instance), a window width of (840 + 60) × 2, or 1,800 HU, will be appropriate. In the mediastinum, fat may measure − 100 HU and the highest density may reach + 100 HU. Therefore, a window width of 400 HU will be satisfactory in most cases. A narrow window width is usually not necessary in the thorax because

of the high natural contrast present. The inaccuracies of CT number determination being always more than ± 10 HU, window widths of less than 160 HU (10 HU for each shade of gray) are unnecessary. The window level should be chosen according to the particular range of densities in the area of interest, usually near the midpoint of that range. The window level affects the size estimation of a structure, particularly in high-contrast body parts such as the lungs. If accurate size measurements are sought, the window level should be placed at a midpoint between the average CT number of the structure to be measured and the average CT number of the surrounding tissue (51,52). For example, the size of a pulmonary nodule measuring 150 HU in lungs that measure − 750 HU will be most accurate at a window level of − 300 HU.

CONSOLE VERSUS HARD-COPY FILM INTERPRETATION

Given the number of window settings at which an examination can be analyzed, we believe that interpretation at the display monitor is preferable to hard-copy interpretation. If interpretation at the console is not possible, hard copies of thoracic examinations should be obtained with at least two sets of window settings: lung settings and mediastinal settings. Hard copies of the examinations are the only practical, long-term records of an examination. Special care should be taken to ensure consistent quality of hard-copy films. Regular densitometric controls are mandatory. Attention to the quality of the cathode ray tube used for generating films is also important (53,54).

MULTIPLANAR RECONSTRUCTION

Coronal, sagittal, and oblique sections can be generated from the data of a series of consecutive axial scans. This rearrangement achieved by computer manipulations can be useful in regions of complex anatomy, such as the hilar and peridiaphragmatic areas (Fig. 12). Multiplanar reconstruction is time-consuming, and experienced interpreters of CT images do not use it often because they can visually reconstruct three-dimensional anatomy by mentally integrating successive CT slices. However, multiplanar reconstructions are helpful in conveying this three-dimensional information to less experienced observers, and sometimes to convince clinicians of the reality of significant but subtle find-

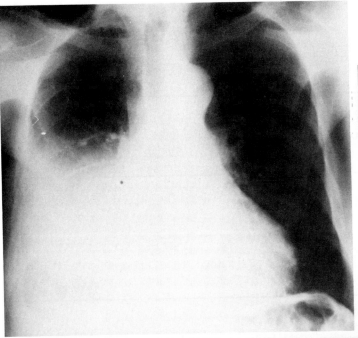

12a, b

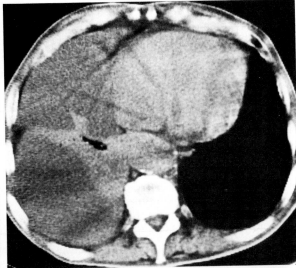

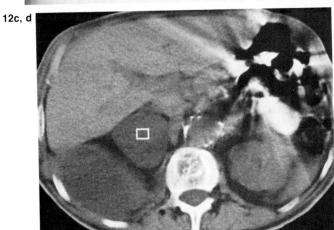

12c, d

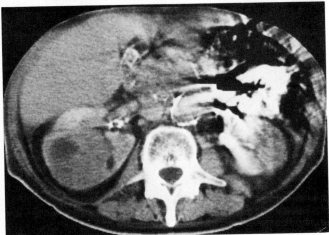

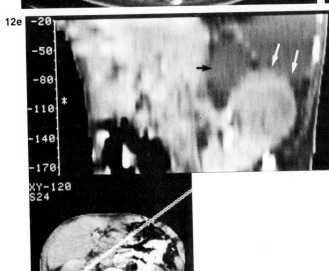

12e

FIG. 12. Multiplanar reconstruction. **a:** PA radiograph shows large right pleural effusion with associated loss of volume in the right lower lobe. **b:** Section through the right lung base shows a large partially loculated pleural fluid collection and collapse of the right lower lobe. **c:** Section through the upper abdomen. Two discrete fluid collections are present in the right side. The exact position of the right hemidiaphragm is uncertain. **d:** Section through the upper pole of the right kidney; there is a large, necrotic mass in the upper pole. **e:** Parasagittal reconstruction through the right side of the chest and abdomen. There is a large pleural fluid collection, inverting the posterior portion of the right hemidiaphragm (white arrows). Additionally, there is a benign renal cyst off the anterior aspect of the upper pole of the kidney (arrow), as well as a necrotic tumor mass in the upper pole. The two fluid collections seen in (c) are clarified by use of this parasagittal reconstruction.

ings made on axial images. Direct coronal CT achieved by placing patients upright in the gantry provides higher-quality images than do computer reconstructions (55).

CT-GUIDED NEEDLE BIOPSY

Biplane fluoroscopic guidance is still the method of choice in thoracic biopsies (56–58). Fluoroscopy allows real-time visualization of the lesion and control of the needle tip at the moment of biopsy. CT is more cumbersome and time-consuming. The needle tip cannot be visually controlled during the biopsy proper.

Computed tomography is mostly used as an adjunct to fluoroscopy to determine the best approach by demonstrating the relationship of vital structures to the lesion, to visualize the relationship of a mass to the fissures in order to avoid puncturing through the fissures, to help avoid bullous changes near lesions, and to indicate the depth of a lesion visible on only one fluoroscopic plane (59,60). CT guidance is used when the lesion cannot be visualized by fluoroscopy because of its location (mediastinal, hilar, and perimediastinal areas, lung apex and near the diaphragm) or if it is very near vital structures.

Particular techniques of biopsy vary with the individual radiologist. A number of key factors should, however, be kept in mind. First, the pleura should not be punctured more than three or four times per procedure. Second, manipulation of the needle should always be done with the patient holding his breath to avoid pleural tears. Third, the patient should be instructed to breathe in a reproducible manner throughout the procedure to avoid respiratory shifts in lesion position. Fourth, since the needle tip cannot be seen during the biopsy itself, it is important that the operator maintain the angles of approach to the lesion during sampling. This is best done by selecting simple angles, such as the vertical or horizontal approaches, and by having aides visually check that the operator is not shifting position.

Technique

Once the best approach is selected, the patient is placed in the appropriate position in the gantry. Supine or prone positioning is preferred because it is more stable and comfortable for the patient. Radiopaque catheters are placed on the skin as markers for measuring angles and determining point of entry. The patient is then scanned and the point of entry is determined on the CT image. The angle from the point of entry to the lesion is mea-

sured. If at all possible, a vertical or horizontal approach is preferred. The measured angle is cut in cardboard. An aide will hold the cardboard during the biopsy to help maintain the appropriate angle of approach. We always use the plane parallel to the scan plane for introducing the needle. If this cannot be done because of intervening ribs, the gantry or the table is tilted to the same degree as the needle. The needle is then advanced at increments of 2 to 3 cm at suspended respiration. Between each advance, a scan of the needle is obtained. Before the scan, the stylet is removed and the needle is obturated with a plastic hub to avoid streak artifacts. To reduce the number of pleural punctures, we try to achieve the proper needle angulation within the chest wall of the patient and before reaching the pleura. In thin patients in whom it is difficult to stabilize the needle in the soft tissues, we first position a shorter, larger-gauge needle, through which our biopsy needle is subsequently passed. The short needle is left in place, thus reducing the number of maneuvers for subsequent passes.

It is important to verify that the scans used include the tip of the needle. If in doubt, scans at slightly different levels should be obtained. Alternatively, the position of the tip of the needle may be estimated on a repeat scanogram, from which the exact level for a transaxial section may be determined.

Short thrusts are used to sample the lesion. To avoid repeating the procedure, specimens are immediately checked by a cytopathologist to determine if good samples were obtained before the patient is removed from the gantry.

EFFICIENT OPERATION OF THE CT SUITE

With the increasing demand for CT services, as well as regulatory limits on CT scanner acquisition and the level of expenses involved, skills that help accommodate large patient loads are useful to the CT radiologist.

With improvements in scan and image reconstruction times, the limiting factors in CT efficiency are no longer technical; they are human. This is compounded by the fact that most scanners are used for head and body applications, as well as for inpatients and outpatients simultaneously. The efficiency of the CT unit is not determined by what happens in the CT suite proper, but by the apparently extraneous factors of patient scheduling, patient handling, and pre-examination planning. The creation of a scheduling grid that takes into account preparation times for the different types of studies is recommended.

The quality of the escort service has an extremely important impact on the efficiency of the CT unit. If escort time cannot be predicted by the CT technologist, significant problems may occur. There will be occasions when no patients will be available for scanning and times when two or three patients may be escorted to the suite simultaneously. In our experience, we have found that the best solution was the creation of a position of "patient handling aide" in the CT suite, a person who has direct control over escort activities. The aide can rapidly become acquainted with the technical requirements of CT scanning, and can start preparing patients on the floors (by bringing contrast solutions to them, for example). The aide frees the technologist from patient handling and from supervision duties outside the scanner room. In a busy department, the creation of an aide position is fully justified. In less busy departments, a clear understanding with the escort service about scheduling CT priorities is very helpful.

Good pre-examination planning remains, however, the most important determinant of CT efficiency. Clear instructions for each study should be given to the technologist before the patient is scanned. All too often, the patient is placed on the table and time is lost in waiting for the radiologist to decide his or her approach. Film jackets and charts should be made available to the radiologist on a systematic basis to help plan the examinations.

SUMMARY AND RECOMMENDATIONS

After reviewing the patient data and defining the role of the CT examination in the evaluation of the particular patient, an estimation of breath holding capacity of the patient should be obtained. Before the patient enters the scanning room, the breathing instructions are explained. Scan time should not be systematically the shortest available for a particular scanner, because very short scan times are usually obtained by decreasing the amount of information collected. Scan times between 5 and 10 sec are adequate for most patients. If the patient cannot hold his or her breath reliably, then the shortest scan time can be used, since respiratory motion will degrade the image to a larger extent than will a very short scan.

The choice of slice thickness is determined by the size and site of the suspected pathology, and the density gradient between this pathology and the surrounding normal tissue. Wide slices are advantageous because of the high natural radiographic contrast of the thorax (Fig. 2). Thick slices help to differentiate vessels from masses (Fig. 3). The amount of patient exposure and examination time is reduced with wide slices. Thinner slices should be used for selected areas where partial volume averaging needs to be reduced. This applies to regions of complex anatomy or pathology such as the hila, to patients with very little mediastinal fat, and to the quantitative analysis of pulmonary nodules. Reducing slice thickness can degrade resolution of low-contrast structures by increasing noise levels. Whereas an exposure of 150 to 250 mAs is adequate for 10-mm sections of the thorax, 300 to 500 mAs may be needed for thinner sections. The radiologist should always verify that proper exposure factors are used in the thorax, which requires less exposure than does the head or abdomen. For routine investigations, spacing of slices by one slice-thickness is usually adequate. Contiguous slices are necessary for occult primary carcinoma and metastatic survey.

Contrast enhancement is generally not needed in thoracic CT. When mediastinal fat is insufficient or when a mass needs to be characterized as vascular, contrast medium should be used. Scanning immediately after injection of the contrast medium is important, in order to better define vascular structures. Redistribution of water-soluble contrast molecules in the extravascular spaces occurs very rapidly, and scans obtained 1 to 2 min after the end of an injection do not reflect vascular distribution but a combination of vascular and extravascular enhancement (Fig. 9). The best vascular enhancement is achieved by bolus injections, with a scanning time that coincides with the bolus transit in the structures examined (Table 1). Extended bolus injections in conjunction with dynamic scanning or a combination of bolus followed by infusion are acceptable alternatives, especially when a large area is being examined. Ideally, all examinations should be reviewed on-line before the patient is removed from the scanner, or at least while he or she is still in the CT suite. The short image reconstruction times now available make this possible. Hard copies of thoracic CT studies should be obtained at two window settings, mediastinal and parenchymal, to allow for reliable film interpretation. Efficient CT performance requires careful planning of each examination and on-line evaluation of the study as it evolves. CT is the most advanced, and usually the last, noninvasive investigative step in the management of patients with thoracic pathology. The radiologist should therefore strive to obtain definite answers by the time the CT examination is ended.

REFERENCES

1. Brooks RA, Di Chiro G. Principles of computer assisted tomography (CAT) in radiographic and radioisotopic imaging. *Phys Med Biol* 21:689–731, 1976
2. McLoud TC, Wittenberg J, Ferrucci JT. Computed tomography of the thorax and standard radiographic evaluation of the chest: a comparative study. *J Comput Assist Tomogr* 3:170–180, 1979
3. Sones PJ, Torres WE, Colvin RS, Meier WL, Sprawls P, Rogers JV. Effectiveness of CT in evaluating intrathoracic masses. *AJR* 139:469–475, 1982
4. Jost RG, Sagel SS, Stanley RJ, Levitt RG. Computed tomography of the thorax. *Radiology* 126:125–136, 1978.
5. Wittenberg J, Fineberg HV, Black EB, et al. Clinical efficacy of computed body tomography. *AJR* 131:5–14, 1978
6. Robbins AH, Pugatch RD, Gerzof SG, et al. Further observations on the medical efficacy of computed tomography of the chest and abdomen. *Radiology,* 137:719–725, 1980
7. Heitzman ER. Computed tomography of the thorax: Current perspectives. *AJR* 136:2–12, 1981
8. Zerhouni EA, Scott W, Baker R, Wharam MD, Siegelman SS. Invasive thymomas: Diagnosis and evaluation by computed tomography. *J Comput Assist Tomogr* 6:92–100, 1982
9. Pugatch RD, Faling LJ, Robbins AH, Snider GL. Differentiation of pleural and pulmonary lesions using computed tomography. *J Comput Assist Tomogr* 2:601–606, 1978
10. Doppmann JL, Brennan MF, Koehler JO, Marx SJ. Computer tomography for parathyroid localization. *J Comput Assist Tomogr* 1:30–36, 1977
11. Mink JH, Bein ME, Sukov R, et al. Computed tomography of the anterior mediastinum of patients with myasthenia gravis and suspected thymoma. *AJR* 130:239–246, 1978
12. Margulis AR, Boyd DP, Axel L. The desirable properties of computed tomography scanners. *Radiology* 134:261, 1980
13. Society for Computed Body Tomography. New indications for computed body tomography. *AJR* 133:115–119, 1979
14. Brooks RA, Di Chiro G. Theory of image reconstruction in computed tomography. *Radiology* 117:561–572, 1975
15. Riederer SJ, Pelc NJ, Chesler DA. The noise power spectrum in computed X-ray tomography. *Phys Med Biol* 23:446–454, 1978
16. Chesler DA, Riederer SJ, Pelc NJ. Noise due to photon counting statistics in computed X-ray tomography. *J Comput Assist Tomogr* 1:64–74, 1977
17. Brooks RA, Di Chiro G. Statistical limitations in X-ray reconstructive tomography. *Med Phys* 3:237–240, 1976
18. Barrett HH, Gordon SK, Hershel RS. Statistical limitations in transaxial tomography. *Comput Biol Med* 6:307–323, 1976
19. Joseph PM. Image noise and smoothing in computed tomography (CT) scanners. *Optic Eng* 17:396–399, 1978
20. Joseph PM, Sadek KH, Schulz RA, Kelcz F. Clinical and experimental investigation of a smoothed CT reconstruction algorithm. *Radiology* 134:507–516, 1980
21. Trefler M, Haughton VM. Patient dose and image quality in computed tomography. *AJR* 137:25–27, 1981
22. Chew E, Weiss GH, Brooks RA, Di Chiro G. Effect of CT noise on detectability of test objects. *AJR* 131:681–685, 1978
23. Hanson K. Detectability in the presence of computed tomographic reconstruction noise. *Proc Soc Photo-Optical Instrumentation Engineers* 127:304–312, 1977
24. Haaga JR, Miraldi F, MacIntyre W, LiPuma JP, Bryan PJ, Wiesen E. The effect of mAs variation upon computed tomography image quality as evaluated in in vivo and in vitro studies. *Radiology* 138:449–454, 1981
25. Meaney TF, Raudkivi U, McIntyre WJ, et al. Detection of low-contrast lesions in computed body tomography: An experimental study of simulated lesions. *Radiology* 134: 149–154, 1980
26. Robbins AH, Pugatch RD, Gerzof SG, Spira R, Rankin SC, Gale DR. An assessment of the role of scan speed in perceived image quality of body computed tomography. *Radiology* 139:139–146, 1981
27. Anderson RE, Radmehr A, Osborn AG, Wing SD. Impact of a "fast" scanner on image quality in pediatric computed tomography. *Radiology* 134:251–252, 1980
28. Alfidi RJ, MacIntyre WJ, Haaga JR. The effects of biological motion on CT resolution. *AJR* 127:11–15, 1976
29. Krudy AG, Doppman JL, Herdt JR. Failure to detect a 1.5 centimeter lung nodule by chest computed tomography. *J Comput Assist Tomogr* 6:1178–1180, 1982
30. Robinson PJ, Jones KR. Improved control of respiration during computed tomography by feedback monitoring. *J Comput Assist Tomogr* 6:802–806, 1982
31. Zimmerman JE, Goodman LR, St. Andre AC, Wyman AC. Radiographic detection of mobilizable lung water: the gravitational shift test. *AJR* 138:59–64, 1982
32. Kuhns LR, Borlaza G. The "twinkling star" sign: An aid in differentiating pulmonary vessels from pulmonary nodules on computed tomograms. *Radiology* 135:763–764, 1980
33. Sage MR. Blood-brain barrier: Phenomenon of increasing importance to the imaging clinician. *AJR* 138:887–898, 1982
34. Kormano M, Dean PB. Extravascular contrast media: The major component of contrast enhancement. *Radiology* 121:379–382, 1976
35. Gardeur D, Lautrou J, Millard JC, Berger N, Metzger J. Pharmacokinetics of contrast media: Experimental results in dog and man with CT implications. *J Comput Assist Tomogr* 4:178–185, 1980
36. Newhouse JH. Fluid compartment distribution of intravenous iothalamate in the dog. *Invest Radiol* 12:364–367, 1977
37. Newhouse JH, Murphy RX. Tissue distribution of soluble contrast: Effect of dose variation and changes with time. *AJR* 136:463–467, 1981
38. Young SW, Turner RJ, Castellino RA. A strategy for the contrast enhancement of malignant tumors using dynamic computed tomography and intravascular pharmacokinetics. *Radiology* 137:137–147, 1980
39. Dean PB, Kivisaari L, Kormano M. The diagnostic potential of contrast enhancement pharmacokinetics. *Invest Radiol* 13:533–541, 1978
40. Ono N, Martinez CR, Fara JW, Hodges FJ. Diatrizoate distribution in dogs as a function of administration rate and time following intravenous injection. *J Comput Assist Tomogr* 4:174–177, 1980
41. Hacker H, Becker H. Time controlled computed tomographic angiography. *J Comput Assist Tomogr* 1:405–409, 1977
42. Cassel DM, Young SW, Brody WR, Muller HH, Hall AL. Radiographic blood pool contrast agents for vascular and tumor imaging with projection radiography and computed tomography. *J Comput Assist Tomogr* 6:141–146, 1982
43. Godwin JD, Webb WR. Dynamic computed tomography in the evaluation of vascular lung lesions. *Radiology* 138:629–635, 1981
44. Glazer GM, Francis IR, Gebarski K, Samuels BI, Sorensen KW. Dynamic incremental computed tomography in evaluation of the pulmonary hila. *J Comput Assist Tomogr* 7:59–64, 1983
45. Reese DF, McCullough EC, Baker HL. Dynamic sequential scanning with table incrementation. *Radiology* 140:719, 1981
46. Korobkin M, Kressel HY, Moss AA, Koehler RE. Computed tomographic angiography of the body. *Radiology* 126:807–811, 1978
47. Young SW, Noon MA, Nassi M, Castellino RA. Dynamic computed tomography body scanning. *J Comput Assist Tomogr* 4:168–173, 1980
48. Godwin JD, Herfkens RL, Skjoldebrand CT, Federle MP, Lipton MJ. Evaluation of dissections and aneurysms of the

thoracic aorta by conventional and dynamic CT scanning. *Radiology* 136:125–133, 1980

49. Gross SC, Barr I, Eyler WR, Khaja F, Goldstein S. Computed tomography in dissection of the thoracic aorta. *Radiology* 136:135–139, 1980

50. Larde D, Belloir C, Vasile N, Frija J, Ferrane J. Computed tomography of aortic dissection. *Radiology* 136:147–151, 1980

51. Passariello R, Salvolino U, Rossi P, Simonetti G, Pasquini U. Automatic contrast media injector for computed tomography. *J Comput Assist Tomogr* 4:278–279, 1980

52. Baxter BS, Sorenson JA. Factors affecting measurements of size and CT number in computed tomography. *Invest Radiol* 16:337–341, 1981

53. Koehler RP, Anderson RE, Baxter B. The effect of computed tomography viewer controls on anatomical measurements. *Radiology* 130:189, 1979

54. Gray JE, Winkler NT. The cathode ray tube (CRT) as a source of "grainy" CT images. *AJR* 135:1100–1101, 1980

55. van Waes PFGM, Zonneveld FW. Direct coronal body computed tomography. *J Comput Assist Tomogr* 6:58–66, 1982

56. Levy JM, Gordon B, Nykamp PW. Computed tomography-guided percutaneous transthoracic lung biopsy. *CT* 2:217–219, 1978

57. Gobien RP, Skucas J, Paris BS. CT-assisted fluoroscopically guided aspiration biopsy of central hilar and mediastinal masses. *Radiology* 141:443–447, 1981

58. Fink I, Gamsu G, Harter LP. CT-guided aspiration biopsy of the thorax. *J Comput Assist Tomogr* 6:958–962, 1982

59. Westcott JL. Percutaneous needle aspiration of hilar and mediastinal masses. *Radiology* 141:323–329, 1981

60. Adler O, Rosenberger A. Computed tomography in guiding of fine needle aspiration biopsy of the lung and mediastinum. *Fortschr Rontgenstr* 133:135–137, 1980

Chapter 2

Aortic Arch and Great Vessels: Normal Anatomy and Variants

Accurate interpretation of mediastinal pathology requires detailed knowledge of normal cross-sectional anatomy, as well as an awareness of the wide range of normal anatomic variants and congenital anomalies that may involve the aortic arch and great vessels. This anatomy has been reviewed by numerous authors (1–5). The significance of recognizing normal anatomy and variants has been emphasized by Baron et al. (6), who, in their evaluation of 71 patients referred for CT examination because of widening of the mediastinum on plain radiographs, have shown that 31 patients (approximately 50%) were found to have a vascular anomaly or abnormality. These included, among others, 14 cases of tortuous great vessels, 10 cases of aneurysmal dilatation of the aorta and its branches, and 6 congenital anomalies of the thoracic vascular system.

The purpose of this chapter is to review normal mediastinal anatomy as a prelude to an in-depth discussion of mediastinal pathology, presented in Chapter 3. Where appropriate, examples of mediastinal pathology will be illustrated in order to reinforce anatomic concepts.

GENERAL PRINCIPLES AND METHODOLOGY

Visualization of mediastinal structures depends on the inherent contrast found between the normal soft tissue density of mediastinal vessels and the surrounding mediastinal fat. Optimal definition requires narrow windows (usually between 300 and 500 Hounsfield units (HU)) with a window level set at soft-tissue density (around 20 to 40 HU). In a majority of cases, sufficient natural contrast is present to define mediastinal structures without the use of intravenous contrast media. Accurate identification of normal anatomic structures and differentiation of pathology depend on recognition of the characteristic morphology of the great vessels as seen in sequential images.

Intravenous contrast medium administration, of course, is especially applicable for definition of the mediastinum, since so much of the anatomy is vascular. Use of contrast agents, however, should be reserved for those cases in which (a) insufficient mediastinal fat is present, making identification of normal structures difficult; (b) confusion may arise concerning differentiation of normal variants or congenital anomalies; or (c) a pathologic process first identified without contrast enhancement is to be further characterized.

Each case should be monitored in progress. In general, 10-mm thick sections taken every 10 or 15 mm are sufficient to define mediastinal anatomy. Thin collimation (usually 5-mm thick sections) should be reserved for difficult cases in which there are problems of spatial resolution between small, adjacent structures. Contrast medium may be administered either as a drip infusion or as a bolus. In the latter case, unless dynamic scanning capability is available, images should be obtained at the level that most needs clarification, easily selected from the precontrast scans. Ordinarily, only two, or rarely three, images will show dense vascular opacification, hence the need for precisely determining the best levels to scan. (For a further analysis of bolus techniques, refer to Chapter 1.)

Recent interest has centered around the potential use of CT pneumomediastinography (7,8). Air within the mediastinum does provide exquisite definition of anatomy (Fig. 1). Additionally, as shown by Sone et al. (8), CT pneumomediastinography has been used successfully to demonstrate with fine detail the pathways of spread of disease between the potential spaces of the mediastinum. Unfortunately, CT pneumomediastinography is invasive, time-consuming, and potentially hazardous; general utilization of this procedure is unwarranted.

ANATOMY OF THE ARCH AND GREAT VESSELS

The anatomy of the aortic arch and great vessels can be conceptualized as a series of characteristic sections. Figure 2 is a schematic drawing of the major arterial and venous structures of the mediastinum in which these characteristic levels have been drawn. In reviewing this anatomy, it is simplest to begin with the aortic arch and proceed upward in a stepwise fashion.

The aortic arch normally has an oblique course extending posteriorly and to the left (Fig. 3a). Anteriorly, the aortic arch lies in front of the trachea and is intimately related to the anteromedial aspect of the superior vena cava on the left side. As the arch extends posteriorly, it lies to the left of the trachea, and, more posteriorly, at the junction of the aortic knob and descending aorta, is intimately related to the esophagus.

At this level, the anterior mediastinum has a triangular configuration, with the apex pointing anteriorly. In a normal adult, following regression of the thymus gland, the anterior mediastinum should contain only fat. (For a full discussion of the thymus, normal and abnormal, see Chapter 3.) The middle mediastinum is also well-defined by fat at this level, bordered posteriorly by the convexity of the trachea, anteriorly by the posterior and posterolateral aspect of the superior vena cava, medially by the arch of the aorta, and laterally by the mediastinal pleural reflections.

Frequently, sections at the level of the aortic arch will also include the arch of the azygos vein (Fig. 3b). The arch of the azygos crosses over the right upper lobe bronchus and courses anteriorly alongside the right wall of the distal trachea to join the superior vena cava. The arch of the azygos usually can be localized to the T5-T6 vertebral body level.

Schnyder and Gamus (9) have called attention to an important space that can be defined at the level of the azygos arch, the pretracheal, retrocaval space (Fig. 3b). This space is limited by the anterior convexity of the distal trachea, the medial wall of the aortic arch, the posterior and posteromedial borders of the superior vena cava, and the medial border of the azygos arch. Normally, the pretracheal, retrocaval space contains mediastinal fat, fibrous connective tissue, and lymph nodes (commonly referred to as azygos nodes). The clinical importance of this space derives from the critical role played by the azygos nodes, which drain the subcarinal and bronchopulmonary–hilar nodes efferently, and are afferent links with the paratracheal and middle mediastinal nodes superiorly. Visualization of these nodes is of critical significance, especially in the evaluation and staging of patients with bronchogenic carcinoma. In the study reported by Schnyder and Gamus, lymph nodes in the pretracheal, retrocaval space were identified in 88% of

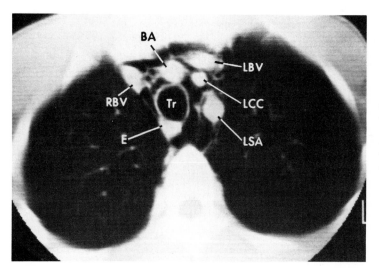

FIG. 1. Post-traumatic pneumomediastinum. Section through the great vessels in a patient with extensive air throughout the mediastinum. Linear markings represent normal fibrous strands. Tr, trachea; E, esophagus; RBV, right brachiocephalic vein; LBV, left brachiocephalic vein; BA, brachiocephalic artery; LCC, left common carotid artery; LSA, left subclavian artery.

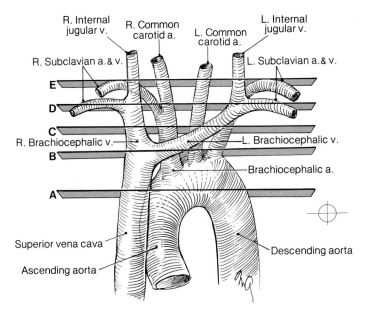

R. Internal jugular v. R. Common carotid a. L. Common carotid a. L. Internal jugular v.

R. Subclavian a.& v. L. Subclavian a.& v.

E
D
C
R. Brachiocephalic v. L. Brachiocephalic v.
B
Brachiocephalic a.
A

Superior vena cava Descending aorta

Ascending aorta

FIG. 2. Schematic drawing of the aortic arch and great vessels. Characteristic levels have been labeled A through E.

127 normal subjects. Only rarely was more than one node present. Of 160 lymph nodes identified, the average diameter was approximately 8 mm (Fig. 3b). The topic of "significant" mediastinal adenopathy will be considered in detail in Chapter 3. For purposes of this discussion, it should be noted that the incidental discovery of mediastinal lymph nodes up to 8 mm in size is frequent in otherwise normal patients.

Above the level of the aortic arch, through most of the superior mediastinum, five vessels can be identified routinely (Fig. 4a; compare with level B, Fig. 2). These include the three major branches of the aortic arch (i.e., the brachiocephalic artery, the left common carotid, and the left subclavian artery) and the left and right brachiocephalic veins. The

brachiocephalic artery is midline, frequently touching the anterior wall of the trachea (Figs. 4a, 5, 6, and 7). The left common carotid artery lies to the left and slightly posterolateral to the brachiocephalic artery; it has the smallest diameter of the three major arteries (Fig. 5). The left subclavian artery, throughout most of its course, is a relatively posterior structure, lying to the left and frequently adjacent to the trachea. Additionally, the lateral border of the left subclavian artery lies adjacent to the mediastinal reflections of the left upper lobe, which it indents in a typically convex fashion (Figs. 4a and 7).

The two brachiocephalic veins have fundamentally different configurations. The right brachiocephalic vein has a nearly vertical course throughout its length; the left brachiocephalic vein has a

3a,b

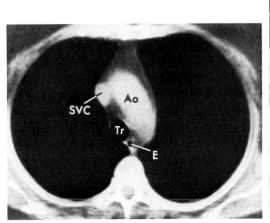
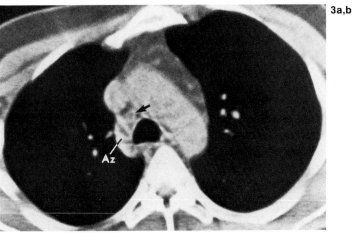

FIG. 3. a: Section through the aortic arch (Ao). SVC, superior vena cava; Tr, trachea; E, esophagus. At this level, the anterior mediastinum has a triangular configuration, with the apex pointing anteriorly. **b:** Section at the level of the azygos arch (Az). A small node can be identified in the pretracheal, retrocaval space *(arrow)*.

4a,b

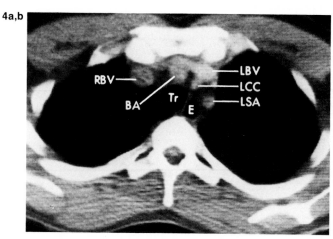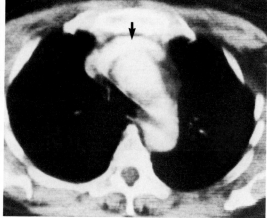

FIG. 4. a: Section through the great vessels. BA, brachiocephalic artery; LCC, left common carotid artery; LSA, left subclavian artery; LBV and RBV, left and right brachiocephalic veins. The horizontal portion of the left brachiocephalic vein serves as a convenient line of demarcation between the anterior mediastinum (prevascular space) and the middle mediastinum. **b:** Section just below the aortic arch. The course of the left brachiocephalic vein is variable *(arrow)*.

longer course, and, inferiorly, courses horizontally as it crosses the mediastinum from left to right (Fig. 4a). The horizontal component of the left brachiocephalic vein is a convenient anatomic landmark, marking the line of demarcation between the anterior mediastinum (the prevascular space) anteriorly and the middle mediastinum posteriorly. The precise configuration of this vein is highly variable. Although generally illustrated at the level of the great vessels (as shown in Fig. 4a), the horizontal component of the left brachiocephalic vein can be found at almost any level of the superior mediastinum, including in front of the aortic arch (Fig. 4b). There is considerable variability in the size of the left brachiocephalic vein. Generally, the veins are structures larger than the corresponding arteries. The left brachiocephalic vein can become markedly distended (Fig. 5). While this is usually a normal variant, marked distension of the left brachiocephalic vein rarely may be an indication of total anomalous pulmonary venous return with drainage to a persistent left-sided vena cava (10). Because of the key role played by the horizontal component of the left brachiocephalic vein in dividing the compartments of the mediastinum, if intravenous contrast medium is employed, it should be given, whenever possible, in a left-sided arm vein. This maximizes visualization of the full length of the left brachiocephalic vein (Fig. 4b).

The right brachiocephalic vein lies anterolaterally and, like the left subclavian artery, is bounded laterally by the mediastinal pleural reflections of the

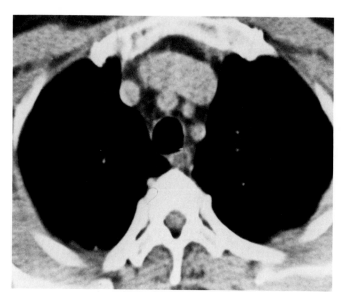

FIG. 5. Section at the level of the great vessels. The brachiocephalic vein is markedly distended, which is, in this case, a normal variant. Marked dilatation of the brachiocephalic vein may denote venous obstruction; more rarely, it may be a sign of total, anomalous pulmonary venous drainage.

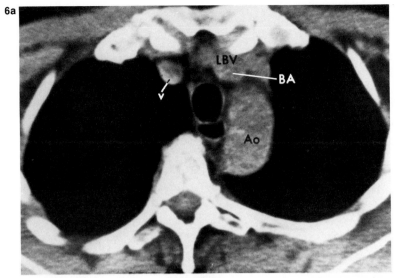

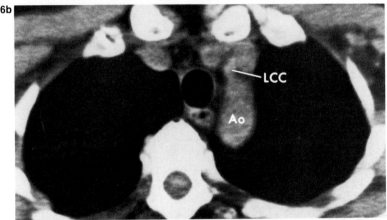

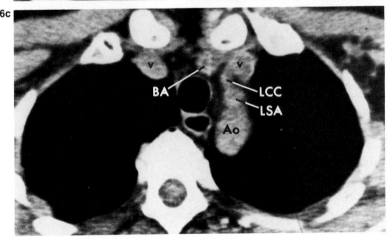

FIG. 6. a, b, c: Sequential images obtained through the aortic arch (Ao). The arch has a general superoposterior configuration; the origins of the great vessels may be identified at different levels. BA, brachiocephalic artery; CC, left common carotid artery; LSA, left subclavian artery; LBV, horizontal component of the left brachiocephalic vein; V, vertical portions of the brachiocephalic veins. The left subclavian artery arises from the posterior portion of the aortic arch, which should not be mistaken for a mediastinal mass (c).

right upper lobe, which it indents in a typically convex fashion (Figs. 4 and 7).

If sequential sections are obtained through the upper portion of the aortic arch, the origins of each of the great vessels can be visualized (Fig. 6). It is important to review this anatomy, since these images, if unfamiliar, may be confused with pathology. The arch of the aorta is not a "flat" structure. Instead, the arch has a general superoposterior configuration, and the three great arteries arise sequentially at different levels. The brachiocephalic artery arises first and at the most caudal level of the arch (Fig. 6a). The left common carotid artery arises next, at a higher level; the left subclavian artery is

7a,b

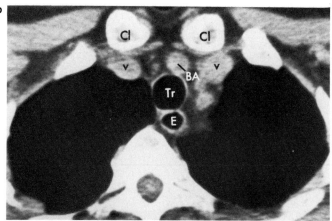
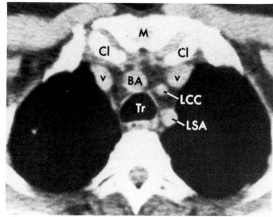

FIG. 7. a, b: Sequential images through the great vessels above the level of the horizontal portion of the left brachiocephalic vein. BA, brachiocephalic artery; LCC, left common carotid artery; LSA, left subclavian artery; Tr, trachea; E, esophagus; V, brachiocephalic veins. (a) is a section through the sternoclavicular joints bilaterally. Cl, clavicular heads; M, manubrium. Note that the amount of air within the esophagus is extremely variable at this level.

the last branch and arises from the posterosuperior portion of the aortic knob (Figs. 6b and c). As sequential images are obtained through the origins of the great vessels, progressively smaller portions of the aortic knob will be visualized posteriorly. At the level of the origin of the left subclavian artery, the posterior portion of the arch should not be confused with a mediastinal mass.

Figures 7a and b are sequential sections through the great vessels above the level of the horizontal portion of the left brachiocephalic vein, and correspond with level C in Fig. 2. The only significant difference in mediastinal anatomy at these levels, as compared with the anatomy illustrated in Fig. 4a, is the position and configuration of the left brachiocephalic vein, which now has a vertical configuration and lies in an anterolateral position (see also Fig. 1).

Above the level of the bifurcation of the brachiocephalic artery, the right subclavian and right common carotid arteries can be identified (Fig. 8; compare with level D, Fig. 2). These vessels are essentially mirror images of the left subclavian and common carotid arteries. The exact position of the bifurcation of the brachiocephalic artery is variable, depending on the length and degree of tortuosity of this vessel (Fig. 8; compare with Fig. 10). In a significant percentage of cases, the brachiocephalic artery bifurcates "late"; in these cases the right subclavian artery will have an oblique course, and if thin sections are not obtained near the thoracic inlet, it may not be visualized at all. When the right common carotid and right subclavian arteries are seen, they normally are found only in sections through the uppermost portion of the superior mediastinum. Visualization of these vessels in a more inferior position, just above the aortic arch, frequently indicates the presence of some type of vas-

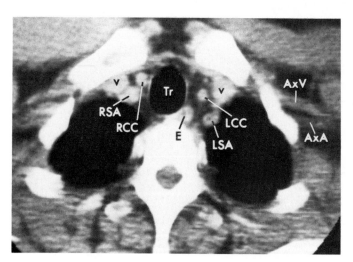

FIG. 8. Section above the level of bifurcation of the brachiocephalic artery. The right subclavian artery (RSA) and right common carotid artery (RCC) are mirror images of the left common carotid artery (LCC) and left subclavian artery (LSA). Tr, trachea; V, brachiocephalic veins. The axillary portion of the left subclavian artery (AxA) and vein (AxV) can be identified posterior to the pectoralis muscles.

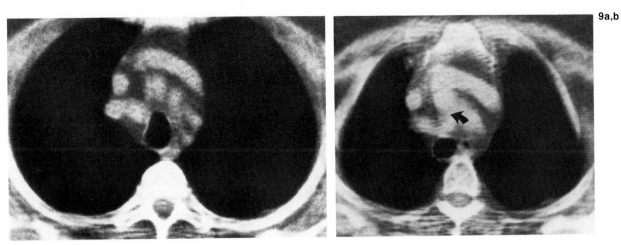

FIG. 9. a: Unenhanced section through the great vessels. The appearance of the great vessels is somewhat atypical; adenopathy cannot be excluded. **b:** Enhanced section at a slightly lower level than shown in (a). There is marked tortuosity of the brachiocephalic artery *(arrow)*, which accounts for the excessive number of rounded structures seen in (a).

cular mediastinal anomaly, usually involving the aortic arch. This has been termed the "four vessel sign" by McLoughlin et al. (11); an example is illustrated in Fig. 23.

Although the great vessels should be recognized by virtue of their characteristic configurations, tortuosity or ectasia of these vessels may present a confusing picture and be easily mistaken as pathologic. Use of intravenous contrast media will almost always resolve this problem (Fig. 9).

The subclavian arteries and veins exit and enter the mediastinum by crossing over the first ribs, behind the proximal portions of the clavicles (Fig. 10; compare with level E, Fig. 2). The subclavian vein lies anterior and the subclavian artery lies posterior to the anterior scalenus muscle, which attaches to the superior border of the first rib. Once it has crossed over the first rib, the subclavian vein courses toward the axilla, which lies behind the pectoralis muscles. This line of continuity is easily

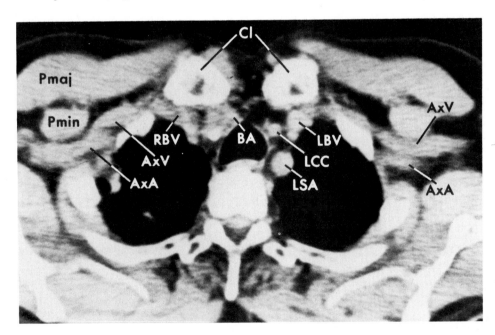

FIG. 10. Section through the sternal notch between the proximal portions of the clavicles (Cl). The subclavian veins cross into the mediastinum by passing over the first ribs, behind the clavicles. There is continuity between the axillary portions of the subclavian veins (AxV), lying posterior to the pectoralis major (Pmaj) and minor muscles (Pmin) and the right and left brachiocephalic veins (RBV and LBV). The subclavian arteries have a more angled, oblique course as they exit the mediastinum, and frequently are not seen crossing the first rib. The axillary portions of the subclavian arteries lie posterior to the corresponding subclavian veins. LSA, mediastinal portion of the left subclavian artery; LCC, left common carotid artery; BA, brachiocephalic artery.

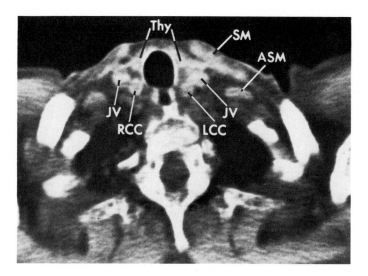

FIG. 11. Section through the thoracic inlet. Thyroid tissue (Thy) surrounds the trachea. RCC and LCC, right and left common carotid arteries; JV, right and left internal jugular veins. These structures are bounded circumferentially by the sternocleidomastoid muscles anteriorly (SM) and the anterior scalenus muscles laterally (ASM); the longus colli muscles lie in the prevertebral area.

traced with CT, allowing differentiation between mediastinal versus axillary venous obstruction. The transition from the mediastinal to the axillary portions of the subclavian arteries is more difficult to visualize because there is a sharper degree of angulation in the course these vessels take as they cross over the first rib (Fig. 2). The axillary portions of the subclavian arteries lie posterior to the corresponding veins (Fig. 10).

The thoracic inlet demarcates the junction between the root of the neck and the superior mediastinum (Fig. 11). It characteristically follows an oblique plane, paralleling the first rib (12). The trachea at this level is surrounded on both sides by the inferior lobes of the thyroid gland; lateral to the trachea, the internal jugular veins and common carotid arteries can be identified. These structures are bounded circumferentially by strap muscles, including the sternocleidomastoid muscles anteriorly, the anterior scalenus muscles laterally, and the longus colli muscles posteriorly in the prevertebral area (Fig. 11).

In our experience, there is some reluctance on the part of many radiologists who are "body" scanners to develop familiarity with the anatomy of the neck. Familiarity with this anatomy is valuable, since disease processes frequently communicate between the upper mediastinum and the neck along well-delineated fascial planes, in particular, those surrounding the trachea (the previsceral fascia).

ANATOMY OF THE AZYGOS, HEMIAZYGOS, AND SUPERIOR INTERCOSTAL VEINS

The anatomy of the azygos, hemiazygos, and superior intercostal venous systems has been described, and is illustrated in Fig. 12 (13–16).

Inferiorly, the azygos and hemiazygos veins represent continuations into the thorax of the left and right ascending lumbar veins. The azygos vein parallels the esophagus to the right, and laterally is in contact with the medial pleural reflections of the right lower lobe, defining the medial border of the azygo-esophageal recess. The azygos vein drains the lower intercostal veins along its route. On the left side, the hemiazygous vein parallels the descending aorta posteriorly, draining the lower intercostal veins on the left side. The hemiazygous vein itself generally drains into the azygos vein via communicating vessels that cross the midline in the vicinity of the T8 vertebral body. Normally, these are almost never seen on CT (44).

Superiorly, the azygos vein terminates by arching over the medial aspect of the right upper lobe bronchus and then coursing anteriorly to join the posterior aspect of the superior vena cava (Fig. 3b). Just prior to the formation of the azygos arch, the azygos vein is joined by the right superior intercostal vein. This vein drains the right second to fourth intercostal veins, and then courses inferiorly in a paraspinal location (Figs. 12 and 13a).

On the left side, the accessory hemiazygos vein continues above the point of termination of the hemiazygos vein (the two are frequently in communication), ascending posterior to the descending aorta. At the level of the aortic arch, the accessory hemiazygos is joined by the left superior intercostal vein (which drains the second to fourth intercostal veins), in approximately 75% of patients (15). The left superior intercostal vein forms a venous arch (also referred to as the arch of the hemiazygos vein) that courses anteriorly around the aortic arch to join the left brachiocephalic vein superiorly (Fig. 13b). On routine radiographs, the left superior intercostal

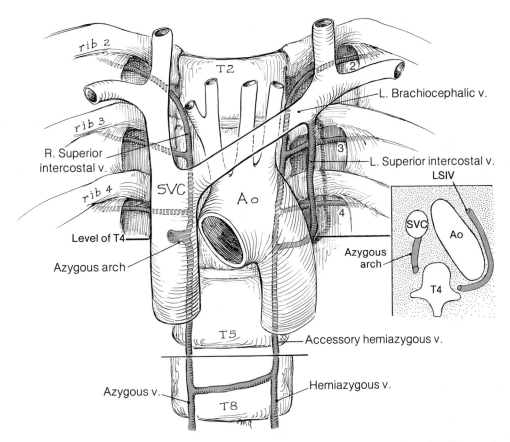

FIG. 12. Schematic drawing of the azygos, hemiazygos, and superior intercostal venous systems. INSET is a schematic cross-section at the level of the aortic arch.

vein is most often seen end-on, adjacent to the aortic knob. Because of its appearance, it has been termed the "aortic nipple," and can be seen in up to 10% of normal patients (15).

The arch of the azygos is well-known radiologically, probably because of the frequent need to differentiate a prominent azygos vein from paratracheal adenopathy. The azygos arch is very variable in dimension (Fig. 3b). Dilatation of the arch may be caused by central venous hypertension (as may occur with right ventricular heart failure), obstruction of the superior or inferior vena cava, or may result from azygos continuation of an anomalous IVC. Idiopathic dilatation of the azygos arch may occur, in which case the arch may be mistaken for a pulmonary lesion (17).

The left superior intercostal vein has a somewhat more variable appearance when seen with CT. Unlike the azygos arch, which is identifiable in nearly 100% of cases, the left superior intercostal vein is only rarely identified (Fig. 13). The course and configuration of the hemiazygos vein and of the left superior intercostal vein as it winds around the aorta and drains into the left brachiocephalic vein are illustrated in Fig. 14. Recognition of this venous

anatomy is important because it is relatively easy to mistake the left superior intercostal vein for pre-aortic adenopathy. As shown in Fig. 14, the left superior intercostal vein frequently has an oblique configuration as it passes around the aortic arch. If this vein should assume a vertical configuration in any portion of its course, the vein will be seen end-on in cross section (Fig. 14c). Differentiation between the left superior intercostal vein and pre-aortic adenopathy is facilitated by close scrutiny of sections obtained above and below the aortic arch in order to visualize the full course of the vein. Administration of intravenous contrast material may be of value, although the degree of opacification of the left superior intercostal vein is often negligible.

The azygos and hemiazygos venous systems are important collateral systems when there is obstruction or interruption of blood flow through either the superior or inferior vena cava. Occasionally, obstruction may occur proximal to the caval system, as shown in Fig. 15.

Dilatation of the azygos and hemiazygos veins is classically associated with anomalies of the inferior vena cava (Fig. 16). This appearance has been reported by numerous investigators (18–20). When

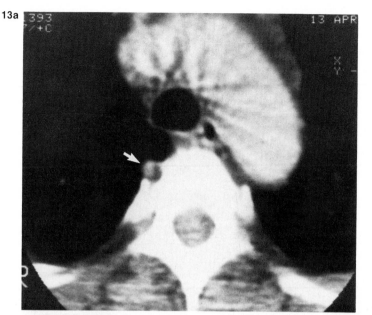

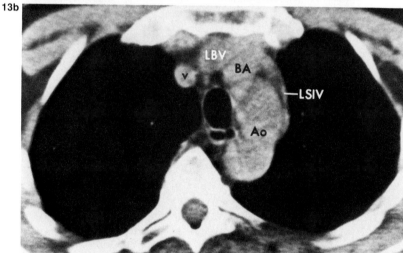

FIG. 13. a: Section through the right superior intercostal vein, which lies in a paraspinal location *(arrow).* **b:** Section through the origin of the brachiocephalic artery (BA) and the posterior portion of the aortic arch (Ao). The left superior intercostal vein (LSIV) courses laterally around the aortic arch to drain into the left brachiocephalic vein (LBV). Superficially, this appearance may mimic an aortic dissection. V, right brachiocephalic vein.

there is developmental failure of the hepatic or infrahepatic (prerenal) segment of the inferior vena cava, blood returns to the heart via the cranial portion of the supracardinal veins, i.e., the azygos and hemiazygos veins. This anomaly has been reported in up to 2% of cases in patients with congenital heart disease undergoing cardiac catherization. The association between azygos continuation and the asplenia and polysplenia syndromes has been well-documented (19). Azygos continuation may also be present in otherwise asymptomatic patients, and in this setting, may be misinterpreted as some other form of pathology, specifically, a right paratracheal mass, a posterior mediastinal mass (if the dilated azygos or hemiazygos vein is identified along the paravertebral pleural reflections), or a retrocrural mass or adenopathy.

The appearance of azygos continuation is easily

defined on CT by the following constellation of findings: enlargement of the arch of the azygos; enlargement of the paraspinal portions of the azygos and hemiazygos veins (especially if confluent at higher sections with the azygos arch); and enlargement of the retrocrural portions of these same veins in the absence of a definable inferior vena cava (Fig. 16b). It should be noted that once an abnormality of the inferior vena cava is diagnosed, careful examination of the abdomen should be performed to further define and clarify its specific nature.

ANOMALIES OF THE AORTIC ARCH AND GREAT VESSELS

To recognize anomalies of the aorta and great vessels it is essential to have some knowledge of embryology. These anomalies are most easily un-

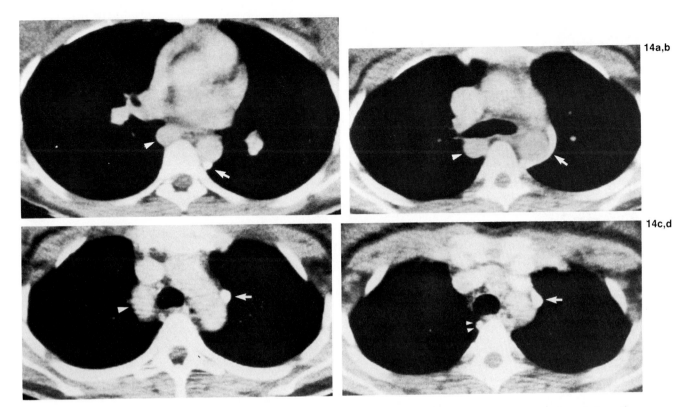

14a,b

14c,d

FIG. 14. Azygos continuation: Left superior intercostal vein. **a–d:** Sequential contrast-enhanced images—from below, then upwards—tracking the course of the accessory hemiazygos vein as it joins the left superior intercostal vein to arch around the aorta and drain into the left brachiocephalic vein *(arrows)*. As the left superior intercostal vein winds around the aorta, it may assume a vertical configuration, in which case it may be mistaken for pre-aortic adenopathy (c). The azygos vein and azygos arch are markedly dilated *(arrowheads)*. The right superior intercostal can be identified in a paraspinal location in (d) *(double arrowhead)*.

derstood if the hypothetical double arch system, described by Edwards (21) as a basic pattern from which all aortic anomalies can be derived, is used (Fig. 17). In this system, there is an aortic arch and a potential ductus arteriosus on each side; the descending aorta is in the midline posteriorly. Interruption of this arch system at different locations can explain the various aortic arch anomalies. These may be divided into three main groups: left aortic arch anomalies, right aortic arch anomalies, and double arch anomalies.

Normally, there is interruption of the hypothetical right arch distal to the right subclavian artery. The right common carotid and subclavian arteries fuse to become the right brachiocephalic artery as the proximal portion of the embryologic right arch becomes incorporated into the left arch. The result is the normal left-sided aortic arch. This series of events is illustrated in Fig. 18.

Left Aortic Arch Anomalies

The most common congenital anomaly of the aorta is an aberrant right subclavian artery originating from an otherwise normal left-sided arch. Theoretically, this occurs when there is interruption of the embryologic right aortic arch between the right common carotid and the right subclavian arteries (21). The right subclavian then originates from the posterior portion of the left-sided arch and crosses the mediastinum obliquely from left to right, lying posterior to the trachea and esophagus (Figs. 17, 19, and 20). Dilatation of the artery at its origin is common. Although the aberrant right subclavian causes an impression on both the trachea and esophagus, symptoms rarely result from this anomaly, and other associated anomalies are never present.

Other left aortic arch anomalies are rare. Left aortic arch associated with a right-sided descending aorta has been reported. This may be associated with an aberrant right subclavian (22). CT is well-suited to detecting this anomaly, as well as other anomalies in the position of the descending aorta.

Right Aortic Arch Anomalies

Numerous variations in the classification of right aortic arch anomalies have been reported (23–25).

15a,b

15c,d

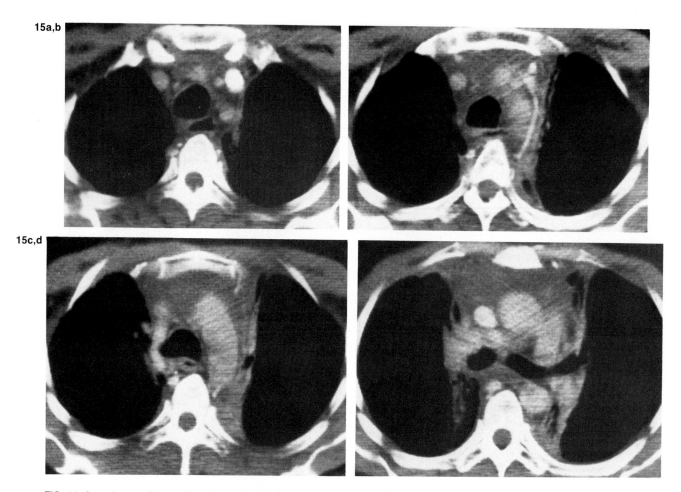

FIG. 15. Lymphoma: Obstruction of the left brachiocephalic vein. **a–d:** Sequential contrast-enhanced sections—from above, then downward—in a patient with mediastinal lymphoma (following radiation therapy). The left brachiocephalic vein is obstructed (and difficult to identify). Contrast medium enters the mediastinum via the proximal portion of the left brachiocephalic vein and then flows through the left superior intercostal vein to reach the hemiazygos vein (c). Contrast medium then passes to the azygos veins and the azygos arch (c) to finally reach the lower portion of the superior vena cava (d).

16a,b

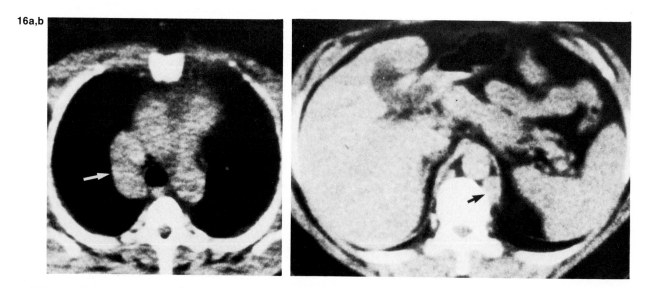

FIG. 16. Azygos continuation of the inferior vena cava. **a:** Section through the azygos arch, which is massively dilated *(arrow)*. **b:** Section through the diaphragmatic crura. There is prominence of the azygos and marked dilatation of the hemiazygos veins *(arrow),* which superficially mimics the appearance of subcrural adenopathy. Although at this level blood preferentially flows through the hemiazygos vein, higher up the blood is routed primarily via the azygos system (a). Note the absence of an identifiable inferior vena cava.

17a,b

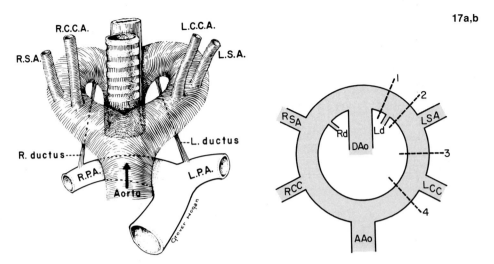

FIG. 17. a: Hypothetical double aortic arch of Edwards. (From: Shuford WH, and Sybers RG. *The Aortic Arch and Its Malformations,* 1974. Courtesy of Charles C Thomas, Springfield, Illinois.) **b:** Schematic representation of embryonic double aortic arch. Normally, there is interruption of the right arch distal to the right subclavian artery. The result is a normal left arch (see Fig. 18). Right aortic arches result when there is interruption of some portion of the left aortic arch. Five potential sites of interruption have been identified. If there is interruption distal to the left subclavian (at either 1 or 2), the result is a right aortic arch with mirror-image branching (types 1 and 2). If there is interruption between the left subclavian and left common carotid arteries (at 3), the result is a right aortic arch with an aberrant left subclavian (type 3). If the arch is interrupted proximal to the left common carotid artery (at 4), the result is a right arch with an aberrant innominate artery (type 4). Finally, interruption may occur both distal to the left subclavian artery and proximal to the left common carotid artery (at both 1 and 4); this results in an isolated left subclavian artery, connected to the left pulmonary artery via the left ductus arteriosus (type 5). DAo, descending aorta; AAo, ascending aorta, LSA, left subclavian artery; LCC, left common carotid artery; Ld, left ductus arteriosus; Rd, right ductus; RCC, right common carotid artery; RSA, right subclavian artery.

Using Edwards' hypothetical double aortic arch model, five potential anomalies can be predicted, although only three are usually described and only two are relatively common (Fig. 17). The type of anomaly encountered will depend on the exact point at which the left aortic arch is interrupted.

The two most common right aortic arch anomalies are right aortic arch with an aberrant left subclavian and right aortic arch with mirror-image branching of the great vessels.

The most common right aortic arch anomaly is a right aortic arch with an aberrant left subclavian (type 3) (23). The sequence of events leading to the malformation is illustrated in Fig. 21. In this case, there is interruption of the left arch between the left common carotid and left subclavian arteries. This leads to an anterior left common carotid artery as the first branch of the ascending aorta, and a retroesophageal left subclavian artery (Fig. 22). The distal portion of the left arch (incorporated into the

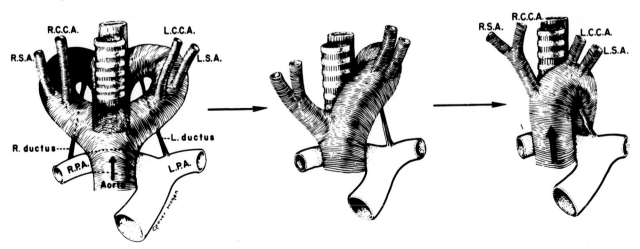

FIG. 18. Hypothesized embryologic development of the normal left arch. The shaded portion of the right arch, distal to the right subclavian artery, is interrupted. (From: Shuford WH, and Sybers RG. *The Aortic Arch and Its Malformations,* 1974. Courtesy of Charles C Thomas, Springfield, Illinois.)

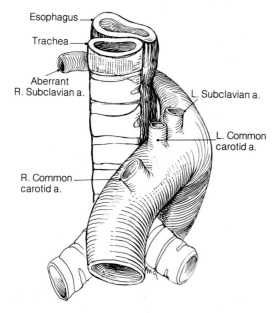

FIG. 19. Schematic representation of an aberrant right subclavian artery.

posterior portion of the right arch) frequently persists and is dilated, the so-called diverticulum of Kommerell. This type of right arch anomaly is only infrequently associated with congenital heart disease.

A right aortic arch with mirror-image branching occurs if the hypothetical left arch is interrupted distal to the left subclavian artery. The left innominate artery then arises as the first branch of the ascending aorta. Most frequently, this interruption is distal to the left ductus arteriosus. The result is a mirror image of normal (Fig. 17). This anomaly is significant because of the well-known association of congenital heart disease (especially tetralogy of Fallot) that is present in nearly 100% of cases (23). The appearance on CT of a right aortic arch with mirror image branching has been reported (26).

In the usual case of right aortic arch with mirror-image branching, interruption of the left arch occurs distal to the ductus arteriosus (type 1). The result is that there is no structure posterior to the trachea or esophagus. More rarely, interruption occurs distal to the left subclavian artery but proximal to the ductus (type 2) (27) (Fig. 17). If the ductus on the left side persists, the result is a true vascular ring, formed by the right-sided aortic arch anteriorly and to the right, and the persistent left-sided ductus, originating from the distal right-sided arch, passing behind the trachea and esophagus and joining the left main pulmonary artery. Symptomatology reflects the degree of constriction caused by the vascular ring. This type of malformation is only rarely

associated with congenital heart disease. While exceedingly rare, the appearance on CT of this anomaly has been reported (28).

Two other right aortic arch anomalies have been described. If the left aortic arch is interrupted proximal to the left common carotid artery, the result is a right aortic arch with an aberrant left brachiocephalic artery (type 4). Its appearance is similar to that of a right arch with an aberrant left subclavian, except that both the left subclavian and left common carotid are "replaced" to the posterior portion of the right arch, and derive from a common trunk.

Finally, the left arch may be interrupted in more than one place. Most typically, interruption occurs both proximal and distal to the left subclavian artery. The result is "isolation of the left subclavian artery" (type 5) (28). The left common carotid artery arises as the first branch of the right-sided aorta. The left subclavian attaches, by a persistent ductus arteriosus, to the left pulmonary artery. Although this anomaly is the third most frequent right aortic arch anomaly, it is rare and has yet to be described with CT (23).

Double Aortic Arch Anomalies

Double aortic arches have been classified into two types, depending on the patency of the arches (29). The most frequent form is a "functional" double aortic arch (type 1). In this case, both arches remain patent; the right common carotid and subclavian arteries arise from the right arch, while the left common carotid and left subclavian arteries arise from the left arch. Both arches join posteriorly to form one descending aorta, which may be midline or, more usually, left-sided. The two arches may be of equal size, although the right arch is generally larger (Fig. 23).

More rarely, a double arch is present, with atresia of some portion of the left arch (type 3) (29). As may be anticipated, there is considerable similarity in appearance between a double aortic arch with atresia of some portion of the left arch and the right aortic arch anomalies. Theoretically, the major difference is that, with double aortic arches, despite atresia, some portion of the left arch persists, and a vascular ring around the trachea and esophagus is present. With right aortic arch anomalies, there is true interruption of the left aortic arch, and a true vascular ring is only rarely formed. Practically, the two may be impossible to differentiate even angiographically, although, as suggested by Gorti et al. (30), a double aortic arch with atresia may be

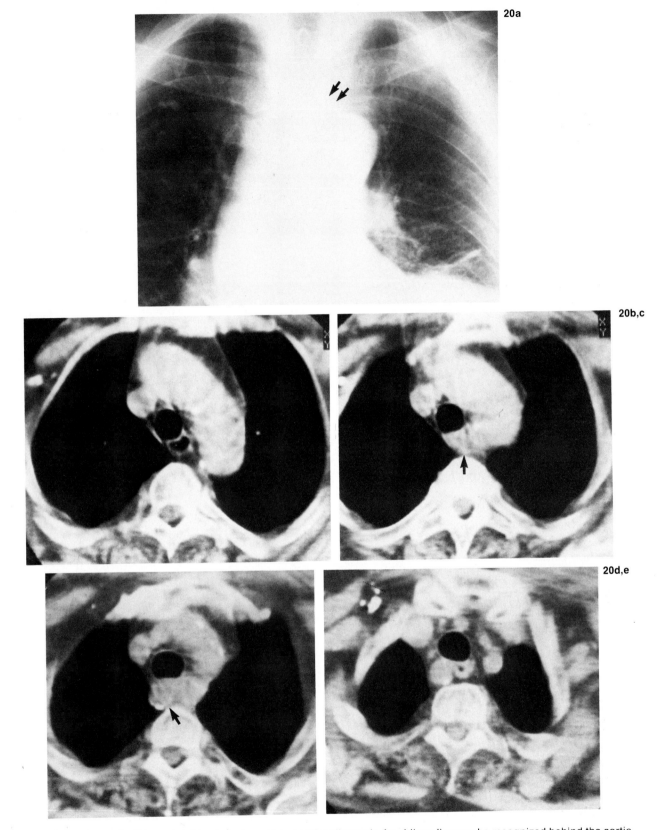

FIG. 20. Left aortic arch: Aberrant right subclavian artery. **a:** PA radiograph. An oblique line can be recognized behind the aortic arch *(arrows)*. **b–e:** Sequential images—from below, then upward—starting at the level of the aortic arch. In (b), the arch is slightly more sagittal than normal. The trachea and esophagus are normal in appearance. In (c), there is an outpouching medially from the posterior portion of the aorta, compressing and narrowing the esophagus *(arrow)*. Slightly higher, a dilated right subclavian artery can be identified, with faint calcification in the wall *(arrow)*. Both the esophagus and, to a lesser degree, the trachea are displaced anteriorly. At a still higher level, the dilated right subclavian artery is easy to identify, more posterior than usual, and at a lower level in the thorax than normal.

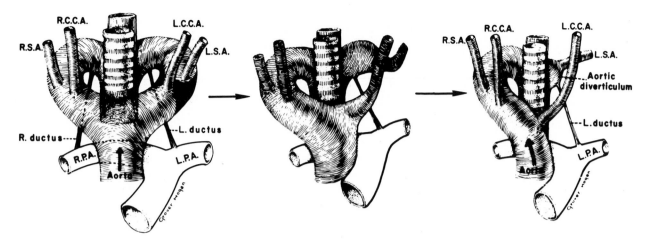

FIG. 21. Hypothesized embryonic development of a right aortic arch with an aberrant left subclavian artery. Abbreviations as in Fig. 17. (From: Shuford WH, Sybers RG. *The Aortic Arch and Its Malformations*, 1974. Courtesy of Charles C Thomas, Springfield, Illinois.)

differentiated from a right aortic arch by noting that (a) double aortic arches cause both a right- and left-sided impression on the esophagram, and (b) with double aortic arches, the left common carotid and left subclavian arteries have independent origins. With right aortic arch anomalies, excepting those with an aberrant subclavian, there is always a left innominate artery.

Care has been taken in this section to present a very detailed description of aortic arch anomalies. This has been done because CT is a potentially invaluable tool in recognizing and classifying those anomalies, and in select cases may obviate the need for further radiologic evaluation. Recognition of aortic arch anomalies can only be expected if the various patterns of anomalies are known in detail. In addition to those anomalies already described, it should be noted that other aortic anomalies, including coarctations, pseudocoarctations, L and D transpositions, and truncus arteriosus, have all been described in the CT literature (6,31).

VENOUS ANOMALIES

In addition to congenital (and acquired) abnormalities of the azygos-hemiazygos venous system, the most common, clinically significant venous anomaly is persistence of the left superior vena cava (32). The left superior vena cava forms from a confluence of the left subclavian and left jugular veins and courses inferiorly in a position analogous to the normal superior vena cava on the right side (Fig. 24). Inferiorly, the left superior vena cava lies anterior to the left hilum and always drains into a markedly dilated coronary sinus (Figs. 25 and 26).

The anatomic course of the left superior vena cava reflects embryologic retention of the left anterior and common cardinal veins and the left horn of the sinus venosus, structures that ordinarily regress. A right superior vena cava may or may not be present.

The clinical significance of this anomaly is minimal unless there is an associated atrial septal defect, with a resultant left-to-right shunt.

THE TRACHEA

Anatomically, the trachea is a cartilaginous and membranous tube that extends from the larynx superiorly (at the level of the sixth cervical vertebra) to the carina (at the level of the fifth thoracic vertebra). There is marked variability in the cross-sectional appearance of the trachea, which normally may appear rounded, oval, or horseshoe-shaped with a flattened posterior wall (33,34). Despite variability in the configuration of the trachea, the tracheal wall is almost always a thin, delicate structure, well-defined internally by the central air column (Figs. 3–10). The position of the trachea will vary, depending on what level sections are obtained through the superior mediastinum. As the trachea courses with a slight anteroposterior obliquity, progressively caudal sections will show the trachea to lie more posteriorly. At all levels, the trachea lies anterior to the esophagus, which usually lies slightly to the left (Figs. 3–10).

Along most of its length, the right wall of the trachea is in contact with the mediastinal pleural reflections of the right upper lobe (Figs. 3a and 4–7). This gives rise to the right paratracheal stripe seen on posterior-anterior (PA) radiographs. Additionally, a potential space exists between the posterior

22a

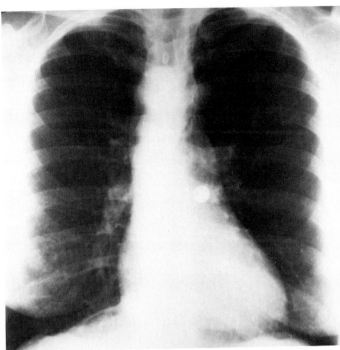

FIG. 22. Right aortic arch: Aberrant left subclavian. **a:** PA radiograph. **b–e:** Sequential sections—from below, then upward—starting at the level of the right-sided aortic arch. The trachea and esophagus are deformed and displaced anteriorly (b,c). There is aneurysmal dilatation of the posterior portion of the aortic arch (c). The left subclavian artery arises from this diverticulum and passes behind the esophagus coursing to the left *(arrow, d)*. The left subclavian artery assumes a normal position at the apex of the mediastinum *(arrow; e)*.

22b,c

22d,e

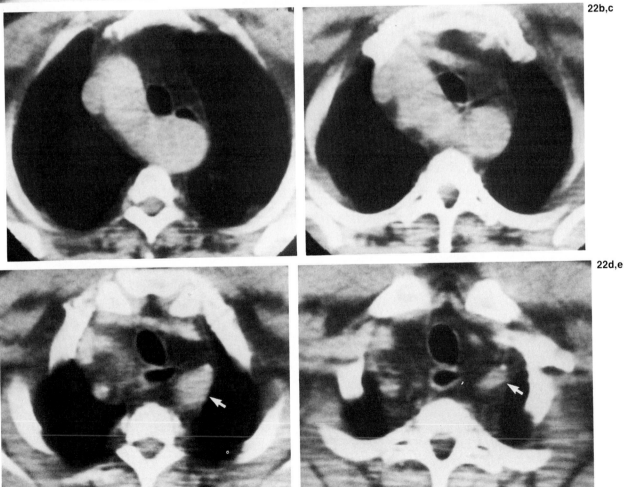

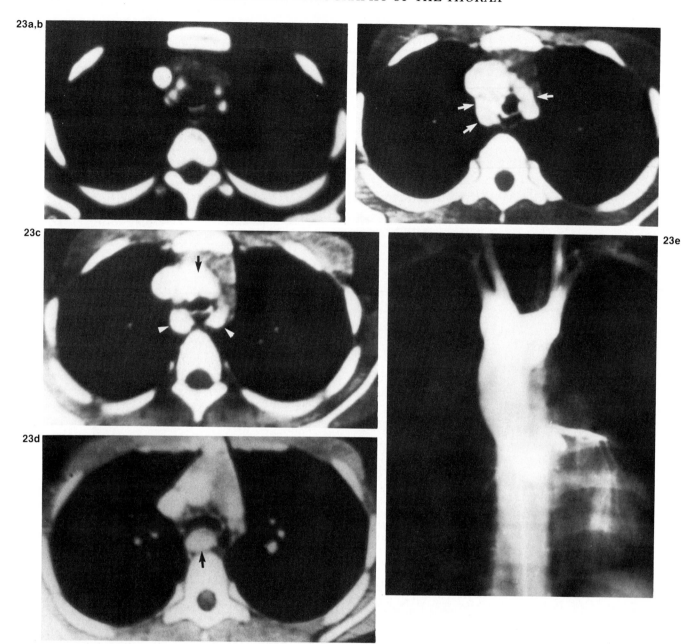

FIG. 23. Double aortic arch. **a–d:** Sequential images—from above, then downward—in a patient with a functional double aortic arch. In (a), all four arteries can be identified at a level more caudal than normal, an important clue to the presence of an arch anomaly. (b) is a section through both arches; the right arch *(two arrows)* is larger than the left arch *(single arrow)*. (c) is a section through the ascending aorta *(arrow)* and the posterior portions of both the right and left arches, which lie behind the trachea and esophagus in close proximity *(arrowheads)*. Below this level, the descending portions of both arches fuse to form one descending aorta *(arrow; d)*. (e) is the corresponding angiogram. (Case courtesy of Ina L. D. Tonkin, M.D., University of Tennessee Center for the Health Sciences. Images obtained by Bennett A. Alford, M.D., University of Virginia Hospital.)

right half of the trachea anteriorly and the right lateral wall of the esophagus medially. This has been called the retrotracheal recess, and is frequently occupied by lung (Fig. 3a). These relationships give rise on lateral radiographs to the posterior tracheal band. Normal and pathological variability in these interfaces has been described by Kittredge (35).

Abnormal variations in the configuration of the trachea are easily defined with CT. Figure 27 is a section at the level of the great vessels in a patient with a saber-sheath trachea. Although described classically as a static deformity consisting of marked coronal narrowing associated with sagittal widening of the trachea, Gamsu and Webb (34) have

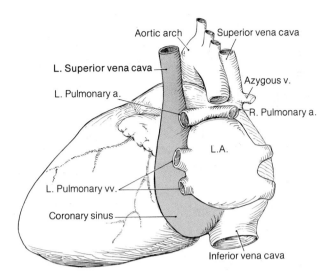

FIG. 24. Schematic drawing of a persistent left-sided superior vena cava, posterior view. The left-sided cava passes in front of the left hilum to drain inferiorly into an enlarged coronary sinus. LA, left atrium.

shown that in two of three patients with this condition examined using CT during a Valsalva maneuver and during forced expiration, there was abnormal narrowing of the tracheal lumen during expiration. This may be significant, since these patients invariably have chronic obstructive pulmonary disease (36).

Tracheal stenosis may also be defined with CT. However, as shown by Gamsu and Webb (34), CT may overestimate both the degree and the length of the stenosis, as compared with tracheograms or endoscopy. Short stenotic segments (i.e., less than 0.5 cm) also prove difficult to define.

Computed tomography is most efficacious in analyzing tracheal neoplasia, both primary and secondary (33,34,37). Despite the presence of air within the tracheal lumen, visualization and definition of tracheal tumors are difficult with routine radiographs, including tomography. This point is illustrated in Fig. 28 (scans of a patient with adenoid-cystic carcinoma). Among primary tracheal neoplasms, adenoid-cystic carcinomas are second only to squamous cell carcinoma in frequency (38). These tumors arise from the tracheobronchial mucous glands, most frequently on the posterolateral wall of the trachea, and they show a marked propensity for local invasion. While endoscopic biopsy can reliably establish the diagnosis, proper preoperative evaluation requires definition of the presence and extent of extraluminal involvement.

25a,b

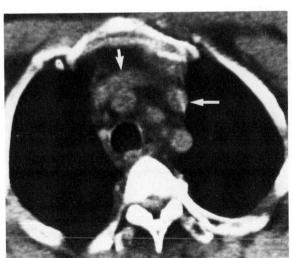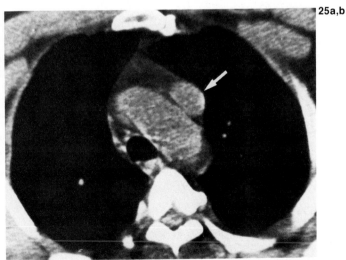

FIG. 25. Persistent left superior vena cava. **a,b:** Sequential images—from above, then downward—of a persistent left-sided vena cava. In (a), the right brachiocephalic vein has a horizontal configuration *(short arrow)* and is joined by a vertically oriented left brachiocephalic vein *(long arrow)*. Note that the left superior vena cava lies anterior to the aortic arch on the left *(arrow; b)*. There is no right-sided vena cava.

26a

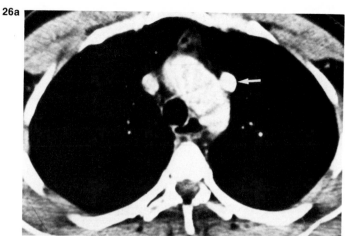

FIG. 26. Double superior vena cava. **a–c:** Sequential images—from above, then downward—starting at the level of the aortic arch. Two vena cava can be identified; the left superior vena cava is opacified *(arrow; a).* Inferiorly, the left vena cava passes anterior to the left hilum as it courses toward the coronary sinus *(arrows; b,c).*

26b,c

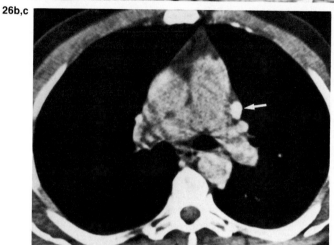
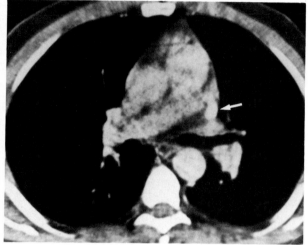

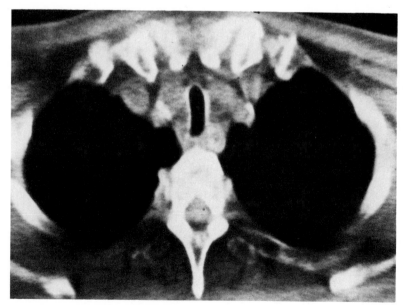

FIG. 27. Saber-sheath trachea. The tracheal lumen has an abnormal configuration, elongated sagittally. There is a high association between this appearance and obstructive lung disease.

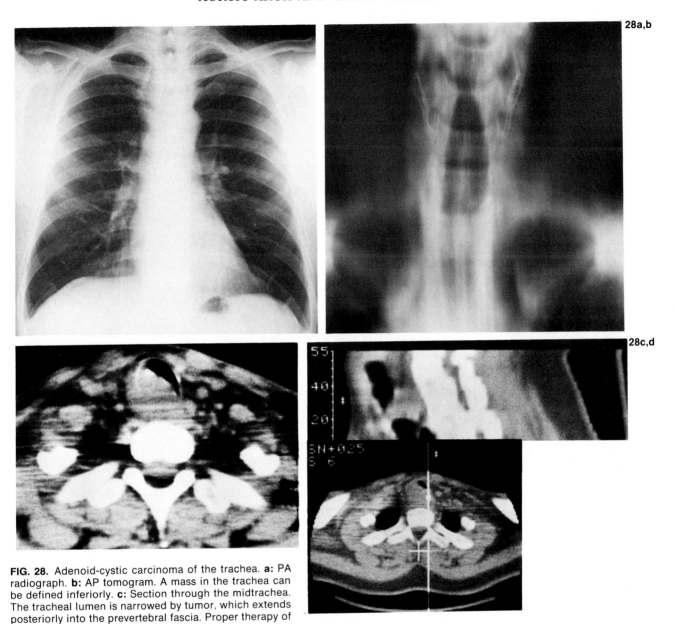

FIG. 28. Adenoid-cystic carcinoma of the trachea. **a:** PA radiograph. **b:** AP tomogram. A mass in the trachea can be defined inferiorly. **c:** Section through the midtrachea. The tracheal lumen is narrowed by tumor, which extends posteriorly into the prevertebral fascia. Proper therapy of these tumors is contingent on defining the true extent of disease, both intra- and extraluminally. **d:** Sagittal reconstruction demonstrates, to good advantage, the true extent of tumor.

This is especially important since recent advances in tracheal surgery have made resection of long tracheal segments possible (39–41).

Secondary neoplastic involvement of the trachea usually results from direct invasion, frequently from esophageal carcinoma. Metastases to the trachea are relatively uncommon, and are usually seen in association with bronchogenic carcinoma.

Mediastinal masses, both benign and malignant, cause displacement of the trachea. The trachea is a relatively flexible structure, allowing for significant deviation without necessarily causing symptoms. A mass adjacent to the trachea *per se* is not good evidence of tracheal involvement; tumor invasion can be diagnosed reliably only when there is marked irregularity of the tracheal wall and/or lumen.

More rarely, inflammatory disease may affect the tracheal wall directly. In our limited experience with this entity, CT disclosed circumferential, uni-

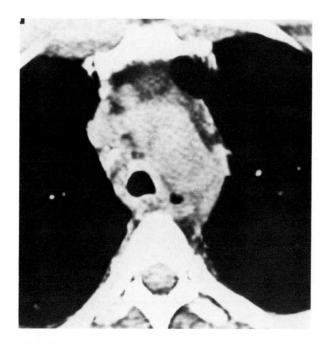

FIG. 29. Tracheal sarcoid. Section through the aortic arch. The trachea is circumferentially thickened; the tracheal lumen is narrowed. Enlarged mediastinal nodes are present as well. Biopsy confirmed tracheal sarcoid. This appearance may be indistinguishable from other infiltrative–inflammatory diseases of the tracheal wall.

form thickening of the entire tracheal wall in a patient with biopsy-proven tracheal sarcoidosis (Fig. 29). It is to be anticipated that other infiltrative–inflammatory diseases of the tracheal wall, such as may result from tuberculosis and amyloidosis, will have a similar appearance (42).

STERNOCLAVICULAR JOINTS AND STERNUM

The sternum and sternoclavicular joints are difficult to evaluate with plain radiographs, mainly because overlying structures are difficult to exclude from view on frontal and oblique projections. The sternoclavicular joints are angled obliquely, making their visualization particularly difficult (Fig. 30).

Figures 31a and b are sequential images through the proximal clavicles and the manubrium, respectively, and correspond with levels A and B in Fig. 30. With the patient's arms held above the head, which is how most CT scans of the thorax are performed, the proximal portions of the clavicles have a steep obliquity and will appear in cross section as elongated or oval structures. The sternal notch is easily defined between the clavicular heads (Fig. 30, level A). The manubrium is the widest part of

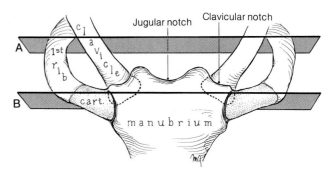

FIG. 30. Schematic drawing of the manubrium and sternoclavicular joints. Characteristic levels are labeled A and B. The sternoclavicular joints are posterior structures.

the sternum and forms the anterior wall of the superior mediastinum. Superiorly, the middle part of the superior border of the manubrium is rounded; this portion is called the jugular notch. To each side of the jugular notch, posteriorly, an indentation in the manubrium can be identified; these are the clavicular notches, which represent the sternal part of the sternoclavicular joints. Sequential scans through the clavicular notches show close approximation of the sternum with the clavicular heads (Fig. 30, level B). Just below this, and somewhat more laterally, a rough projection in the contour of the manubrium can be defined, representing the point of articulation between the sternum and the first costal cartilage.

The value of CT in assessing lesions of the sternoclavicular joints and sternum has been documented by Destouet et al. (43). In their series of 17 patients with sternoclavicular abnormalities, CT demonstrated pathology better, or provided additional diagnostic information in the majority of cases. These included six cases of sternoclavicular joint dislocation, two cases of nonspecific synovitis and osteoarthritis, and two cases of osteomyelitis. Depiction of tumor involvement is particularly easy to assess with CT (Fig. 32).

SUMMARY

Radiologic evaluation of the mediastinum has undergone a profound change since the advent of CT. The superior resolution of mediastinal structures provided by cross-sectional images makes the thorough knowledge of normal mediastinal anatomy necessary, as well as familiarity with the wide range of normal variants and anomalies.

As pointed out in the beginning of this chapter, vascular anomalies and variants represent a signifi-

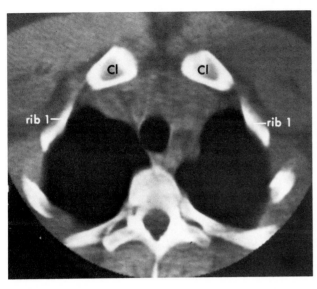
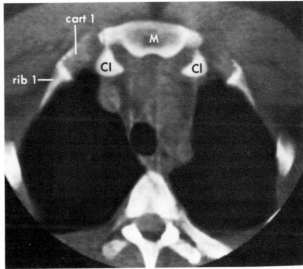

FIG. 31. a: Section at the level of the sternal notch, imaged with bone window settings. **b:** Section through the sternoclavicular joints. The clavicular heads articulate with the manubrium (M) posteriorly. The costal cartilage of the first ribs articulates with the sternum anteroinferiorly. Cl, proximal clavicles; cart 1, first costo-chondral junction.

cant clinical problem in plain-film interpretation. These frequently cause mediastinal widening and/or masses that previously required more definitive evaluation, either angiographic or surgical. It is not an overstatement to suggest that identification of these variants and exclusion of more significant pathology have been the greatest benefits derived from CT. For this reason, considerable attention has been paid in this chapter to the various vascular anomalies, in particular those affecting the aortic

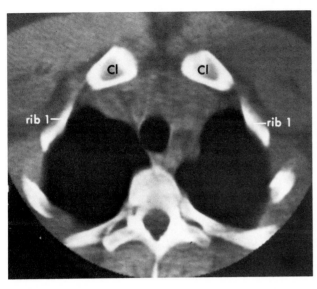

FIG. 32. Invasive thyroid carcinoma. Section through the sternum in a patient with invasive thyroid cancer. The degree of sternal involvement is easily assessed.

arch, since these are the most complex and the easiest to misdiagnose. Wherever possible, the anatomy has been reinforced with illustrative pathology. A more in-depth consideration of mediastinal disease is presented in Chapter 3.

REFERENCES

1. Heitzman ER, Goldwin RL, Proto AV. Radiological analysis of the mediastinum utilizing computed tomography. *Semin Roentgenol* 13:277–292, 1978
2. Jost RG, Sagel SS, Stanley RJ, Levitt RG. Computed tomography of the thorax. *Radiology* 126:125–136, 1978
3. Crowe JK, Brown LR, Muhn JR. Computed tomography of the mediastinum. *Radiology* 128:75–87, 1978
4. Hyson EA, Ravin CE. Radiographic features of mediastinal anatomy. *Chest* 75:609–613, 1979
5. Chasen MH, LaMasters DL. A mini-atlas of computed coronal and sagittal pixel tomography of the mediastinum. *Med Radiogr Photogr* 57:(3), 1981
6. Baron RL, Levitt RG, Sagel SS, Stanley RJ. Computed tomography in the evaluation of mediastinal widening. *Radiology* 138:107–113, 1981
7. Mitsuoka A, Kitano M, Ishii S. Technical note: Gas-contrasted computed tomography of the mediastinum. *J Comput Assist Tomogr* 5:588–590, 1981
8. Sone S, Higashihara T, Morimoto S, et al. Potential spaces of the mediastinum: CT pneumomediastinography. *AJR* 138:1051–1057, 1982
9. Schnyder PA, Gamus G. CT of the pretracheal retrocaval space. *AJR* 136:303–308, 1981
10. R. Moncada, personal communication. Loyola University, Chicago, IL, U.S.A.
11. McLoughlin MJ, Weisbrod G, Wise DJ, Yeung HPH. Computed tomography in congenital anomalies of the aortic arch and great vessels. *Radiology* 138:399–403, 1981
12. Reede DL, Bergeron T, McCauley DI. CT of the thyroid and

of other thoracic inlet disorders. *J Otolaryngol* 11:349–357, 1982

13. Smathers RL, Buschi AJ, Pope TL, Brenbridge AN, Williamson BR. The azygos arch: Normal and pathologic CT appearance. *AJR* 139:477–483, 1982

14. Friedman AC, Chambers E, Sprayregen S. The normal and abnormal left superior intercostal vein. *AJR* 131:599–602, 1978

15. Ball JB, Proto AV. The variable appearance of the left superior intercostal vein. *Radiology* 144:445–452, 1982

16. Lane EJ, Heitzman ER, Dinn WM. The radiology of the superior intercostal veins. *Radiology* 120:263–267, 1976

17. Rockoff SD, Druy EM. Tortuous azygos arch simulating a pulmonary lesion. *AJR* 138:577–579, 1982

18. Allen HA, Haney PJ. Case report: Left-sided inferior vena cava with hemiazygos continuation. *J Comput Assist Tomogr* 5:917–920, 1981

19. Breckenridge JW, Kinlaw WB. Azygos continuation of the IVC. *J Comput Assist Tomogr* 4:392–397, 1980

20. Churchill RJ, Wesby G, Marsan RE, Moncada R, Reynes CJ, Love L. Case report: Computed tomographic demonstration of anomalous inferior vena cava with azygos continuation. *J Comput Assist Tomogr* 4:398–402, 1980

21. Edwards J. Anomalies of derivatives of the aortic arch system. *Med Clin North Am* 32:925–949, 1948

22. Dominguez R, Oh KS, Dorst JP, Young LW. Left aortic arch with right descending aorta. *AJR* 130:917–920, 1978

23. Shuford WH, Sybers RG, Edwards FK. The three types of right aortic arch. *Am J Roentgenol Radium Ther Nucl Med* 109:67–74, 1970

24. Felson B, Palayew MJ. The two types of right aortic arch. *Radiology* 81:745–759, 1963

25. Stewart JR, Kincaid OW, Edwards JE. *An Atlas of Vascular Rings and Related Malformations of the Aortic Arch System.* Springfield, IL, Charles C. Thomas, 1964

26. Webb WR, Gamus G, Speckman JM, Kaiser JA, Federle MP, Lipton MJ. CT demonstration of mediastinal aortic arch anomalies. *J Comput Assist Tomogr* 6:445–451, 1982

27. Eichelberger RP, Long SI, Maulsby GO. Type IIIA1B right aortic arch: Angiographic and computed tomographic evaluation. *CT* 4:241–244, 1980

28. Nath PH, Castenada-Zuniga W, Zollikofer C, et al. Isolation of a subclavian artery. *AJR* 137:683–688, 1981

29. Shuford WH, Sybers RG, Weens HS. The angiographic features of double aortic arches. *AJR* 116:125–140, 1972

30. Garti IJ, Aygen MM, Levy MJ. Double aortic arch anomalies: Diagnosis by countercurrent right brachial arteriography. *AJR* 133:251–256, 1979

31. Gaupp RJ, Fagan CJ, Davis M, Epstein NE. Case report: Pseudocoarctation of the aorta. *J Comput Assist Tomogr* 5:571–573, 1981

32. Webb WR, Gamsu G, Speckman JM, Kaiser JA, Federle MP, Lipton MJ. Pictorial essay: Computed tomographic demonstration of mediastinal venous anomalies. *AJR* 139:157–161, 1982

33. Kittredge RD. Computed tomography of the trachea: A review. *CT* 5:44–49, 1981

34. Gamsu G, Webb WR. Computed tomography of the trachea: Normal and abnormal. *AJR* 139:321–326, 1982

35. Kittredge RD. The right posterolateral trachea band. *J Comput Assist Tomogr* 3:348–354, 1979

36. Greene R. "Saber-sheath" trachea: Relation to chronic obstructive pulmonary disease. *AJR* 130:441–445, 1978

37. Naidich DP, McCauley DI, Siegelman SS. Computed tomography of bronchial adenomas. *J Comput Assist Tomogr* 6:725–732, 1982

38. Houston HE, Payne WS, Harrison EG, Olsen AM. Primary cancers of the trachea. *Arch Surg* 99:132–140, 1969

39. Jensik RJ, Faber LP, Brown CM, Kittle CF. Bronchoplastic and conservative resectional procedures for bronchial adenoma. *J Thorac Cardiovasc Surg* 68:556–565, 1974

40. Ross JAT. Techniques in the surgical repair of tracheal stenosis. *Otolaryngol Clin North Am* 12:893–899, 1979

41. Dedo HH, Fishman NH. Laryngeal release and sleeve resection for tracheal stenosis. *Ann Otol Rhinol Laryngol* 78:285–296, 1969

42. Hof DG, Rasp FL. Spontaneous regression of diffuse tracheobronchial amyloidosis. *Chest* 76:237–239, 1979

43. Destouet JM, Gilula LA, Murphy WA, Sagel SS. Computed tomography of the sternoclavicular joint and sternum. *Radiology* 138:123–128, 1981

44. Smathers, RL, Lee, JKT, Heiken, JP. Clinical image. Anomalous preaortic interazygous vein. *J Comput Assist Tomogr* 7:732–733, 1983

Chapter 3

Mediastinum

The value of thoracic CT is greatest in the study of the mediastinum. With conventional radiography, pathologic processes cannot be detected unless they produce a contour abnormality of the lung–mediastinal interface. With its superior contrast resolution, CT readily distinguishes vessels, lymph nodes, and masses from the surrounding fat. The transaxial plane of CT imaging is well-suited to the investigation of the mediastinal structures, most of which are oriented perpendicularly to the axial plane. Confusing radiographic appearances due to superimposition of different structures are readily resolved. The site of origin and extent of lesions are clearly depicted. With CT, the traditional radiologic "blind spots" of the thoracic inlet, the intrapericardial vessels, and the diaphragmatic crura are no longer difficult to evaluate (1).

The indications for mediastinal CT can be subdivided into two broad categories:

(1) To better define an abnormality detected by plain chest roentgenography. The chest radiograph remains the screening procedure of choice in the thorax. When a mediastinal abnormality is suspected, CT should be the next procedure; it has replaced conventional tomography (2,3). With CT, the radiologist easily recognizes normal variations and benign conditions, such as abnormal fat accumulations or water-containing cysts (4,5). If a pathologic condition is present, CT can precisely define its site of origin (vessels versus nodes versus adjacent lung) and direct further investigations (5,6).

(2) To more critically evaluate the mediastinum in patients with an established clinical problem. CT may be indicated in these patients because of its high detection sensitivity. Radiographically occult pathology can be readily detected, which helps the staging, treatment planning, and follow-up of patients with known neoplasia, as well as the management of conditions potentially associated with a mediastinal abnormality, such as a thymoma in myasthenia gravis or an ectopic parathyroid adenoma in surgically resistant hyperparathyroidism.

Classically, the mediastinum is divided into several anatomic compartments. This facilitates interpretation of the conventional radiographic manifestations of mediastinal pathology (7). Although some entities are more commonly seen in certain subcompartments, most pathologic processes can express themselves in all. Furthermore, CT can separately visualize the basic mediastinal anatomic components: fat, lymph nodes, veins and arteries, airways, thymus, esophagus, and the paraspinal tissues.

For these reasons, this chapter is organized so that each of these components is discussed separately; this provides a more unified and clinically relevant look at mediastinal CT than would the traditional compartmental approach.

TECHNIQUE

The chest radiograph should always serve as the guide to the CT study. With bulky masses, interspacing of slices by one slice width is adequate and can be supplemented by additional contiguous slices in selected areas.

A slice thickness of 10 mm is generally sufficient. Thinner slices are required for the assessment of smaller abnormalities, in areas where anatomic structures are not oriented perpendicularly to the scan plane (such as the aortopulmonary window), and when mediastinal fat is lacking (see Fig. 5, Chapter 1).

In the majority of cases, contrast medium administration is unnecessary. Contrast medium is used only if an abnormality needs to be differentiated from surrounding vessels or if mediastinal fat is insufficient. Discrimination of vascular from nonvascular structures is best achieved with bolus injections of 20 to 25 cc of contrast agent, with scanning timed to coincide with the passage of contrast medium in the vessels near the abnormality. For studies of extended areas using contrast agents, a bolus injection followed by a rapid infusion is the best alternative (see Chapter 1). Dynamic scanning should be used for analysis of contrast medium transit, and is especially valuable in aortic dissection.

MEDIASTINAL FAT

Fat is specifically recognized by its low CT numbers, which vary from -70 to -130 Hounsfield units. Fat is normally present in the mediastinum and the amount of it may increase with age. Normal fat is unencapsulated and equally distributed throughout the connective tissue matrix of the mediastinum. Most of the fat in the anterior mediastinum is contained within the fibrous skeleton of the involuted thymus. The contours of the mediastinum are not affected by normal amounts of fat.

Abnormalities of fat distribution can be diffuse, as in lipomatosis, or focal, as in lipomas or fat-containing transdiaphragmatic hernias.

Mediastinal Lipomatosis

Lipomatosis is a benign condition in which overabundant amounts of histologically normal, unen-

capsulated fat accumulate in the mediastinum. The excess deposition is most prominent in the upper mediastinum, with resulting smooth mediastinal widening on chest radiographs and convex-bulging pleuromediastinal interfaces on CT images (Fig. 1). Tracheal compression or displacement is uniformly absent (8–10). Less commonly, fat will also accumulate in the cardiophrenic angles and paraspinal areas (11,12). The fat in lipomatosis should appear homogeneously lucent. If inhomogeneity is noted, superimposed processes such as mediastinitis, hemorrhage, tumor infiltration, postradiation fibrosis, and postsurgical changes should be considered. Lipomatosis may be associated with simple obesity or Cushing's syndrome, but these factors are absent in up to one-half of cases (13). The diagnosis, therefore, should not be excluded in the absence of predisposing factors. CT is the definitive diagnostic modality for this entity, which is now diagnosed with surprising frequency.

The rare entity of *multiple symmetrical lipomatosis* may mimic the appearance on CT of simple lipomatosis, but often produces compression of surrounding structures, in particular the trachea, and does not involve the anterior mediastinum, cardiophrenic angles, or paraspinal regions. In addition, periscapular lipomatous masses are almost always present (14).

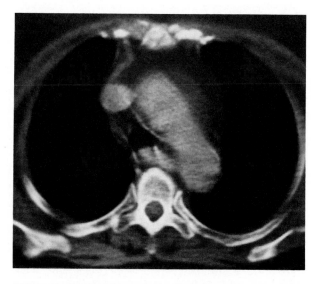

FIG. 1. Mediastinal lipomatosis. Excess amounts of normal-appearing, homogeneous fat in the upper mediastinum is the typical presentation of lipomatosis. This 52-year-old patient had no history of obesity, steroid therapy, or Cushing's syndrome. The study was performed as part of the workup of a newly discovered intra-abdominal lymphoma. Note the laterally bulging pleuromediastinal interface and the absence of tracheal or vascular displacement.

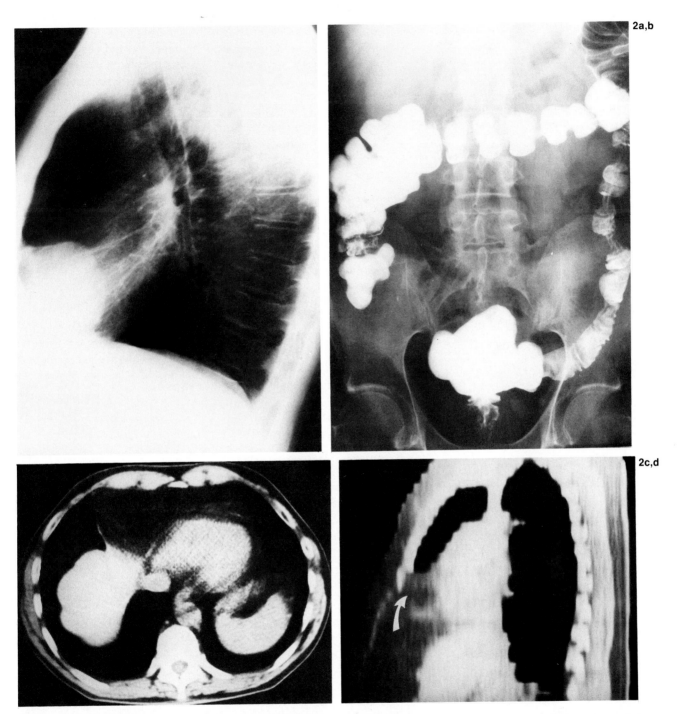

2c,d

FIG. 2. Morgagni hernia, containing omental fat only. A 65-year-old male with incidentally discovered right cardiophrenic angle mass. The mass was diagnosed as a lipoma. At surgery, a Morgagni hernia containing omental fat was found. **a:** Lateral chest radiograph. **b:** Barium enema. **c:** Axial CT image, near diaphragm. **d:** Sagittal reconstruction through mass. The lateral view of the chest best demonstrates the cardiophrenic angle mass. The barium enema shows the absence of colonic displacement, which should not exclude the diagnosis of hernia. On the axial CT image, fine linear densities are noted within the right-sided fatty mass. We presume that they represent omental vessels, and, when seen, should suggest the proper diagnosis of omental hernia. The sagittal reconstruction through the foramen clearly demonstrates the discontinuous diaphragm and the continuity of the thoracic fatty mass with the abdominal fat *(arrow).*

Fatty Masses

In the large majority of cases, the discovery of the fatty nature of a mass indicates benignancy. In our experience, most fatty masses are seen in the peridiaphragmatic areas and they most often represent herniation of abdominal fat. True lipomatous tumors are much less common.

Fatty Herniations

There are several direct connections between the abdomen and mediastinum that permit passage of intra-abdominal fat into the thorax.

Omental fat can herniate through the foramen of Morgagni to create the appearance of a cardio-phrenic angle mass, almost always located on the right side (15). The omentum is freely mobile and does not always carry the transverse colon with it into the hernia. Fine linear densities can sometimes be seen within herniated omental fat and probably represent omental vessels. When seen within a fatty mass, these linear densities should suggest fat herniation rather than a lipoma (Fig. 2).

Fat herniation through the foramen of Bochdalek occurs most often on the left side, since the liver prevents its occurrence on the right.

Herniation of perigastric fat through the phrenicoesophageal membrane surrounding and fixating the esophagus to the diaphragm is the first step in the pathogenesis of hiatus hernias. The herniated fat can extend along the aorta and widen the paraspinal line (Fig. 3) or it can appear as a retrocardiac mass (Fig. 4). Multiplanar reconstructions are sometimes helpful for demonstrating the connections of the fatty hernia with abdominal fat (Figs. 2 and 4).

Lipomas

Mediastinal lipomas are uncommon tumors (16). They are soft, and do not produce compressive symptoms unless they are large enough to compress surrounding structures. They may or may not be encapsulated. Although they contain variable amounts of fibrous septa, they appear to have homogeneously low CT numbers. Their boundaries are smooth and sharply defined, with no blurring, thickening, or invasion of surrounding structures (Fig. 5). If inhomogeneity, higher CT numbers than usual, poor demarcation, or invasion of the surrounding structures are seen, a benign lipoma cannot be confidently diagnosed. A superimposed process should be suspected, with consideration

3a,b

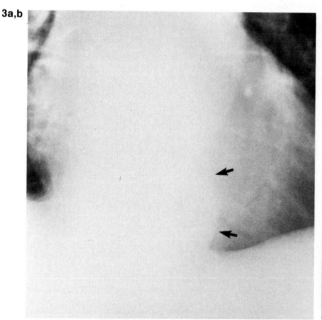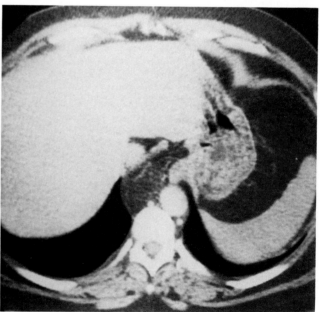

FIG. 3. Lesser omental fat herniation through esophageal hiatus. A 56-year-old male with paraspinal line widening on chest radiographs. **a:** PA chest radiograph. **b:** CT at level of esophageal hiatus. The bulging paraspinal line could be due to a number of causes *(arrows)*. CT demonstrates a fatty structure accounting for the radiographic abnormality. Note again the linear densities within the fatty mass, a clue to its omental origin. The esophageal hiatus is also much wider than usual. In the pathogenesis of hiatus hernia, perigastric fat displacement into the mediastinum, because of an incompetent phrenicoesophageal membrane, is thought to be the first step, and is best detected with CT.

4a,b

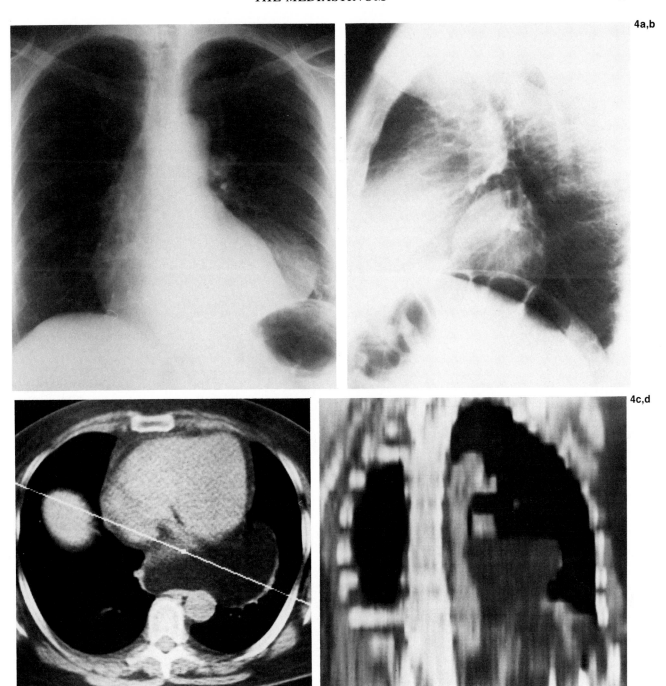

4c,d

FIG. 4. Large paraesophageal omental hernia. A 39-year-old female with dysphagia. **a,b:** PA and lateral radiographs. **c:** CT scan at level of mass. **d:** Oblique reconstruction through axis of line seen in (c). A large, smooth retrocardiac mass is identified. The axial CT image shows an entirely fatty mass. Note again the faint linear densities within the mass, most probably representing omental vessels. A planar reconstruction shows the true intra-abdominal origin of the mass, found at surgery to represent omental fat extending into the mediastinum via a large esophageal hiatus. Peridiaphragmatic fatty masses are much more likely to represent hernias containing fat than lipomas.

given to the rare possibility of a liposarcoma or lipoblastoma (17–19) (Fig. 6). Inhomogeneous fatty masses of the anterior mediastinum raise the possibility of a fat-containing teratoma or a thymolipoma (20) (Fig. 7).

MEDIASTINAL LYMPH NODES

In autopsy series, the average number of mediastinal nodes is 64 (21). Almost 80% of the nodes are located immediately adjacent to the tracheo-

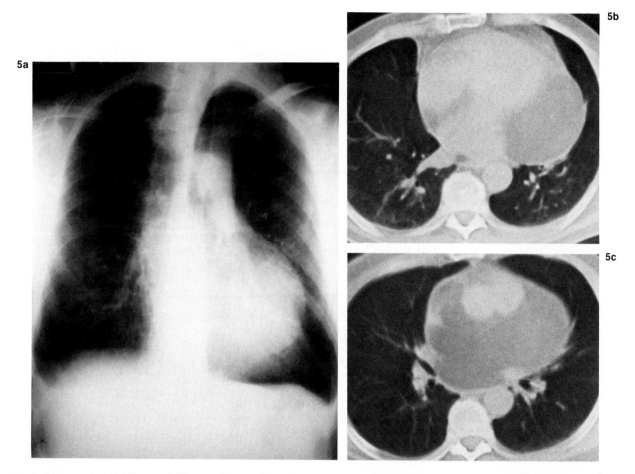

FIG. 5. Large pericardial lipoma. A 65-year old asymptomatic male with a large paracardiac mass incidentally discovered on chest radiography. **a:** PA chest radiograph. **b** and **c:** CT sections at level of mass. An entirely fatty mass with homogeneously low CT numbers is identified. Its margins are smooth and well-defined. The vascular structures are clearly separated from the mass. Although minimal displacement of normal structures is seen, the benign appearance on CT led to conservative management; 5 years after diagnosis the patient remains asymptomatic.

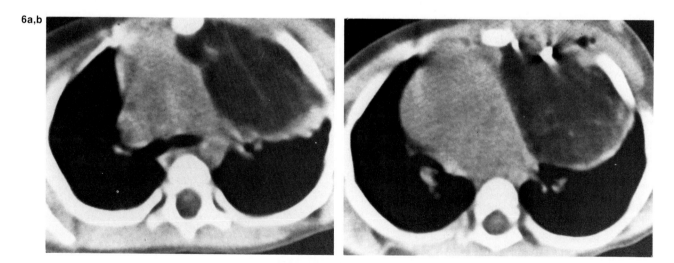

FIG. 6. Lipoblastoma. An 8-month-old male with large mass discovered on chest radiograph. **a** and **b:** CT scans show a large mass with low CT numbers compatible with a fatty tumor. The suggestion of chest wall invasion anteriorly in (b), the patient's age, and the minimal inhomogeneity would be unusual for a simple lipoma. Surgery was therefore recommended. A lipoblastoma, a rare benign tumor of childhood made of immature adipose tissue with rapid growth and local recurrence potential, was removed.

7a,b

7c,d

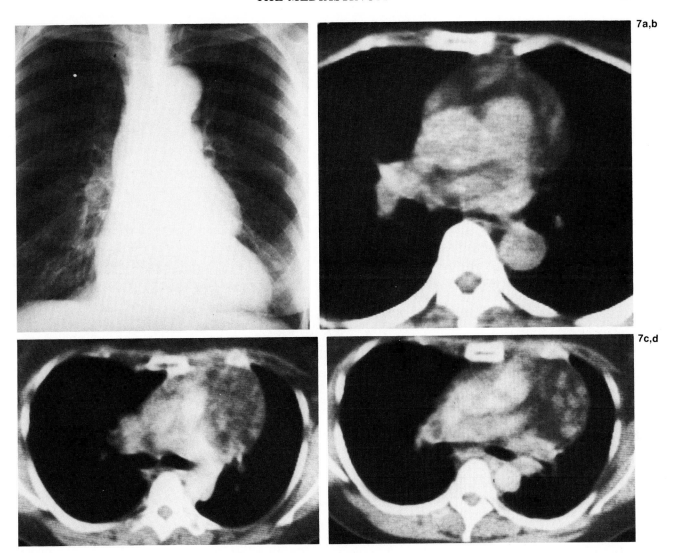

FIG. 7. Thymolipomas. **a** and **b:** A 71-year-old asymptomatic female. PA chest radiograph (a). A smooth mass deforms the contour of the left heart border. CT at level of mass (b). The mass is mostly fatty, but areas of soft-tissue density are identified within it. It is therefore unlikely to represent a simple lipoma. However, its sharp borders, the lack of compression of the nearby vessels, and its location point to a benign lesion. Thymolipoma is a benign fatty tumor of the thymus that is usually of no clinical consequence. No surgery was performed. **c** and **d:** Another example of thymolipoma in a 51-year-old female. Note again the inhomogeneous appearance of the mass (c). Note in (d) the round areas of increased density which were found to represent lymph nodes on pathologic examination. No thymic tissue was identified.

bronchial tree and drain the lungs. Several systems of anatomic classification of the mediastinal nodes have been proposed (7), and are all based on the location of the nodes. In addition, nodes can be characterized as visceral when they drain a thoracic organ, or parietal if they drain the chest wall or the diaphragm.

The most generally used classification is that of Rouviere (22), which will be briefly presented here with slight modifications. The nodes can conveniently be divided into three groups:

(i) Anterior mediastinal nodes.
   (a) Internal mammary nodes. These lie parallel to the internal mammary arteries. They are parietal and drain the anterior chest wall, anterior diaphragm, and the medial portion of the breasts.
   (b) Visceral nodes. These lie in the fatty tissues anterior to the large vessels and include the "ductus" node(s) or "aortopulmonary window" node(s), which drains the left upper lobe.
   (c) Cardiophrenic angle nodes.
(ii) Middle mediastinal nodes. This is the largest visceral group and comprises:
   (a) The tracheobronchial nodes or hilar nodes, subdivided into upper and lower

groups according to their location relative to the hila.

(b) The paratracheal nodes, which are subdivided into right, left, and anterior chains; they drain the upper hilar nodes. The lowest node(s) on the right is the azygos node(s).

(c) The bifurcation or subcarinal nodes, which are located beneath the carina; they drain the lower groups of hilar nodes, and preferentially drain into the right paratracheal chain.

(iii) Posterior mediastinal nodes.

(a) Paravertebral chains. These parietal nodes lie in the proximal intercostal space adjacent to the vertebrae and drain the posterior chest wall, parietal pleura, and vertebrae.

(b) Periesophageal nodes. Located anteriorly around the esophagus and lower aorta, they drain the posterior diaphragm and pericardium, esophagus, and medial aspect of the lower lobes. They communicate with the thoracic duct, subcarinal, intra-abdominal, para-aortic, and celiac axis nodes.

Extensive and complex intercommunications exist among the various groups of lymph nodes. Anatomic classifications do not allow the radiologist to infer the origin of any pathologic process from the location of affected nodes. Different flow patterns, including backflow, can occur because of nodal obstruction secondary to previous inflammation and scarring. Left lower lobe tumors produce contralateral, without ipsilateral, nodal involvement in up to 25% of cases. In mediastinoscopic series, however, contralateral, with ipsilateral, involvement is as common for right-sided tumors as for left-sided tumors (23). The pathways of lymphatic involvement should best be thought of as variable, and not be given too much diagnostic value. For the purposes of CT interpretation, it is more important to classify mediastinal nodes according to their accessibility to the various tissue sampling techniques currently available (Table 1).

With CT, nodes appear as round, oval, or triangular soft-tissue densities against the lower-density background of mediastinal fat. They are often found in clusters of two or three (Fig. 8). The ability to see nodes is directly correlated with the amount of mediastinal fat present. Interpretation of contiguous

TABLE 1. *Nodal accessibility*

Transcervical mediastinoscopy
  Right paratracheal nodes to level of azygos arch
  Anterior paratracheal nodes to level of bifurcation
  Left paratracheal nodes to aortic arch

Anterior mediastinotomy
  Right or left internal mammary nodes
  Anterior mediastinal nodes
  Aortopulmonary window nodes

Thoracotomy
  All nodes

Needle biopsy (percutaneous and transtracheobronchial)
  All nodes

CT scans is always necessary to differentiate nodes from vessels.

With state-of-the-art scanners, normal nodes can be seen in a large percentage of patients. In a large series of normal volunteers, azygous nodes were identified in 88% of the patients. The average size of the nodes was 5.5 ± 2.8 mm. The maximal size of normal nodes ranged from 10 to 14 mm and appeared to increase with the age of the subject (24). Normal nodes larger than 2 cm are rare in the mediastinum and uncommon in the hila.

The manifestations on CT of nodal pathology are simple and nonspecific. Four stages can be recognized in nodes involved by neoplastic as well as non-neoplastic diseases. (a) Normal node. The internal nodal architecture cannot be analyzed with CT. If no enlargement is present, pathology cannot be suspected or excluded with certainty. (b) Enlargement. With further progression of the disease, the nodes enlarge. Enlargement is recognized by direct measurement of the cross section of affected nodes or because of bulging mediastinal contours, such as the normally concave azygo-esophageal recess. However, caution should be exercised to avoid overdiagnosing subcarinal adenopathy in children and young adults in whom the azygo-esophageal recess may be convex normally (25). The margins of nodes may lose their sharp definition and the surrounding fat may increase in density. These changes may be due to extension of the primary process through the nodal capsule or to an associated fibrotic or inflammatory reaction. (c) Coalescence. With further progression, the pathologic process may "burst" through the capsules of several adjacent nodes and fuse to form a single larger mass. (d) Diffuse spread. The connective tissue and fat may be diffusely invaded, with no recognizable nodes or focal mass (Fig. 9).

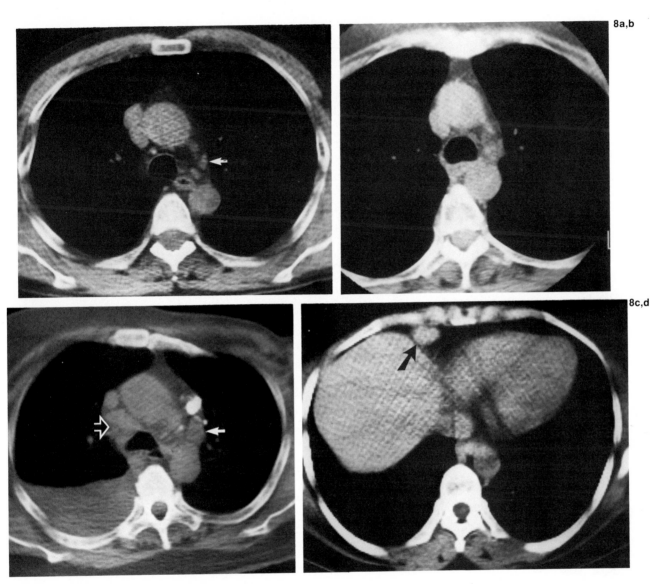

FIG. 8. Mediastinal nodes. A combination of cases is presented to illustrate normal and abnormal nodes in different anatomic locations. **a:** Normal "aortic pulmonary window" nodes are usually found in clusters of two or three. They are clearly seen in this case because there is a sufficient amount of surrounding fat. Their borders are smooth and sharply demarcated *(arrow).* **b:** False-negative aortic pulmonary window nodes in a patient with esophageal carcinoma. A cluster of small nodes is identified. Their appearance and size are similar to those of normal nodes, but metastatic disease was found at surgery. False-negative results with normal-sized nodes are common with esophageal carcinoma but uncommon in lung cancers, in which a negative CT study of the mediastinum (all nodes less than 1 cm in size) is at least as reliable as mediastinoscopy in predicting the absence of metastatic disease. **c:** True-positive nodes. A calcified node is seen in the anterior mediastinum. A larger (2 × 3 cm) node is seen in the aortic pulmonary window *(solid arrow).* Large nodes are also present in the pretracheal retrocaval space on the right side *(open arrow).* At autopsy, all these nodes, including the calcified one, demonstrated metastatic involvement. The aortic pulmonary window node would have been accessible by a left anterior mediastinotomy or needle biopsy. The right-sided paratracheal nodes would have been reachable by transcervical mediastinoscopy. **d–f:** Cardiophrenic angle nodes. A patient with Hodgkin's disease. These nodes are located anteriorly in the cardiophrenic recesses, which may extend over the liver. Thus, cardiophrenic nodes may superficially seem to be intra-abdominal. There are three groups of nodes in this region: The right, illustrated in (d), the left in (e), and the median or subxyphoid in (f) *(arrows).* The median group of nodes is within normal limits in this case.

FIG. 8 continued on next page.

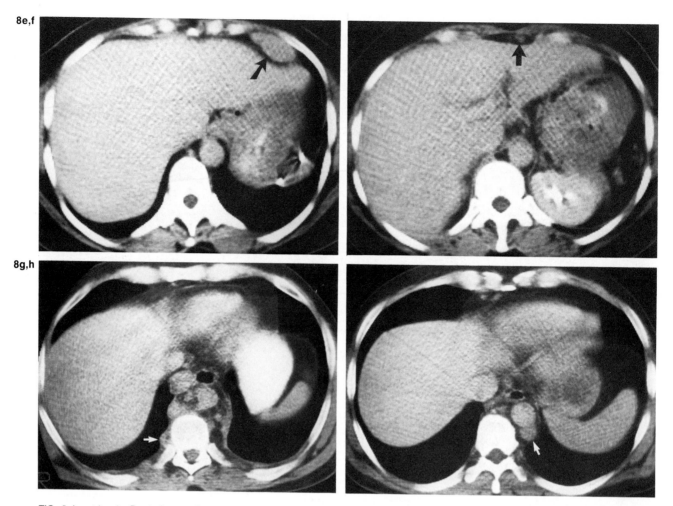

FIG. 8 *(cont.).* g,h: Posterior mediastinal nodes. A 60-year-old male with histiocytic lymphoma. There are paravertebral chains of lymph nodes lying in the proximal intercostal space, adjacent to the vertebrae *(arrow).* Para-aortic nodes are seen in the retrocrural area also and are connected to the paravertebral nodes, as well as to higher para-aortic and periesophageal nodes, as seen in (h). Incidentally noted are small median cardiophrenic nodes.

Granulomatous Diseases

Infectious

The mediastinal lymph nodes are affected by the primary phase of granulomatous infections such as tuberculosis or histoplasmosis. Enlarged nodes with focal lung infiltrate (the GHON complex) is the typical presentation. In the majority of cases, spontaneous regression occurs, often leading to calcification of the affected nodes. Even densely calcified nodes are not inactive and can be involved with other processes, such as metastatic disease, at a later time. In infants, children, and young adults, progression of the disease can lead to symptomatic adenitis, which may require investigation with CT.

One or more groups of enlarged regional nodes, most commonly the right paratracheal, may be seen, but most often a single mass with poorly defined margins is identified (Fig. 9). This mass, due to the fusion of several affected nodes, is initially associated with periadenitis, and later heals by fibrous encapsulation and calcification. These masses are intimately adherent to the surrounding mediastinal structures, and no clear cleavage plane is seen with CT (Fig. 9). Fibrous healing may lead to complications such as vena caval or airway obstruction (26). In rare instances, the fibrosis is not self-limited, but progressively encases all mediastinal structures to result in "mediastinal collagenosis," with replacement of the low-density mediastinal fat by higher-density fibrous tissue and sometimes diffuse calcification (Fig. 10). Histoplasmosis is the most commonly identified etiology but in the majority of cases the cause is not discovered (27).

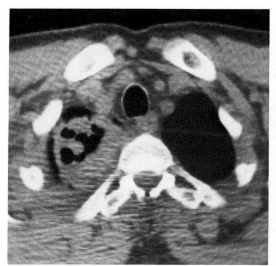
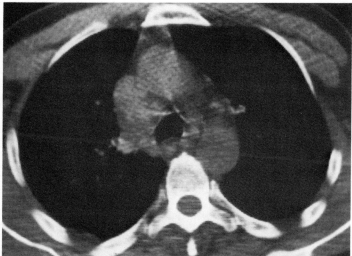

9a,b

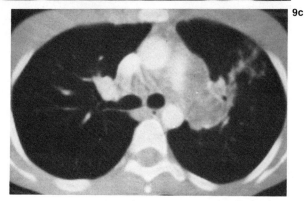

9c

FIG. 9. Mediastinal nodes and tuberculosis. **a:** A 36-year-old male with a large cavity in the right upper lobe that proved to be tuberculous. **b:** Lower section shows enlarged right paratracheal nodes that have lost their margins and fused into a single nodal mass. This appearance is indistinguishable from that of metastatic nodes, as illustrated in Fig. 8c, and demonstrates the nonspecificity of the CT findings. **c:** A 19-year-old female with biopsy-proven mediastinal tuberculosis. A large mass is seen in the aortopulmonary window and is distinguished from vessels on this contrast-enhanced (bolus) study. The intramediastinal margins of the mass are indistinct, and the entire mediastinal connective tissues are of the same density, suggesting that the disease has reached the stage of diffuse spread [as opposed to the local regional nodal involvement seen in (b)]. This appearance could more properly be designated "mediastinitis." A peripheral lung infiltrate is also seen, probably representing the initial pulmonary localization of the disease.

Sarcoidosis

Computed tomography has a limited role in the diagnosis and management of patients with sarcoidosis. This multisystem granulomatous disease is most often detected on routine chest radiography. Bilateral hilar adenopathy, often accompanied by right paratracheal adenopathy in an asymptomatic patient, is the typical presentation (28). Random sampling of bronchial walls and lung parenchyma through the fiberoptic bronchoscope has simplified the procurement of tissue for the diagnosis of sarcoidosis (29). When bronchoscopic biopsies fail, the older methods of scalene node biopsy or mediastinoscopy may be used. In this context, CT provides a map of the affected nodes and shortens procedure time.

With CT, nodes appear moderately enlarged in sarcoidosis. Their margins are well-defined. The nodes do not usually coalesce into a single mass as they do in other granulomatous diseases and lymphomas. As opposed to granulomatous infectious diseases, sarcoidosis involves more than one regional group of nodes, most often symmetrically. In our experience, in most cases, nodal enlargement is seen in all mediastinal compartments. Classically, with conventional radiography, sarcoidosis is said to spare anterior mediastinal nodes. With CT, however, enlarged anterior mediastinal nodes are detected regularly (Fig. 11).

In rare instances, asymmetric involvement of hilar or mediastinal nodes raises the possibility of an infectious or neoplastic etiology. This asymmetry is probably due to asynchronous regression of sarcoidosis in the affected nodes.

Lymphomas

Mediastinal lymph node involvement is a common manifestation of disseminated lymphoma and is the most common intrathoracic manifestation of all lymphomas. Hodgkin's disease is the lymphoma that most commonly presents with adenopathy limited to the mediastinum (30). Only 11% of histiocytic lymphomas are purely mediastinal (31). Lym-

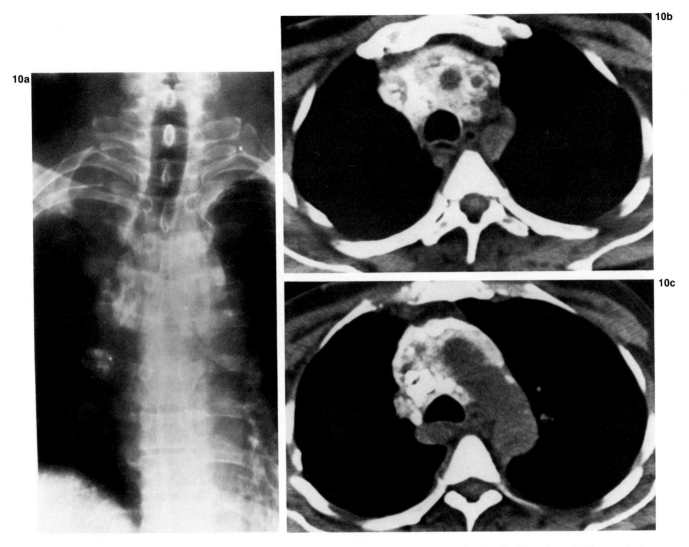

FIG. 10. Healed mediastinitis from histoplasmosis. After diffuse mediastinal involvement, healing by fibrosis and diffuse calcification may be seen, as in this case.

phomatous masses are most commonly found in the anterior mediastinum because up to 40% of patients with Hodgkin's disease, which is the most common intrathoracic lymphoma, present with an anterior mediastinal mass. Histiocytic lymphoma is more apt to localize in the middle mediastinum (31). Although they are suggestive of the type of lymphoma, localization patterns are not specific enough to have a significant role in diagnosis.

The appearance on CT of lymphomatous nodes is not distinctive. The size and appearance of the nodes span the entire spectrum, from well-defined nodes to diffuse extensive involvement (Fig. 12). CT plays a major role in the diagnosis, staging, treatment-planning, and follow-up of these patients. The precise guidance offered by CT combined with a wider availability may make needle biopsy a via-

ble alternative to mediastinoscopy, anterior mediastinotomy, or thoracotomy in these patients.

CT mapping helps in radiotherapy planning and surgical resection. As a follow-up modality, CT assesses treatment responses and permits readjustment of therapy when needed. Complete return to normalcy after successful therapy does not always occur. Follow-up CT studies may demonstrate persistently enlarged nodes, even though they contain no viable tumor tissue. These "sterilized" nodes pose a diagnostic and therapeutic dilemma (32). Cytologic evaluation is notoriously difficult, if not impossible, after irradiation, which complicates the problem. Serial CT examinations to determine relative changes may be the best approach in these patients. Recurrence or failure should be considered only if another increase in size occurs.

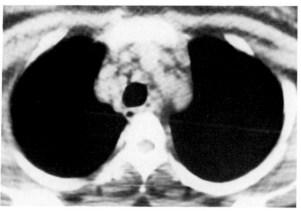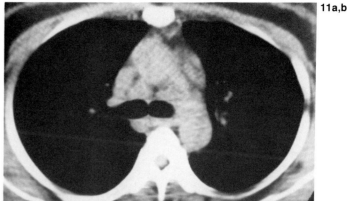

11a,b

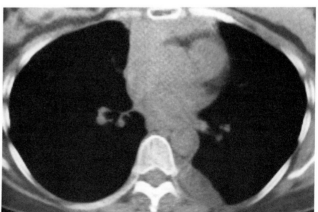

11c

FIG. 11. Mediastinal nodes and sarcoidosis. A 33-year-old female with proven sarcoidosis. Enlarged nodes are seen in all regions of the mediastinum. **a:** Right and left paratracheal nodes. **b:** Anterior mediastinal and anterior carinal nodes. **c:** Subcarinal and hilar nodes. The azygo-esophageal recess is normally concave medially. In this case, it is convex—a reliable clue to the presence of subcarinal adenopathy (except in young patients in whom the recess may normally be convex). In sarcoidosis, the nodes are moderately enlarged. In our experience, their margins are well-defined, and adjacent nodes do not fuse to form a larger mass, as they do in other conditions. Also noted is symmetrical involvement of all nodal chains and the frequent presence of anterior mediastinal as well as subcarinal adenopathy.

Metastatic Nodes

Metastases to mediastinal lymph nodes from extrathoracic malignancies are rare. In a review of 1,071 cases of extrathoracic neoplasms, only 25 (2.3%) had evidence of hilar or mediastinal adenopathy (33). The extrathoracic tumors most likely to metastasize to the mediastinum originate from the head and neck, genitourinary tract, breasts (with a predilection for the internal mammary nodes), and skin with malignant melanoma.

The great majority of nodal mestastases originate

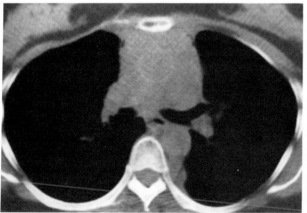

12a,b

FIG. 12. Diffuse mediastinal involvement by histiocytic lymphoma. **a:** The normal low density of the mediastinal connective tissue has been replaced by a diffuse process of soft-tissue density. The ascending aorta is barely recognizable. **b:** The tumor has extended inferiorly to the base of the heart, the azygo-esophageal recess, and the paraspinal region on the left side. As with granulomatous infections and metastatic disease, lymphomas can evolve from solitary enlarged nodes to fusion of regional nodes to diffuse invasion of the perinodal soft tissues by extension through the nodal capsules.

from within the thorax, primarily the lungs and esophagus. Compared with other noninvasive techniques, CT can better delineate the local extent of lung tumors as well as visualize the mediastinal nodes. CT provides unsurpassed guidance for radiotherapy planning for unresectable tumors (34).

Contrary to an earlier report that noted a false-negative rate of 28% in demonstrating nodal invasion, current studies with state-of-the-art scanners demonstrate a high accuracy for CT in the detection of nodal metastases (35,36). Thus, lung cancer staging has become an important application for mediastinal CT. The radiologist needs to be familiar with the total issue of lung cancer staging in order to better interpret CT findings. Salient points will be reviewed and illustrated.

Mediastinal CT and Lung Cancer Staging

Thoracotomy with total resection of the neoplasm is the modality of choice for curing patients with non-oat cell carcinoma of the lung. Historically, the cure rates for surgery have been disappointing. The 5-year survival rates are at most about 30%, presumably because of poor patient selection (37). Operative mortality is high. In one study of 421 patients, surgical mortality was 11% and 5-year survival was 13% (38). Median survival may not be significantly longer with surgery. In one series, the median survival for surgically treated patients was 22 months, compared to 19 months in nonsurgically treated patients (39). These results indicate that surgery is ineffective in improving outcome when the disease cannot be entirely removed. Unfortunately, at the time of presentation, up to 50% of the patients with lung cancer already have direct extrapulmonary extension, regional nodal involvement, or distant metastases. Methods to segregate these patients from the patients with curable disease should therefore improve the results of surgical resection and prevent unnecessary surgical morbidity and mortality. This selection process takes into account three major factors: (a) The

TABLE 2. *The clinical staging of cancer: definitions of T, N, and M categories for carcinoma of the lung*[a]

T (primary tumors)

T0	No evidence of primary tumor.
TX	Occult tumor with positive cytology.
TIS	Carcinoma *in situ*.
T1	A tumor that is 3.0 cm or less in greatest diameter, surrounded by lung or visceral pleura and without evidence of invasion proximal to a lobar bronchus at bronchoscopy.
T2	A tumor more than 3.0 cm in greatest diameter, or a tumor of any size that either invades the visceral pleura, or which has associated atelectasis or obstructive pneumonitis extending to the hilar region. At bronchoscopy, the proximal extent of demonstrable tumor must be within a lobar bronchus or at least 2.0 cm distal to the carina. Any associated atelectasis or obstructive pneumonitis must involve less than an entire lung, and there must be no pleural effusion.
T3	A tumor of any size with direct extension into an adjacent structure, such as the parietal pleura or chest wall, the diaphragm, or the mediastinum and its contents; or a tumor demonstrable bronchoscopically to involve a main bronchus less than 2.0 cm distal to the carina; or any tumor associated with atelectasis or obstructive pneumonitis of an entire lung or pleural effusion.

N (regional lymph nodes)

N0	No demonstrable metastasis to regional lymph nodes.
N1	Metastasis to lymph nodes in the peribronchial or the ipsilateral hilar region, or both, including direct extension.
N2	Metastasis to lymph nodes in the mediastinum.

M (distant metastasis)

M0	No distant metastasis.
M1	Distant metastasis.

[a] Each case must be assigned the highest category of T, N, and M that describes the full extent of disease in that case.

From ref. 41.

physiologic status of the patient—age, cardiovascular status, and pulmonary function evaluation determines the surgical risk or operability. (b) The biological characteristics of the tumor—squamous cell carcinoma offers the best surgical cure potential and can be resected even in the presence of ipsilateral mediastinal node involvement (40). Large cell carcinoma, adenocarcinoma, and oat cell carcinoma (in that order) have progressively poorer prognoses. Oat cell carcinoma is generally considered a nonsurgical tumor. (c) The anatomic extent of the tumor—tumor extent is classified in stages that help define prognosis and technical resectability. The American Joint Committee for Cancer Staging—TNM System has become the standard staging system (41). Interpretation of the CT examinations of patients with lung cancer should be based on a working knowledge of the TNM System (Tables 2 and 3).

Tumor extent (T).

Since total resection offers the best hope for cure, an effort should be made to avoid false-positive readings. The CT study should show gross, definite evidence of mediastinal, parietal, pleural, or chest wall invasion before it can be considered to indicate a T3 lesion. Simple contact of the tumor with or without thickening of the pleuromediastinal interface should be considered indeterminate. Frank "interdigitation" of tumor tissue with the normal mediastinal structures should be seen, preferably within 2 cm of the carina, to positively diagnose mediastinal invasion (Fig. 13).

Regional lymph node involvement (N).

Computerized tomography is the only noninvasive method that provides direct visualization of mediastinal nodes. Size, shape, and margins of nodes can be evaluated, but there is no morphologic appearance specific for metastatic adenopathy. Fortunately, nodal size is a reasonably accurate guide for the assessment of metastatic disease.

Using 1 cm or less as the upper limit of normal, recent series have found a 3–7% false-negative rate in detecting nodal metastases (36,42,43). Since metastatic disease does not always enlarge lymph nodes, CT assessment will always be associated with a false-negative group of patients (44).

Even though a definite cutoff size for normal nodes cannot be defined, the false-negative rates of less than 10% obtained with current scanners, using 1 cm as a limit, compare favorably with the false-negative rates of mediastinoscopy, which vary between 5% and 35%. Using 2 cm as the lower limit

TABLE 3. *The clinical staging of cancer: stage grouping in carcinoma of the lung*

Occult carcinoma TX N0 M0	An occult carcinoma with positive cytology but without other evidence of the primary tumor or evidence of metastasis to the regional lymph nodes or distant metastasis.
Stage I TIS N0 M0	Carcinoma *in situ*.
T1 N0 M0 T1 N1 M0 T2 N0 M0	A tumor that can be classified T1 without any metastasis or with metastasis to the lymph nodes in the peribronchial and/or ipsilateral hilar region only, or a tumor that can be classified T2 without any metastasis to nodes or distant metastasis.
Stage II T2 N1 M0	A tumor classified as T2 with metastasis to the lymph nodes in the peribronchial and/or ipsilateral hilar region only.
Stage III[a] T3 with any N or M N2 with any T or M M1 with any T or N	Any tumor more extensive than T2, or any tumor with metastasis to the lymph nodes in the mediastinum, or with distant metastasis.

[a] Note: Stage III lesions are considered unresectable.
Based on the Report of the American Joint Committee for Cancer Staging and End Results Reporting, Chicago, 1973.

13a,b

13c,d

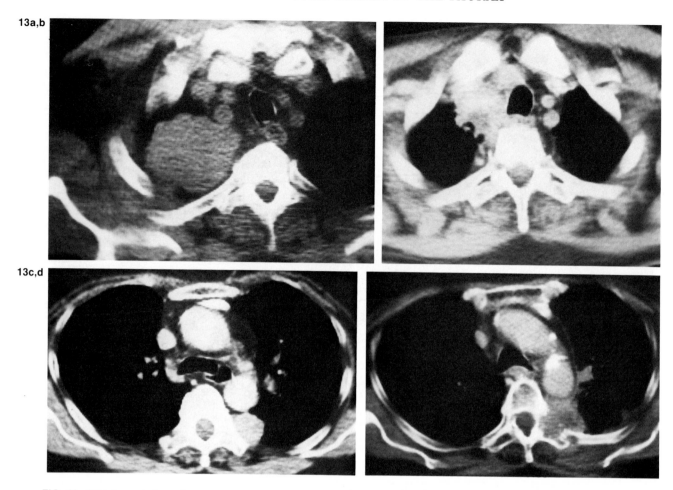

FIG. 13. CT interpretation of tumor extent (T). A series of cases are presented and should be correlated with Table 2. **a:** T2 squamous cell carcinoma of right upper lobe. The tumor is larger than 3 cm. Although it abuts the chest wall and mediastinal pleura, caution should be exercised so that invasion is not diagnosed, because no definite destruction is seen. At surgery a resectable lesion was found. **b:** T3 squamous cell carcinoma of right upper lobe. As opposed to A, the mediastinal–tumor interface is irregular and blurred. The mediastinal fat is definitely invaded. **c:** Adenocarcinoma of left lower lobe. The tumor is in contact with the chest wall and vertebral body, but no definite invasion is seen. This should be interpreted as a T2 lesion. **d:** Same case as (c). The patient was inoperable. Six months later, the tumor has grown to destroy the adjacent bony structures, making it a definite T3 lesion at this time.

for definitely malignant nodes, no false-positives occurred in a series of 98 patients (36).

In a single study in Scandinavia of 35 patients with non–oat cell carcinoma, 17 patients had nodes larger than 1 cm, but intranodal tumor was found in only two (42). To date, this is the only study with such disappointing results. The upper limit of normal size may be dependent on the prevalence of granulomatous diseases in a given population. In our experience in the northeast portion of the United States, false-positive diagnoses definitely occur in fewer than 10% of cases.

The greatest overlap between normal and malignant nodes is in the 1–2 cm range. Above 2 cm, metastatic involvement is the rule. Anecdotal cases of enlarged nodes due to causes other than metastatic disease have occurred, but they are not com-

mon enough to significantly decrease the predictive value of discovering a node larger than 2 cm.

Classically, mediastinoscopy and anterior mediastinotomy are used to sample mediastinal nodes. These techniques are not without risks, and are limited to certain groups of mediastinal nodes (see Table 1). The subcarinal and posterior mediastinal nodes are inaccessible by these techniques but are easily visualized with CT when they are abnormal. CT can be used as a roadmap to select the most appropriate approach to tissue sampling by pointing out the location of the largest nodes, which are most likely to harbor tumor. CT can also be used to guide percutaneous or transtracheobronchial needle biopsies. In our experience, nodes smaller than 1 cm are not easy to sample by any technique. During mediastinoscopy or anterior mediastinotomy, the

13e,f

13g,h

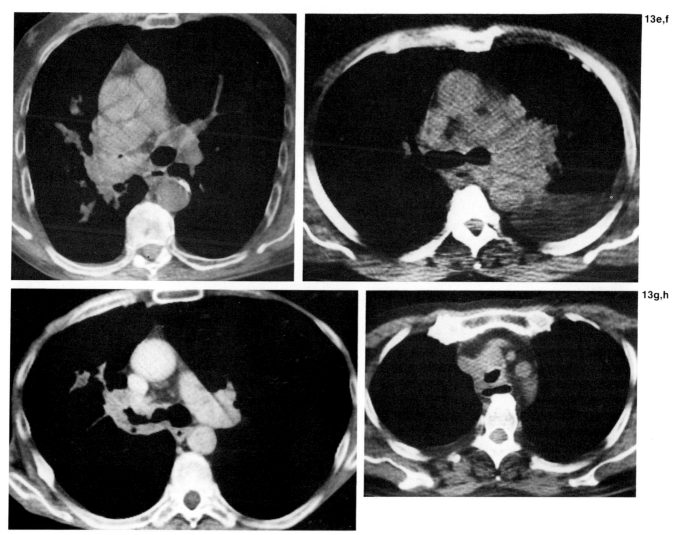

FIG. 13 (cont.). e: Right hilar squamous cell carcinoma. The right main-stem bronchus is almost totally occluded. The tumor extends into the subcarinal space. This lesion was interpreted as a T3, unresectable. At surgery, however, total resection with sleeve reconstruction of the trachea was possible. Some cases are difficult to classify as T2 or T3. Furthermore, surgical therapy for squamous cell carcinomas tends to be more aggressive. **f:** Left hilar adenocarcinoma. Enlarged mass with definite extension into the mediastinal soft tissue and large pleural effusion make this lesion a definite T3. **g:** Squamous cell carcinoma of right upper lobe bronchus. The tumor extends to the right main-stem bronchus to well within 2 cm of the carina, and should be interpreted as a T3 lesion. **h:** Primary squamous cell carcinoma of the trachea. Such a lesion is unresectable by definition. Invasion of the peritracheal soft tissue is present.

surgeon does not have the advantage of the "panoramic" view offered by CT and can never be sure that a particular node he or she is palpating or seeing corresponds to a node shown by CT.

In our experience, the main effect of CT staging has been to reduce the number of negative mediastinoscopies and anterior mediastinotomies by avoiding them in most patients having negative CT examinations (no nodes over 1 cm in size). Over an admittedly limited period, we have not observed a decrease in the number of attempted curative thoracotomies which turn out to have positive nodes in the mediastinum.

Based on the above considerations, we have developed a set of practical guidelines, summarized in Table 4.

Distant metastases (M).

Routine CT of the brain, liver, and upper abdomen in the staging of small cell carcinoma is of little value because, in this nonsurgical disease, CT is limited to radiotherapy planning and treatment-response evaluation (45). The management of non–oat cell carcinoma is, on the other hand, affected by the discovery of distant metastases. In autopsy series,

TABLE 4. *Guidelines for CT interpretation of mediastinal nodes in staging of bronchogenic carcinoma*

Nodal size (mm)	Patients in category[a] (%)	Interpretation	Recommendation
0–5	10	Negative	Surgery
5–10	20	Negative	Surgery (Except for patients with borderline operability in whom tissue confirmation may be required)
10–20	35	Indeterminate	Node sampling with CT guidance (Except for squamous cell carcinoma with only low ipsilateral nodes where surgery is directly performed)
>20	35	Positive[b]	No surgery (Except for patients with good operability in whom tissue confirmation may be required)

[a] These percentages are approximate and based on personal data.
[b] Positive hilar nodes do not contraindicate surgery but may make pneumonectomy rather than simple lobectomy necessary.

metastases to the adrenal gland from lung cancer can be found in up to 38% of patients (46). By weight, the adrenals have the highest incidence of metastatic disease of any organ. In a clinical series of 110 patients, adrenal masses were found in 11 patients, and in 5 patients they were the only site of metastasis (47). Because of the high incidence of adrenal involvement, we routinely extend scanning to the adrenals when mediastinal CT is negative. Metastatic masses to the adrenals tend to be larger than 2 cm. Smaller masses are more likely to represent nonfunctioning cortical adenomas, which are benign tumors of the adrenals discovered more frequently since the advent of CT. Patients should not be prevented from undergoing surgery solely on the basis of an adrenal mass. Needle-biopsy confirmation is recommended in these cases. At this point, no other CT study has proven to be definitely beneficial as a routine screening procedure in the management of patients with lung cancer, and none is performed unless there is a clinical suspicion of specific organ involvement.

MEDIASTINAL VESSELS

Normal appearance and congenital variations of mediastinal vessels are discussed in Chapter 2.

Arteries

Tortuosity of Vessels

Excessively tortuous arteries may produce abnormalities of mediastinal contours indistinguishable from masses or aneurysms on chest radiographs (48). CT is the most elegant and rewarding procedure for the demonstration of the innocuous nature of the radiographic abnormality. The most commonly encountered example of this problem is buckling of the innominate artery, which produces a convex right superior pleuromediastinal line. Buckling occurs in 17% of patients with hypertension and/or arteriosclerosis (Fig. 14) (48).

Aneurysms

Aneurysms are more common than dissections in the thoracic aorta, but acute aneurysmal rupture does not occur as frequently. Contrast-enhanced CT can demonstrate all the gross pathologic features of aortic aneurysms, i.e., dilatation, intraluminal thrombi, displacement or erosion of adjacent structures, and perianeurysmal thickening and hemorrhage (49). The majority of aortic aneurysms are secondary to arteriosclerosis, which explains the

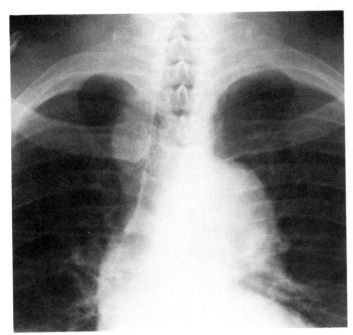

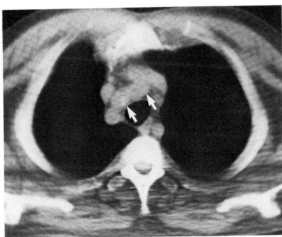

14a,b

FIG. 14. Buckling of innominate artery. **a:** Chest radiograph shows a convex, right superior pleuromediastinal interface. **b:** CT scan at level of convex contour identifies the innominate artery *(arrows)*, which is almost parallel to the scan plane at this level due to its excessive tortuosity.

high frequency of mural calcifications found with CT.

A minimal diameter of 4 cm should be measured before diagnosing aneurysmal dilatation of the thoracic aorta (50). The maximal diameter of the aneurysm correlates with the incidence of rupture, which ranges from 2% for diameters of less than 5 cm to more than 50% for aneurysms larger than 10 cm (51).

The most common error made in estimating vascular diameter occurs with markedly tortuous vessels running obliquely to the CT slice. Additional problems may occur with poor vascular enhancement due to slow infusion or delayed scanning, with subsequent failure to demonstrate the vascular nature of an aneurysmal mass, or when a saccular aneurysm is entirely clotted and may simulate a mass despite good enhancement. The latter problem occurs also with angiography. In rare instances, some nonvascular lesions may be enhanced as much as adjacent vessels and mimic aneurysms, especially if scanning is not performed immediately after bolus injection of contrast medium (Figs. 9 and 10, Chapter 1).

CT is the most appropriate modality for follow-up of aneurysms. An increasing diameter is readily detected with serial scans and helps prompt a surgical decision. This is especially valuable in post-traumatic aneurysms, which have a high incidence of rupture. Traumatic aneurysms occur most commonly at the level of the ligamentum arteriosum, just distal to the subclavian artery (60%). They may also occur near the aortic hiatus of the diaphragm (20%), and in the ascending aorta (20%). A minority of these patients survive long enough to reach a hospital, and angiography is the procedure of choice in the acute phase. If the angiogram is negative and the patient unstable, CT may still be of value because, in the early post-traumatic phase, a definite aneurysm may not yet be formed, even though significant damage to the aorta has occurred and periaortic hemorrhage, detectable only by CT, would be the only sign present. After a few days, an aneurysm may develop and can be readily detected by CT as well as by angiography. CT may then be used as a surveillance modality in patients in whom surgery may be relatively contraindicated, or if a major artery such as the anterior spinal artery of Adamkiewickz arises from the traumatic aneurysm (52).

Aortic Dissection

Computed tomography can reliably diagnose or exclude aortic dissection. The specific diagnosis of dissection with CT rests on (a) the demonstration of medially displaced intimal calcifications and (b) the visualization of the intimal flap. The latter requires high-quality contrast enhancement and patent true and false lumina. Secondary signs are the presence of a long segment of aortic dilatation, deformity, and narrowing of the true lumen. In chronic dissection, thickening with enhancement of the aortic wall may also be noted (53).

A noncontrast-enhanced scan is always performed first to detect displaced intimal calcifications. Cross-sectional imaging permits accurate measurement of the distance between outer wall and calcified intima when the aorta runs perpendicular to the CT slice. A contrast-enhanced study then follows, preferably with bolus injections supplemented by rapid dynamic scanning in the areas of highest suspicion. Dynamic scanning is necessary to visualize differential flow between true and false lumen, a finding pathognomonic of dissection. Flow-related artifacts may mimic dissection and are best recognized with dynamic scanning (54).

Unlike angiography, CT has the advantage of demonstrating periaortic hemorrhage into the mediastinum or extrapleural space, findings highly suggestive of dissection. Like angiography, CT has difficulty showing dissection when the false lumen is entirely clotted, in which case distinction from a fusiform aneurysm with a laminated thrombus against the wall may be difficult. In dissection, the residual lumen is most often narrowed, eccentric, and deformed, whereas aneurysms have a larger, round or oval lumen (Fig. 15).

A laminated thrombus is distinctly unusual in ascending aortic aneurysms, and when it is seen in the ascending aorta or arch, it is more suggestive of dissection.

Several well-defined problems and pitfalls in the diagnosis of dissection should be recognized:

1. Insufficient contrast enhancement may lead to failure to detect intimal flaps.
2. The left innominate vein running anterior to the arch and the left superior intercostal vein running parallel to the arch may simulate the appearance of a flap in the arch (see Figs. 4b and 13b, Chapter 2).
3. Streak artifacts mimicking intimal flaps are common in the ascending aorta.
4. Pseudodisplacement of intimal calcifications due to partial volume averaging occur, particularly in the aortic arch.
5. Thickened pleura may mimic chronic dissection.
6. The higher physical density of contrast medium leads to laminar, gravity-dependent flow in the descending aorta, simulating the appearance of differential flow in a false lumen (55,56).

Patients who survive their initial dissection are prone to redissection, extension of dissection, aortic aneurysm, and aortic rupture. CT has proven valuable in detecting these complications (57) (Figs. 15 and 16). Interestingly, a totally thrombosed false lumen appears to correlate well with a favorable response to medical therapy (54).

CT Versus Angiography in Aortic Dissection

There is some controversy as to what the proper diagnostic procedure should be in patients suspected of having aortic dissection. CT can demonstrate most of the features of dissection, but cannot reliably detect occlusion of major aortic branches. Such occlusions are a major determinant in surgical therapy. Hence, angiography is often required in addition to CT. Because of the large cumulative doses of contrast agent used in these studies and the additional expenses of performing both, criteria to select the most appropriate procedure in the individual case need to be developed. An appreciation of the issues involved in managing patients with dissection is the best guide in such a choice.

Dissection of the aorta most often presents as a clinical catastrophe, sometimes difficult to distinguish from myocardial infarction or pulmonary embolization. An insidious onset is, however, not infrequent. The chest radiograph usually demonstrates a widened aortic shadow; rarely, it may remain normal. Dissection is most common in the ascending aorta, and proximal extension of the dissection to affect the aortic valve or rupture into the pericardium is the main pathophysiologic mechanism of death in these patients. Therefore, the presence of intrapericardial blood is an ominous finding that can be made with CT and that should be sought in all cases by carefully examining the pericardium (58) (Fig. 16).

De Bakey Type I (dissection involving the entire arch) and Type II (dissection involving ascending aorta only) have better prognoses with surgery, mainly because reinforcement of the aortic wall prevents proximal extension. In follow-up studies of operated patients, the false lumen is often seen to remain patent, which suggests that prevention of proximal extension by suturing or grafting rather than closure of the primary tear of the dissection is the main beneficial effect of surgery (57). Type III (dissection involving the descending aorta only) does not carry the risk of proximal extension and is

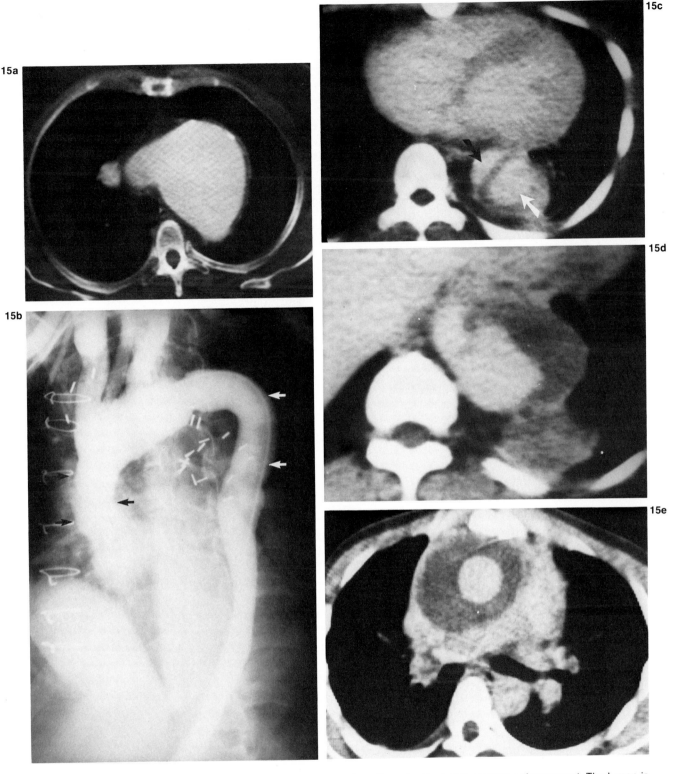

FIG. 15. Aneurysm and dissection. **a:** Typical fusiform aneurysm of aortic arch after bolus contrast enhancement. The lumen is large. No mural thrombus is seen. Laminated thrombi are very unusual in aneurysms of the ascending aorta and arch. The calcified intimal plaques are not medially displaced. **b–d:** A 69-year-old patient had a Type I dissection (extending from ascending to descending aorta). Surgery had been performed twice: first, to place a synthetic graft in the ascending aorta and, second, to place a graft in the proximal descending aorta. The patient was readmitted because of progressive back pain and labile blood pressure. **b:** Angiogram. The ascending aortic graft *(black arrows)* and the descending aortic graft *(white arrows)* are clearly seen. The catheter is in the true lumen, which is narrowed in the lower thoracic aorta because of dissection and secondary compression by the false lumen. **c:** CT after bolus contrast enhancement. The false lumen (almost always located posterolaterally) is patent *(white arrow)*. The true lumen *(black arrow)* is much narrower. The intimal flap is identified between the two lumina. **d:** Lower CT section. The large false lumen now appears partially clotted. Furthermore, a hematoma is seen outside the confines of the aorta due to rupture of the false lumen, not detected with angiography (courtesy of Dr. Robert Woolfitt, Eastern Virginia Medical School, Norfolk General Hospital, Norfolk, Virginia). **e:** Appearance of surgically corrected aneurysm of the ascending aorta in a 35-year-old male with Marfan's syndrome. The prosthetic graft is opacified by contrast media and lies within an enlarged thrombus-filled ascending aorta. CT is valuable in the follow-up of patients' status post aortic surgery to demonstrate stability as well as rule out postsurgical leakage.

16a,b

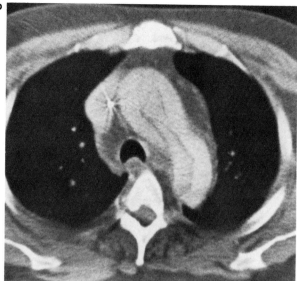 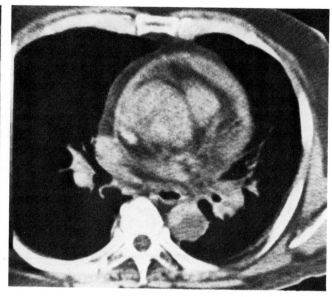

FIG. 16. Complications of dissection. CT sections in a 66-year-old male with sudden onset of deep abdominal pain radiating to the substernal region, and absent lower extremity pulses. **a:** Intimal flaps recognized as linear lucencies within the aortic arch confirm the clinical diagnosis of dissection. The true lumen is the central area between the two flaps. **b:** The dissection extends to the descending aorta, confirming the diagnosis of Type I dissection. The false lumen is clotted at this level. The true lumen is crescent-shaped and narrowed. In the pericardium, a dense effusion is seen. At surgery, a hemopericardium was evident. Proximal extension into the aortic valve apparatus, with rupture into the pericardium, is the major cause of death in the acute phase in patients with Type I and II dissections (courtesy of Dr. Moulay Meziane, with permission, ref. 58).

best treated medically by reducing peak systolic pressure to allow healing. Occlusion of major aortic branches and rupture of the aorta itself are the other main determinants of outcome in patients with dissection. Angiography demonstrates better than can CT the relationship of the dissection to the aortic valve, as well as the status of the major aortic branches—two important factors in deciding a surgical approach. Based on the preceding considerations, angiography should be the procedure of choice in patients who are potential candidates for initial surgery, that is, patients with clinical suspicion of Stage I or II acute dissection with (a) evidence of proximal extension, such as signs of significant aortic regurgitation, congestive heart failure, signs of pericardial tamponade, or recurrent arrhythmias or right bundle branch block; (b) signs of major aortic branch occlusion, such as neurologic deficits suggesting cerebral ischemia or persistent oliguria; or (c) medical therapy failure, as evidenced by intractable chest pain or persistent elevated blood pressure (59).

In the acute phase, CT is best reserved for patients responding rapidly to medical therapy (within 4 hr) and without any of the above signs, or for patients with an uncertain diagnosis of dissection. The main pitfall to avoid in such cases is to "economize" on contrast medium dosage under the as-

sumption that the patient may need an angiogram later. Only negative studies of the highest quality can reliably exclude dissection. If the patient cannot cooperate for the study or if there are severe constraints on the amounts of contrast medium to be used, angiography may be more appropriate.

Three percent of patients with dissection die immediately, 20% in 24 hr, and 50% at the end of the first week. At 1 year, only 10–20% of patients are still alive. Fifteen percent of the patients with dissection develop saccular aneurysms that require surgical therapy. Given these statistics, there is, undoubtedly, a role for CT in the monitoring of all these patients after the acute phase and particularly during the first week.

ACQUIRED VENOUS ABNORMALITIES

Venous obstruction due to extrinsic processes is easily detected with CT. Most often there is direct visualization of the cause of obstruction. Indirect signs such as collateral circulation in the veins of the chest wall or azygos vein are useful. Venous enlargement alone should not be relied on as a sign of obstruction, because it is dependent on the respiratory cycle or a Valsalva maneuver, and sometimes represents a normal variant.

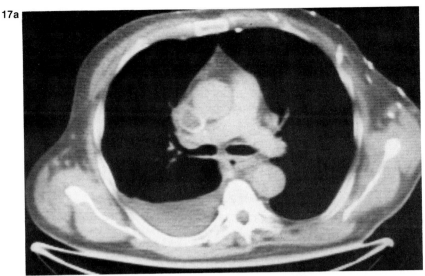

FIG. 17. Superior vena caval thrombosis. **a:** Patient with carcinoma of the pancreas and spontaneous thrombosis of the superior vena cava. The classical signs are present: enlargement of the vein, lucent center, rim enhancement, and collateral circulation through superficial veins in the chest wall. **b:** Normal patient with scan taken during contrast agent injection. Flow phenomena due to mixing of opacified and nonopacified blood may simulate the appearance of venous thrombosis. **c:** Superior vena caval syndrome due to tumor invasion and thrombosis. The thrombosed vein is recognized by its location and enhancing wall.

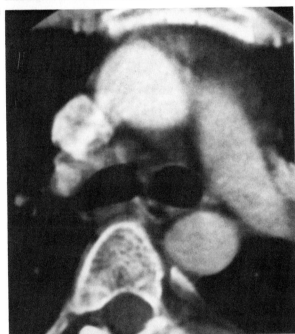

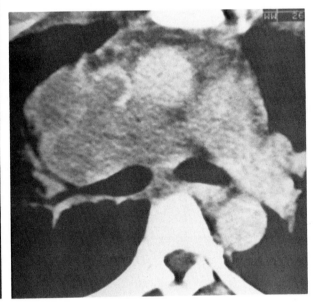

Intrinsic obstruction due to thrombosis is becoming more common due to the increasing use of central venous catheters, larger-bore catheters for hyperalimentation, and the increasing number of procedures involving passage of tubes into the upper body veins. These include Swan-Ganz catheterization, pacemaker placement, and intravenous digital angiography. The classical signs on CT of venous thrombosis are (a) enlargement of the vein, (b) a lucent center, and (c) enhancing vein wall on contrast-enhanced studies (60) (Fig. 17).

A fresh thrombus can be initially as dense as flowing, contrast-enhanced blood and may be missed. Caution should be exercised so venous thrombosis is not diagnosed on scans obtained during or immediately after a bolus injection of contrast agent, since flow phenomena may mimic filling defects in mediastinal veins (54) (Fig. 17).

THYMUS

Normal Thymus

Computed tomography offers an opportunity to view the thymus with much greater clarity than is provided by plain chest roentgenography or standard chest tomography. One must be aware that

(a) thymic morphology changes drastically with aging, and (b) in younger individuals (particularly those under age 25), there is a wide variation in the "normal" size and weight of the thymus gland. Knowledge of the various normal appearances of the thymus helps in the interpretation of CT studies of the anterior mediastinum. The thymus is a bilobed structure fused at its apex near the thyroid gland and smoothly molded to the anterior aspect of the great vessels. It occupies the thyropericardic space of the anterior mediastinum and extends down to the base of the heart. The thymus is very rarely found in an ectopic location, usually the neck.

On conventional radiographs, the thymus seems largest in the neonate and young infant. In fact, the average weight of the thymus is 22 ± 13 g at birth and increases progressively to reach a maximum at puberty of 34 ± 15 g (61). The impression of a large thymus at younger ages stems from a higher ratio of thymic size to chest size.

Beginning at puberty, a phase of rapid involution takes place over a period of 5 to 15 years. The process of thymic involution is essentially one of progressive replacement of atrophied thymic follicles by fatty tissue. The proportion of thymic tissue to fat decreases progressively to become negligible after age 60 (62,63). In an autopsy series of 20 patients over 60 years of age with myasthenia gravis, no thymus could be recognized on gross examination and only 11 had any thymic remnant seen histologically (63).

The appearances on CT of the thymus can be summarized as follows:

1. Birth to puberty. The thymus entirely fills the anterior mediastinum. It has a CT density equal to or slightly higher than muscle. Its borders are convex laterally. In this age group, it usually appears triangular or vaguely bilobed and molds the anterior aspect of the mediastinal vessels. Fat is notably lacking in this age group.
2. Puberty to 25 years. During this phase of involution, fat appears in the anterior mediastinum. The thymus can now be recognized as a distinct triangular or bilobed structure. Formerly convex, its borders are now flat or concave laterally. Its CT density decreases to less than that of muscle.
3. Over 25 years. With further involution, the well-defined soft-tissue-density structure previously recognized as the thymus will no longer be seen. Islands of soft-tissue density over the background of more abundant fat are

noted. The speed and degree of involution are variable from subject to subject, and occasionally the thymus may still be recognized as an individual structure up to age 40. Finally, the anterior mediastinum appears entirely fatty. Most of the anterior mediastinal fat is contained within the fibrous skeleton of the thymus and may have a CT density slightly higher than that of subcutaneous fat (Fig. 18).

Normal CT measurements have been defined for the thymus (64). The most meaningful is the thickness measured as the largest distance across the long axis of the gland on the CT image (Fig. 18). Before age 20, 1.8 cm is the maximum normal for thickness, and 1.3 cm thereafter.

Abnormal Thymus

Thymic Enlargement

Since the thymus may weigh as much as 45–50 g in some normal younger individuals, it is difficult to certify mild degrees of thymic enlargement. However, when the thymus is manifested as a mediastinal mass readily detectable on plain chest roentgenography in older children or young adults, it can be considered to be enlarged. Hyperthyroidism is a condition that may be responsible for thymic enlargement (61). Less common associations are acromegaly, Addison's disease, and children recovering from burns (65). Occasionally, a thymus weighing over 50 g will be biopsied or resected in a teenaged subject (largely because malignant lymphoma cannot be excluded) only to discover an enlarged thymus with a normal histologic appearance.

Thymic Hyperplasia

Thymic germinal hyperplasia is a term used by pathologists to describe a gland that demonstrates numerous, active, lymphoid germinal centers in the medulla (61). Although lymphoid follicles are often present in the medulla of the normal thymus, particularly in younger individuals, in myasthenia gravis the thymus often exhibits a distinctive proliferation of germinal centers. Is it possible to use CT to detect this condition? This question has not been definitively answered. Castleman and Norris (66) have shown that, in myasthenia gravis, total thymic weight of glands with germinal hyperplasia does not differ significantly from that in normal controls. In-

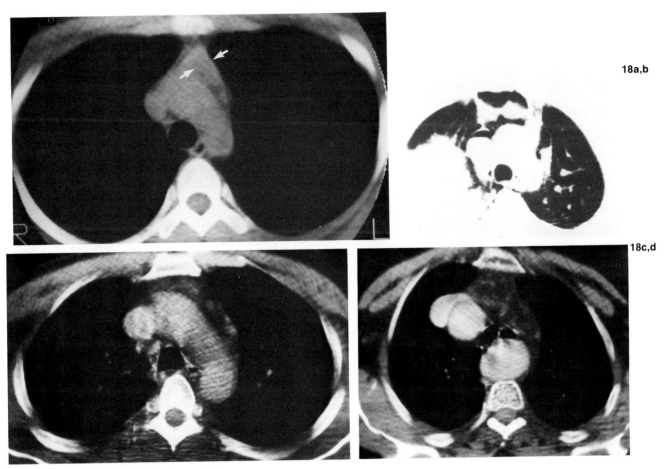

18a,b

18c,d

FIG. 18. Thymus: normal variations with age. **a:** A 19-year-old female. The thymus appears triangular and occupies most of the anterior mediastinal space. Thickness measurements are most useful and are taken as indicated between the *arrows*. **b:** An 18-year-old with traumatic pneumomediastinum. The thymus is visualized as a bilobed structure with soft tissue connections between the two lobes. **c:** A 47-year-old. Rapid involution with fatty replacement occurs normally after puberty, but the speed of the involution is variable. After age 40, the anterior mediastinum is usually of homogeneous fat density. Islands of residual thymic tissue are still present in this normal subject. **d:** A 71-year-old. Most of the anterior mediastinal fat is contained within the thymic fibrous skeleton, which in some patients will remain visible through life (as illustrated in this patient) with linear densities identified within the anterior mediastinal fat.

deed, we have noted several cases in which a thymus appearing entirely normal on CT proved to contain germinal hyperplasia. It is our impression, however, that glands with hyperplasia most frequently appear larger than do those of age-matched controls. We would theorize that although total thymic weight is normal, glands with hyperplasia have delayed fatty involution, and hence the volume of fat-free thymic tissue visualized by CT exceeds the usual age standards. At the present time, there are inadequate data on cases of thymic hyperplasia and normal controls to test this hypothesis. Thymomas are rare before age 20. In patients aged 20–30, it may not be possible to distinguish between thymic hyperplasia (with a slightly enlarged gland) and a small thymoma.

Thymoma

If glandular enlargement is grossly asymmetric (the left lobe is normally larger than the right and the gland is always slightly asymmetric) or if a lobular contour is seen, a thymic mass should be suspected. The most common primary thymic tumor is thymoma. This designation is limited to neoplasms originating from the thymic epithelium (67). On CT, thymoma appears as a homogeneous soft-tissue density, oval, round, or lobulated mass, and usually sharply demarcated. Most often the tumor grows asymmetrically to one side of the anterior mediastinum (Fig. 19). The tumor usually enhances homogeneously after contrast medium injection. It may contain calcium but not commonly. Thirty percent of

19a,b

19c,d

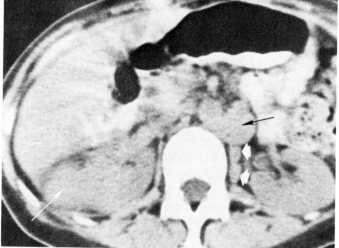

19e

FIG. 19. The spectrum of thymoma. **a:** Benign thymoma. Tumor is sharply demarcated from surrounding structures and is of homogeneous density. **b:** Invasive thymoma. The tumor has an irregular, lobulated contour. Poor definition of the interface between the tumor and the chest wall due to invasion is noted. Invasive thymomas grow by contiguous spread, and a tongue of tumor tissue extends along the pleuromediastinal surface on the left side and reaches the para-aortic–paraspinal area. From there it can extend superiorly **(c)** or inferiorly **(d)** along the diaphragm and crus *(white arrows)* [to be compared with the normal crus *(black arrows)*]. **e:** Further contiguous extension may lead to tumor growth into the retroperitoneum via the aortic or esophageal hiatus. Tumor implants are identified by *arrows.*

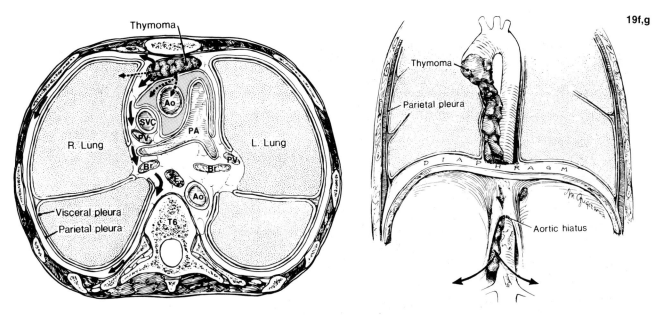

FIG. 19 (cont.). f,g: The pattern of spread of invasive thymomas is graphically represented. In cross-section (f), the tumor can directly invade surrounding structures *(broken arrows)* or insinuate itself between the chest wall or mediastinum and the parietal pleura *(solid arrows)*. Once the para-aortic–paraspinal area is reached (g), inferior extension through the aortic or esophageal hiatus can occur. With CT, such extension can be seen reliably and the study should always be extended to the upper abdomen. Ao, aorta; PA, pulmonary artery; PV, pulmonary vein; Br, bronchus; E, esophagus; SVC, superior vena cava. (Figs. 19d, e, f, and g are reprinted from ref. 69.)

thymomas are malignant. The histological appearance of thymoma does not allow a reliable differentiation between benign and malignant thymoma. The presence of tumor growth into or through the capsule determines malignancy. Malignant thymoma rarely metastasizes outside the thorax. This neoplasm grows to invade local structures and spreads by contiguity along pleural reflections, usually on one side of the chest cavity only (67–69). Thus, "invasive" is a more appropriate designation than "malignant" for this tumor.

Invasive thymomas can be classified into three stages: Stage I, intact capsule or growth within capsule only; Stage II, pericapsular growth into mediastinal fat; and Stage III, invasive growth of surrounding organs and pleural implants at a distance from primary mass. Surgery is indicated in all three stages, with supplemental radiotherapy in Stage II and radiotherapy plus chemotherapy in Stage III (68).

With CT, caution should be used to avoid overdiagnosing invasion. As with other tumors, direct contact and absence of cleavage planes are not reliable criteria to predict invasion.

Invasive thymomas growing along pleural surfaces can reach the posterior mediastinum and extend downward along the aorta to involve the crus of the diaphragm and the retroperitoneum. These areas are "hidden" in conventional studies, but CT excells at demonstrating these sites of involvement (69) (Fig. 19). A full CT examination of the thorax extended to the upper abdomen should be performed in these patients. CT provides invaluable guidance for the radiotherapist and chemotherapist to adjust their treatment plans.

Thymus and Myasthenia Gravis

The association of thymic pathology and myasthenia gravis is the clinical issue most relevant to thymic imaging.

Cures and remissions can be observed in patients with myasthenia gravis following thymic removal with or without a thymoma (70). To date, there is no convincing evidence to suggest that systematic removal of the thymus, whether normal or abnormal, improves outcome in patients who are medically well-controlled. When medical therapy fails, it is generally agreed that surgery is indicated, regardless of thymic status.

Thymoma occurs in 15% of patients with myasthenia gravis. The patients most likely to benefit from thymomectomy, in terms of disease control, are young females with a disease of short duration. Older patients rarely benefit from thymomectomy. However, because thymoma is invasive in 30% of cases, surgical removal is indicated in all patients to eliminate the risk of malignancy, regardless of the effect of the surgery on the course of myasthenia.

The role of the radiologist, then, is to segregate patients with thymoma who should undergo surgery from others. The apparent difficulty in this task would be in distinguishing hyperplasia from thymoma. Sixty-five percent of patients with myasthenia gravis have thymic hyperplasia. This problem is compounded by the normally large thymic size in patients less than 25 years old. However, thymomas are extremely rare in this population, and, unless very obvious, we would not make this diagnosis in this age group (71). Over the age of 40, the diagnosis on CT of thymoma usually poses no problem. In the intermediate range, from 25 to 40 years, the thymus may normally be present, and, unless a definite mass-like structure is seen, which is usually the case, a definite diagnosis cannot be made. It should be noted that invasive thymomas, our main concern, are such slow, locally growing tumors having no potential for distant metastasis that, if in doubt, follow-up CT examinations can be safely recommended.

A positive diagnosis on CT of hyperplasia is not very relevant to clinical decision-making, since poor clinical response determines the need for thymic resection regardless of the presence of hyperplasia. Hyperplasia cannot reliably be excluded either, because it is a purely histologic diagnosis and the gland is not always enlarged. In a recent series, 50% of the thymuses called normal on CT turned out to be hyperplastic at surgery (71).

Differential Diagnosis of Thymoma

Most primary mediastinal neoplasms present in the anterior mediastinum and need to be differentiated from thymomas.

Lymphoma

Hodgkin's lymphoma, particularly the nodular sclerosing type, is the most common lymphoma of the anterior mediastinum. Differentiation from thymoma, in particular invasive thymoma, is difficult. Both lesions are of homogeneous soft-tissue density on CT. They may be lobulated and have poorly defined margins. Classically, it is said that calcifications can be seen in thymoma, but never in untreated lymphoma. In our experience, calcification in a thymoma is unusual and this differential

sign is not often helpful. Anterolateral extension of thymomas behind the parietal pleura to produce a thickened extrapleural space on CT is common (Fig. 19). This may also occur with Hodgkin's disease either directly or through involvement of the internal mammary nodes (Fig. 20). The best differential features we have observed between lymphoma and thymoma are that (a) the presence of adenopathy elsewhere in the mediastinum is rarely, if ever, seen with thymoma, and (b) the pleural implants, especially when seen at several separate locations (in particular along the aorta and near the aortic hiatus), are most suggestive of thymoma. Leukemia and non-Hodgkin's lymphoma may also localize to the anterior mediastinum and pose the same differential diagnostic problem.

Germ Cell Tumors

Sometimes classified with thymic tumors, it is now generally accepted that germ cell tumors arise from primitive germ cells that have arrested their embryological migration in the mediastinum. Most cases occur during the second to fourth decades of life. They comprise dermoid cysts, benign and malignant teratomas, seminomas, embryonal carcinomas, endodermal sinus tumors, and choriocarcinoma. Fewer than 20% are malignant. Dermoid cysts and benign teratomas form the great majority of these lesions, and malignant teratoma is by far the most common of the malignant germ cell tumors. There is a strong preponderance of males in the group with malignancies, whereas benign lesions show equal sex distribution.

Dermoid cysts, which are said to contain ele-

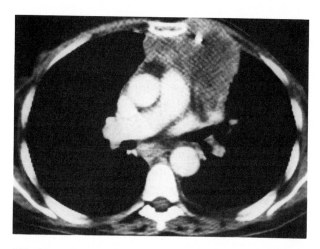

FIG. 20. Hodgkin's lymphoma. A large anterior mediastinal mass with direct invasion of the chest wall is indistinguishable from an invasive thymoma.

ments of the ectodermal layer of germ cells only, and benign teratoma, said to contain elements of all three germinal layers, have overlapping manifestations on CT. They are well-demarcated, and their benign character is suggested by this feature. Encapsulation, sometimes with an enhancing rim, is the rule. Calcifications are seen in one-third to one-half of cases. The mixture of CT densities within the mass is varied; when fat is present, the proper diagnosis can be strongly suspected, but only half demonstrate fat (72). The fluids within the cystic parts of the tumors also vary in their CT density and may reach soft-tissue density (Fig. 21).

Typically, teratomas contain a variable admixture of tissues that exhibit CT numbers in the range of fat, soft tissue, and calcium. This pleiomorphic appearance is an important clue to the etiology of the lesion and makes possible its differentiation from thymoma and lymphoma (Fig. 22). Malignant teratoma seems to be distinguishable from its benign counterpart in most cases. Its borders are poorly defined, and the tumor molds and compresses surrounding structures.

The other germ cell tumors are much less common. In the few documented cases imaged by CT, no specific features are noted. These lesions appear as homogeneous soft-tissue-density masses indistinguishable from lymphoma or thymoma (Fig. 22).

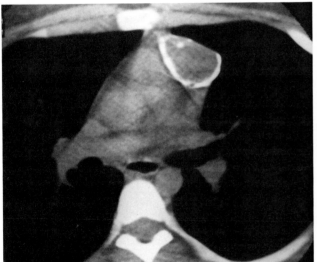
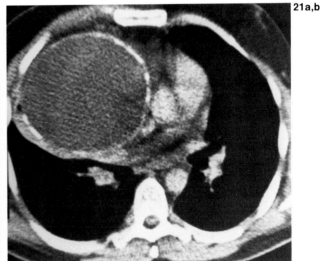

21a,b

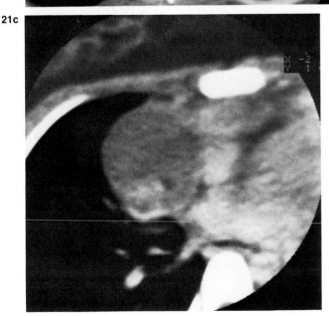

21c

FIG. 21. The benign germ cell tumors. Benign germ cell tumors comprise 80% of all germ cell tumors. **a:** Dermoid cyst incidentally discovered on chest radiography. The mass is of homogeneous soft-tissue density, with a dense rim of calcification. At surgery, the lesion was found to be cystic. **b:** Benign cystic teratoma. This large mass was incidentally discovered. The contents measure in the range of water density. Note again a rim of calcification, commonly seen in these lesions. **c:** Benign teratoma. Small well-defined mass with areas of soft tissue, calcium, and fat density.

22a,b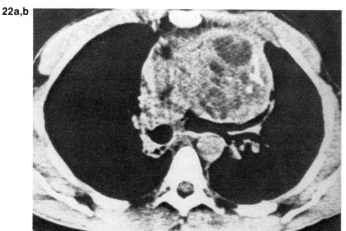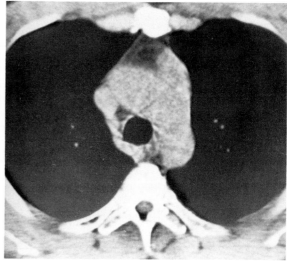

FIG. 22. Malignant germ cell tumors. **a:** Malignant teratoma. The pleiomorphic character of the lesion with solid, cystic, fatty, and calcified areas is typical of malignant teratoma, as illustrated in this case. **b:** Malignant dysgerminoma. This tumor is indistinguishable from thymoma or lymphoma.

Thymolipoma

This is a rare, benign, intrathymic neoplasm that may grow down to involve the cardiophrenic angles and, as a rule, is asymptomatic. On CT, the tumor appears to be almost entirely fatty, with some areas of inhomogeneity. It does not compress or invade surrounding structures (Fig. 7).

Thyroid Masses

Intrathoracic extensions of thyroid tissue constitute a significant percentage of mediastinal lesions. They usually represent direct contiguous growth of a goiter into the mediastinum. Such lesions are almost always connected to the thyroid gland, even though the mass may appear to be separated from the thyroid on nuclear studies (73). Truly ectopic mediastinal thyroids are extremely rare. In approximately 80% of cases, the thyroid mass arises anteriorly from a lower pole or isthmus of the gland and extends into the thyropericardic space in front of the trachea. In approximately 20% of cases, the mass arises posteriorly from a lower lobe and extends into the mediastinum posterior and lateral to the trachea and major vessels, most commonly on the right side.

With CT, most of these masses have a suggestive appearance, probably because as goiters they show (a) inhomogeneous densities, with small, cystic-appearing areas, curvilinear calcium deposits, and areas of high density presumably due to the iodine content of the gland (fat has not been reported in these lesions and is a differential feature from teratomas); (b) marked enhancement after contrast media injection, sometimes to the point of simulating a vascular lesion; (c) demonstration of a communication with the thyroid gland when contiguous sections are extended to include the neck; and (d) prolonged contrast enhancement of the gland (73); this sign is due, presumably, to the thyroid actively trapping the iodine contained in the contrast medium.

Other Masses

Rarely, a thymic cyst with dense fluid may simulate a thymoma. Simple lymphangiomas and hemangiomas, composed of capillary-sized, thin-walled channels, may also appear as solid masses. Cavernous and cystic lymphangiomas or hemangiomas demonstrate a more complex anatomy, with cystic and solid areas allowing their differentiation from thymomas (74).

One pitfall in the diagnosis of thymoma is the presence of an unusually high pulmonary artery in front of the aortic arch, duplicating the appearance of a thymoma (75) (Fig. 23).

Parathyroid Adenoma

Ninety percent of normal or abnormal parathyroid glands are located near the thyroid gland. Their precise localization and number are variable.

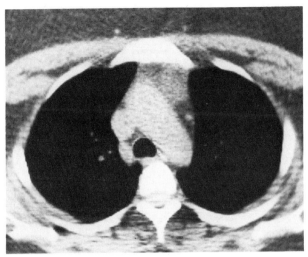 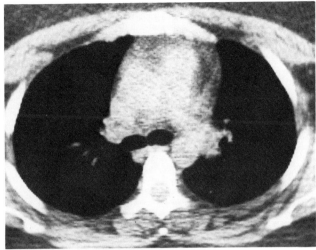

FIG. 23. High main and left pulmonary arteries simulating a thymoma. **a:** An apparent anterior mediastinal mass is seen in this patient with myasthenia gravis. A thymoma was diagnosed, but none was found at surgery. **b:** A lower section reveals that the "mass" represents a high-positioned, main pulmonary artery, which was partially imaged in the CT slice in (a). This CT pitfall should be recognized and can be avoided by interpretation of the CT scans in sequential order.

Most parathyroid adenomas are found in the inferiorly located group of parathyroid glands, which, importantly, are also the least constant in location. Ten percent of parathyroid glands are ectopic. Sixty-two percent of the ectopic glands are located in the anterior mediastinum, 30% are embedded within thyroid tissue, and 8% are found in the posterior-superior mediastinum (76). The anterior mediastinal parathyroid adenomas are intimately connected with the thymus gland. Islands of parathyroid tissue carried to the anterior mediastinum by the descending thymus during embryologic development is the accepted theory that explains the presence of mediastinal parathyroid adenomas. In patients with documented primary hyperparathyroidism, surgical neck exploration to remove the parathyroid tissues is curative in 90% of cases. In the group of patients in whom surgery fails, a higher than normal percentage of ectopic glands is seen. Ectopia is therefore a significant cause of surgical failure. Almost 50% of these patients will have mediastinal parathyroid glands; two-thirds of these glands will be located in the superior mediastinum, particularly in the posterior aspect near the tracheoesophageal groove, and one-third in the lower anterior mediastinum (77). With CT, the parathyroid adenomas vary in size from 0.3 to 3 cm. They are usually homogeneous in density, unless their vascular supply has been compromised at surgery, in which case they may appear cystic. In the anterior mediastinum they are indistinguishable from small thymic remnants, small thymomas, or small nodes, and

are found in the expected location of the thymus (Fig. 24).

With state-of-the-art scanners, the neck and mediastinum can be examined with high accuracy. CT is definitely indicated in the minority of patients in whom surgery has failed to control the hyperparathyroidism. Initially, with older scanners, CT was not thought to be helpful before the initial surgical exploration of the neck because of cost considerations (77). More recently, it has become apparent that CT can reduce the operating time (itself a significant cost factor) by pinpointing the location of adenomas that are potentially difficult to find (78). This is especially helpful in the posterior-superior mediastinum, where half of the missed adenomas are subsequently found that could have been resected at the time of the first surgical operation if the surgeon had known of their presence (79).

MEDIASTINAL CYSTS

Excluding significant pathology by demonstrating the fatty or vascular nature of a roentgenographic abnormality is one of the most important functions of mediastinal CT. Likewise, when a benign cyst can be confidently diagnosed, unnecessarily invasive action can be avoided. With CT, most benign cysts can be recognized as such and managed conservatively if asymptomatic.

Mediastinal cysts are of congenital origin and include bronchogenic, duplication, neurenteric, and pleuropericardial cysts.

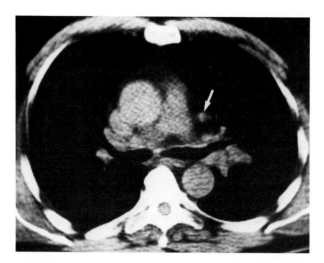

FIG. 24. Ectopic parathyroid adenoma. A 45-year-old patient with hyperparathyroidism not responding to surgical therapy. The CT scan reveals a small, 0.5-cm density in the anterior mediastinum *(arrow)*. At surgery, a small parathyroid adenoma was found. Mediastinal parathyroid adenomas are found in the usual location of the thymus. They are difficult to distinguish from small nodes or residual thymic tissue.

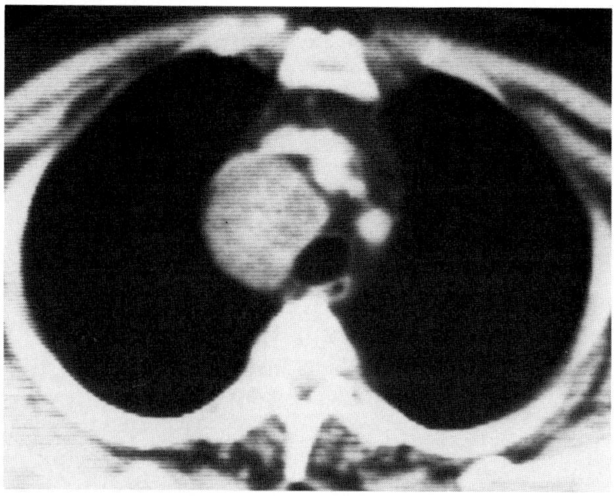

FIG. 25. Bronchogenic cyst. A right paratracheal smooth mass with high-density contents is identified. A solid tumor could not be excluded. At surgery, a bronchogenic cyst with thick mucoid contents was removed. Approximately one-half of all bronchogenic and duplication cysts may have higher-than-water-density fluid contents.

Bronchogenic Cysts

Bronchogenic cysts arise from primitive bronchi and are lined by a columnar epithelium. They contain fluid that ranges in color from clear to milky white to brown, with variable viscosity. This variable fluid composition explains the different CT densities observed in bronchogenic cysts. Half of these cysts are of water density. In the other half, the CT density can vary from a low soft-tissue range to higher-than-muscle density, presumably because of thick cyst contents (80) (Fig. 25). When dense, bronchogenic cysts are indistinguishable from solid lesions. Most bronchogenic cysts are located along the right paratracheal wall, or near the carina in the middle or middle-posterior mediastinum. They are sharply marginated unless infected. They are usually in contact with the carina and may deform it slightly. These cysts rarely can be seen in other locations, such as the anterior mediastinum, the low posterior mediastinum, or in the lung itself. Significantly, these lesions fail to enhance following contrast administration.

Duplication Cysts

Duplication cysts arise from the foregut and are sometimes grouped with bronchogenic cysts as "broncho-esophageal cysts." They are lined by gastrointestinal tract mucosa. They are usually lo-

cated in the posterior mediastinum in a paraspinal location. They are most often connected to the esophagus, and are sometimes found within its wall. Their appearance on CT is indistinguishable from that of bronchogenic cysts, except for their location.

Neurenteric Cysts

These rare lesions are connected to the meninges through a midline defect in one or more vertebral bodies. They are also often connected to the esophagus. The appearance on CT of the cyst itself is the same as that of duplication cysts, but the presence of the vertebral abnormality points to the diagnosis.

Pleuropericardial Cysts

These cysts, representing defects in the embryogenesis of the coelomic cavities, are most often located in the cardiophrenic angles or lower aspect of the pericardium. Their appearance is usually diagnostic of their cystic nature. They are sharply marginated, and have low CT numbers. Pleuropericardial cysts, however, are not always round; they may assume different shapes. When small, they can sometimes be confused with enlarged cardiophrenic angle nodes.

Differential Diagnosis of Mediastinal Cysts

Differentiation of an uncomplicated congenital cyst from other cystic encapsulated lesions, such as abscesses, old hematomas, or rare cystic lymphangiomas or hemangiomas, relies on the clinical presentation, the location, and the appearance on CT of the cyst.

Uncomplicated congenital cysts are typically asymptomatic. Cystic masses of the anterior mediastinum are rarely due to congenital cysts, but are more likely related to a cystic tumor or a thymic cyst. Abscesses, hematomas, and cystic tumors commonly demonstrate thick walls, with septa on occasion, and mixed-density fluids (Fig. 26). Anterior meningoceles may closely resemble congenital cysts, but careful examination of adjacent sections should demonstrate the intraspinal connection of the mass through a neural foramen.

ESOPHAGUS

When sufficient posterior mediastinal fat is present, the esophagus can be adequately visualized with CT. The esophagus is in intimate contact anteriorly with the posterior aspect of the trachea, the left main-stem bronchus, and left atrium. The esophagus is bordered by the aorta on the left and the azygos vein on the right. Intraluminal air is a common and normal finding with CT.

The apparent thickness of the esophagus is normally variable and dependent on the state of distention. There is no reliable way to maintain a constant distention of the esophagus. We have tried to use effervescent products, as well as diluted contrast agents, to achieve a reliable distention of the esophagus, but these techniques are not sufficiently reproducible. As a general guideline, a thickness of 3 mm or more should be considered abnormal (81).

The manifestations on CT of esophageal disease are (a) dilatation; (b) thickening of the wall; (c) asymmetry in wall thickness; (d) loss of periesophageal fat planes; (e) invasion of surrounding organs; and (f) periesophageal adenopathy.

Asymmetry of wall thickness is a reliable sign of pathology. Wall thickening is, however, nonspecific, and we do not attempt to differentiate benign from malignant disease with CT. Benign disease is more likely to be limited to the esophageal wall, with clear fat planes seen around the esophagus. Early carcinomas limited to the mucosa or wall would, however, look identical (Fig. 27). Once a diagnosis of malignant disease is estab-

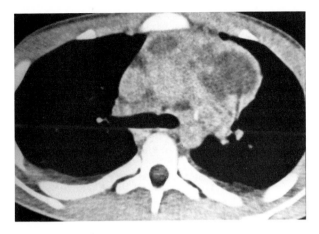

FIG. 26. Mediastinal abscess. A patient with infectious pericarditis extending into the mediastinum proper to form an abscess. The mass is complex, partially cystic, with thick and irregular walls and poor margination.

lished, usually by endoscopy, CT can be used to define the extent of the disease. In this application, CT was found to be sensitive in detecting extraesophageal extension of the carcinoma (82). A word of caution should be said about using the absence of periesophageal fat planes as a sign of invasion. Patients with esophageal carcinoma are often cachectic and lack normal fat planes. Previous surgery or radiation therapy can also blur the margins of the esophagus. Lastly, the frequency of periesophageal involvement in this disease is so high that it is difficult to determine whether CT can, indeed, reliably detect invasion solely on the basis of fat plane disappearance. Extraesophageal extension of carcinoma is present in more than 80% of patients at the time of initial diagnosis, and probably explains the high predictive value of poor fat planes in this disease (whereas for other neoplasms, invasion can be reliably diagnosed only when destruction of a nearby structure is seen).

Certainly, CT can provide exquisite depiction of the tumor to guide radiotherapy. If no extraesophageal disease is demonstrated, resectability may be suggested (82). In this regard, it should be remembered that periesophageal nodes can drain inferiorly to the retroperitoneal nodes, in particular the celiac group. Thus, when investigating the esophagus for malignant disease, the upper abdomen should also be examined (Fig. 28). CT, however, appears insensitive in detecting nodal metastases from esophageal carcinoma. In a study of 52 patients, 28 had no evidence of adenopathy with CT, but 12 of these patients had positive nodes, and of 43 metastatic lymph nodes sampled, only 3 were

27a,b

27c,d

27e,f

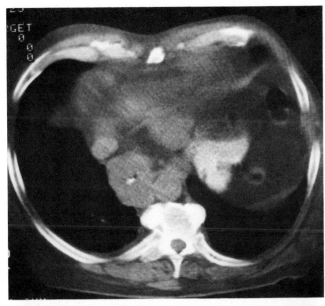

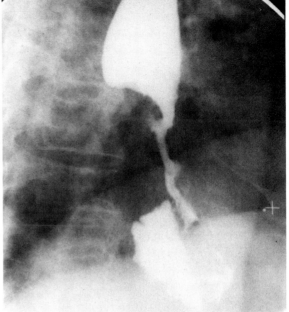

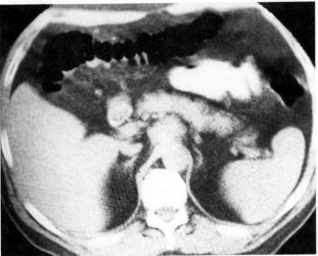

FIG. 28. Esophageal carcinoma. **a:** Large tumor of lower esophagus with marked lobulated thickening. Note good preservation of fat planes. **b:** Esophagram demonstrating the large lower esophageal carcinoma. **c:** Upper abdominal section. Celiac axis adenopathy due to metastatic disease is identified. The CT study should be extended to the upper abdomen for carcinoma of the esophagus.

larger than 7 mm (83). CT would be of great value if patients with resectable esophageal carcinoma could be reliably distinguished from the large majority of patients with unresectable disease at presentation. The resolution of this problem awaits further experience.

PARASPINAL REGIONS

The richness of neural tissue in the paravertebral areas explains the frequent paraspinal location of

neurogenic tumors. Thirty percent of such tumors are malignant. Neural tumors are usually of soft-tissue density, but they may be of lower density, presumably because of the high amounts of lipids in neural tissue and the relative proportion of neural tissue to fibrous tissue in the individual tumor (84). Benign tumors classically are sharply marginated and homogeneous (Fig. 29). Smooth pressure changes in the adjacent vertebral bodies or ribs may be seen. The intraspinal component of "dumbbell"

FIG. 27. Benign and malignant esophageal disease. **a–c:** A 57-year-old male with dysphagia. In (a), there is marked concentric thickening of esophagus, with slightly irregular margins. In (b), asymmetric thickening is seen, inferior to (a). In (c), a benign-appearing ulcer is identified in a barium esophagram. Moderate narrowing due to scarring is also present. At endoscopy, chronic esophagitis, benign ulcer, and the diagnosis of Barrett's esophagus were confirmed. **d–f:** A 65-year-old male with dysphagia. In (d) and (e), concentric thickening of esophageal walls is seen, with smoother outer margins than in (a) and (b). In (f), barium esophagram shows typical appearance of esophageal carcinoma. CT cannot reliably differentiate benign from malignant esophageal disease.

29a,b

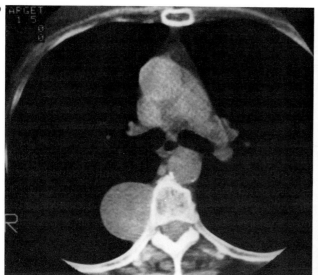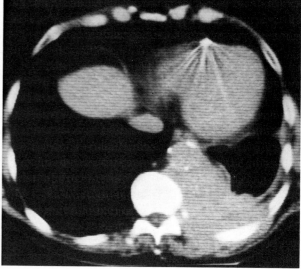

FIG. 29. Neurogenic tumors. **a:** Benign neurofibroma. Typical appearance and location. **b:** Malignant neurofibrosarcoma. The tumor has invaded the chest wall, which it molds.

neurofibromas is readily identified with CT. Malignant neurogenic tumors tend to mold the paraspinal areas and have poorly defined borders. The paraspinal areas are also rich in elements of the reticuloendothelial systems, which explains the frequent paravertebral localization noted in patients with extramedullary hematopoiesis [a phenomenon most commonly seen in conditions associated with chronic bone marrow deficiency, particularly thalassemia (Fig. 30)]. Lymphomas may, likewise, be present in these regions and simulate malignant neurogenic tumors or extramedullary hematopoiesis. Infectious involvement of the spine may lead to the development of paraspinal abscesses, most commonly seen with tuberculosis (Fig. 31). The paraspinal mediastinal regions are in direct communication with the retroperitoneum via the aortic and esophageal hiatus. Diseases can spread between the thorax and abdomen by direct extension along this route, as demonstrated by invasive thymomas (Fig. 19). Lymphatic and neural communications through the hiatus explain the common finding of lymphomatous or neurofibromatous masses extending across it into the mediastinum (Figs. 8 and 33, Chapter 10). Inflammatory masses, such as pancreatic pseudocysts, can similarly invade the paraspinal mediastinal regions (Fig. 31).

SUMMARY

Analysis of the abnormal mediastinum is the most common indication for the use of thoracic CT. The superb density resolution of CT permits the differ-

entiation of benign fatty and cystic processes of the mediastinum from adenopathy, solid tumors, and vascular lesions. CT has totally replaced conventional tomography as the procedure of choice in the investigation of the mediastinum. True fatty tumors of the mediastinum are not as common as diffuse lipomatosis or herniations of abdominal fat through the diaphragm. A lesion of pure-fat density, with well-defined margins, is almost invariably benign. Chest roentgenographic abnormalities due to tortuous vessels are readily explained using CT. Like-

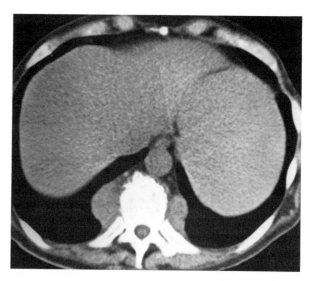

FIG. 30. Extramedullary hematopoiesis. A 35-year-old patient with myelofibrosis. Large paraspinal masses in the region of the paravertebral nodal chains are identified. The spleen is markedly enlarged.

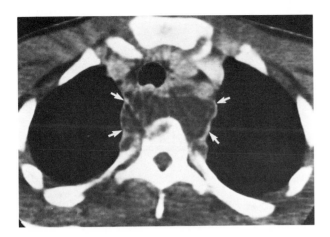

FIG. 31. Paraspinal tuberculosis abscesses. A large anterior and bilateral paraspinal collection is present in association with minimal destruction of the vertebral body. (Courtesy of Dr. Margaret Whelan, New York University Medical Center, New York, New York, with permission.)

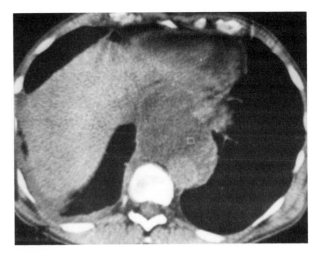

FIG. 32. Mediastinal pseudocyst. A lower mediastinal cystic mass is seen, representing direct extension of a pancreatic pseudocyst through the aortic hiatus.

wise, asymptomatic mediastinal cysts can be safely managed conservatively when CT confirms their fluid content and demonstrates smooth walls.

With state-of-the-art scanners, normal lymph nodes can be visualized in a high percentage of cases. There is no reliable size criterion separating normal from abnormal nodes. The prevalence of granulomatous diseases in a given population will affect the "normal" nodal size. Metastatic disease does not always enlarge affected nodes. Neoplastic as well as inflammatory processes can lead to lymph node enlargement, fusion of several nodes, and, lastly, diffusion outside the nodes into the connective tissues of the mediastinum.

With CT, all mediastinal lymph nodes can be examined, and, when found to be enlarged (over 1 cm), the most appropriate method of tissue sampling can be selected. Mediastinal CT plays an increasingly important role in the staging of lung cancer. To date, we can safely conclude that a negative CT examination of the mediastinum is a reliable indication of resectability, and should preempt the use of mediastinoscopy and mediastinotomy in the majority of cases. Nodes larger than 2 cm are very probably involved with metastatic disease in patients with lung cancer, but unless other contraindications to surgery exist, tissue confirmation may still be required.

With proper contrast enhancement, CT is reliable in distinguishing vascular from nonvascular structures. Furthermore, aneurysms and dissections of the thoracic aorta are clearly depicted. However, clinical considerations should determine the choice of CT or angiography in the initial evaluation of patients with suspected vascular pathology.

Computed tomography is the most accurate noninvasive procedure used to define the extent of mediastinal neoplasms, and it is invaluable in guiding therapy. Processes frequently missed by conventional radiography, such as thymomas or ectopic parathyroid adenomas, are most sensitively detected with CT. In myasthenia gravis, to date, the main role of CT is in detecting thymomas and in prompting their surgical resection because of their malignant potential. In younger patients, it may be difficult to differentiate thymic hyperplasia from a thymoma, but in this age group, thymomas are rare.

With CT, benign and malignant processes of the esophagus cannot be reliably differentiated. Wall thickening is the most common and least specific finding. In diagnosed cases of esophageal carcinoma, CT helps assess the extent of the disease outside the esophageal lumen. Since a very high percentage of patients with esophageal cancer have unresectable disease at the time of diagnosis, the true test of the usefulness of CT in these patients would be to reliably identify the minority of patients with resectable lesions. At this point, further experience is required to answer this question. Although the total impact of CT on the management and outcome of patients with thoracic malignancies involving the mediastinum is not yet fully defined, it is nonetheless evident that CT has become the most valuable diagnostic method of investigation of the mediastinum, second only to the standard chest roentgenogram.

REFERENCES

1. Heitzman ER. Computed tomography of the thorax: Current perspectives. *Am J Roentgenol* 136:2–12, 1981
2. Mintzer RA, Malave SR, Neiman HL, Michaelis LL, Vanecko RM, Sanders JH. Computed vs conventional tomography in evaluation of primary and secondary pulmonary neoplasms. *Radiology* 132:663–659, 1979
3. Sones PJ, Torres WE, Colvin RS, Meier WL, Sprawls P, Rogers JR, Jr. Effectiveness of CT in evaluating intrathoracic masses. *Am J Roentgenol* 139:469–475, 1982
4. Jost RG, Sagel SS, Stanley RJ, Levitt RG. Computed tomography of the thorax. *Radiology* 126:125–136, 1978
5. Crowe JK, Brown LR, Muhm JR. Computed tomography of the mediastinum. *Radiology* 128:75–87, 1978
6. Baron RL, Levitt RG, Sagel SS, Stanley RJ. Computed tomography in the evaluation of mediastinal widening. *Radiology* 138:107–113, 1981
7. Heitzman ER. *The Mediastinum: Radiologic Correlations with Anatomy and Pathology.* St. Louis, C.V. Mosby, 1977
8. Lee WJ, Fattal G. Mediastinal lipomatosis in simple obesity. *Chest* 70:308–309, 1976
9. Koerner HF, Sun DIC. Mediastinal lipomatosis secondary to steroid therapy. *Am J Roentgenol Rad Ther Nucl Med* 98:461–464, 1966
10. Price JE, Rigler LG. Widening of the mediastinum resulting from fat accumulation. *Radiology* 96:497–500, 1970
11. Bein NE, Mancuso AA, Mink JH, Hansen GC. Computed tomography in the evaluation of mediastinal lipomatosis. *J Comput Assist Tomogr* 2:379–383, 1978
12. Streiter ML, Schneider HJ, Proto AV. Steroid-induced thoracic lipomatosis: Paraspinal involvement. *Am J Roentgenol* 139:679–681, 1982
13. Homer JM, Wechsler RJ, Carter BL. Mediastinal lipomatosis. *Radiology* 128:657–661, 1978
14. Enzi G, Biondetti PR, Fiore D, Mazzoleni F. Computed tomography of deep fat masses in multiple symmetrical lipomatosis. *Radiology* 144:122–124, 1982
15. Rohlfing BM, Korobkin N, Hall AD. Computed tomography of intrathoracic omental herniation and other mediastinal fatty masses. *J Comput Assist Tomogr* 1:181–183, 1977
16. Keely JG, Vana AJ. Lipomas of the mediastinum, 1940–1955. *Int Abst Surg* 103:312–322, 1956
17. Cohen WN, Seidelmann FE, Bryan PJ. Computed tomography of localized adipose deposits presenting as tumor masses. *Am J Roentgenol* 128:1007–1011, 1977
18. Schweitzer DL, Aguam AS. Primary liposarcoma of the mediastinum. *J Thorac Cardiovasc Surg* 741:83–97, 1977
19. Rubin E. Case of the winter season. *Semin Roentgenol* 13:5–6, 1978
20. Mendez G, Isikoff MB, Isikoff SK, Sinner WN. Fatty tumors of the thorax demonstrated by CT. *Am J Roentgenol* 133:207–212, 1979
21. Beck E, Beattie EJ, Jr. The lymph nodes in the mediastinum. *J Int Coll Surgeons* 29:247–251, 1958
22. Rouviere H. *Anatomie des Lymphatiques de l'Homme.* Paris, Masson et Compagnie, 1932
23. Goldberg EM, Shapiro CM, Glicksman HS. Mediastinoscopy for assessing mediastinal spread in clinical staging of lung carcinoma. *Semin Oncol* 1:205–215, 1974
24. Schnyder PA, Gamsu G. CT of the pretracheal retrocaval space. *Am J Roentgenol* 136:303–308, 1981
25. Onitsuka H, Kuhns LR. Dextroconvexity of the mediastinum in the azygo-esophageal recess: A normal variant in young adults. *Radiology* 135:126, 1980
26. Goodwin RA. Disorders of the mediastinum. In: *Pulmonary Diseases and Disorders,* ed. by AP Fishman. New York, McGraw-Hill, 1980, pp 1482–1486
27. Goodwin RA, Nickell JA, Des Pres RM. Mediastinal fibrosis complicating healed primary histoplasmosis and tuberculosis. *Medicine* 51:227–246, 1972
28. Siltzbach LE. Sarcoidosis. In: *Pulmonary Diseases and Disorders,* ed. by AP Fishman, New York, McGraw-Hill, 1980, pp 889–907
29. Teirstein AS, Chuang MT, Choy AR, Miller A. Fiberoptic bronchoscopy in the diagnosis of sarcoidosis. *Mt Sinai J Med* 44:740–744, 1977
30. Filly R, Blank M, Castellino RA. Radiographic distribution of intrathoracic disease in previously untreated patients with Hodgkin's disease and non-Hodgkin's lymphoma. *Radiology* 120:277–281, 1976
31. Burgener FA, Hamlin D. Intrathoracic histiocytic lymphoma. *Am J Roentgenol* 136:499–504, 1981
32. Libshitz HJ, Jing BS, Wallace S, Logothetis CJ. Sterilized metastases: A diagnostic and therapeutic dilemma. *Am J Roentgenol* 140:14–19, 1983
33. McLoud TC, Kalisher L, Stark P, et al. Intrathoracic lymph node metastases from extrathoracic neoplasms. *Am J Roentgenol* 131:403–407, 1978
34. Emami B, Melo A, Carter BL, Munzenrider JE, Piro AJ. Value of computed tomography in radiotherapy of lung cancer. *Am J Roentgenol* 131:63–67, 1978
35. Underwood GH Jr, Hooper RG, Axelbaum SP, Goodwin DW. Computed tomography scanning of the thorax in staging of bronchogenic carcinoma. *N Engl J Med* 300:777–778, 1979
36. Baron RL, Levitt RG, Sagel SS, White MJ, Roper CL, Marbarger JP. Computed tomography in the preoperative evaluation of bronchogenic carcinoma. *Radiology* 145:727–732, 1982
37. Mittman C, Bruderman I. Lung cancer: To operate or not? *Am Rev Respir Dis* 116:477–496, 1977
38. Weiss W, Cooper DA, Boucot KR. Operative mortality and five year survival rates in men with bronchogenic carcinoma. *Ann Intern Med* 71:59–65, 1969
39. Boucot KR, Cooper DA, Weiss W. The role of surgery in the cure of lung cancer. *Arch Intern Med* 120:168–175, 1967
40. Kirsh MM, Kahn DR, Gago O, et al. Treatment of bronchogenic carcinoma with mediastinal metastases. *Ann Thorac Surg* 12:11–21, 1971
41. Beahrs HO, Myers MH, eds. *Manual for Staging Cancer,* 2nd edition. Philadelphia, J.B. Lippincott, 1983
42. Lewis JW, Madrazo BL, Gross SC, et al. The value of radiography and computed tomography in the staging of lung carcinoma. *Ann Thorac Surg* 34:553–557, 1982
43. Rea HH, Shevland JE, House AJS. Accuracy of computed tomographic scanning in assessment of the mediastinum in bronchial carcinoma. *J Thorac Cardiovasc Surg* 81:825–829, 1981
44. Ekholm S, Albrechtsson U, Kugelberg J, Tylen U. Computed tomography in preoperative staging of bronchogenic carcinoma. *J Comput Assist Tomogr* 4:763–765, 1980
45. Poom PY, Feld R, Evans WK, Yeoh JL, McLoughlin ML. Computed tomography of the brain, liver and upper abdomen in the staging of small cell carcinoma of the lung. *J Comput Assist Tomogr* 6:963–965, 1982
46. Glomset DA. The incidence of metastases of malignant tumors to the adrenals. *Am J Cancer* 32:57–61, 1938
47. Sandler MA, Pearlberg JL, Madrazo BL, Girschlag KF, Gross SC. Computed tomographic evaluation of the adrenal gland in the preoperative assessment of bronchogenic carcinoma. *Radiology* 145:733–736, 1982
48. Schneider HJ, Felson B. Buckling of the innominate artery simulating aneurysm and tumor. *Am J Roentgenol* 83:1106, 1961
49. Godwin JD, Herfkens RL, Skiödebrand CG, Federle MP, Lipton MJ. Evaluation of dissections and aneurysms of the thoracic aorta by conventional and dynamic scanning. *Radiology* 136:125–133, 1980
50. Egan TJ, Neiman HL, Herman RJ, Malave SR, Sanders JH. Computed tomography in the diagnosis of aortic aneurysm dissection or traumatic injury. *Radiology* 136:141–146, 1980
51. Fomon JJ, Kurzweg FT, Broadaway RK. Aneurysms of the aorta: A review. *Ann Surg* 165:557–563, 1967

52. Harrington DP, Barth KH, White RI Jr, Brawley RK. Traumatic pseudoaneurysm of the thoracic aorta in close proximity to the anterior spinal artery: A therapeutic dilemma. *Surgery* 87:153–156, 1980

53. Heiberg E, Wolverson M, Sundaram M, Connors J, Susman M. CT findings in thoracic aortic dissection. *Am J Roentgenol* 136:13–17, 1981

54. Godwin JD, Webb RW. Contrast-related flow phenomenon mimicking pathology on thoracic computed tomography. *J Comput Assist Tomogr* 6:460–464, 1982

55. Dimsmore RD, Willerson JT, Buckley MJ. Dissecting aneurysm of the aorta. *Radiology* 105:567–575, 1972

56. Godwin JD, Breiman RS, Speckman JM. Problems and pitfalls in the evaluation of thoracic aortic dissection by computed tomography. *J Comput Assist Tomogr* 6:750–756, 1982

57. Godwin JD, Purley K, Herfkens RJ, Lipton MJ. Computed tomography for follow-up of chronic aortic dissections. *Radiology* 139:655–660, 1981

58. Meziane MA, Fishman EK, Siegelman SS. Computed tomographic diagnosis of hemopericardium in acute dissecting aneurysm of the thoracic aorta. *J Comput Assist Tomogr* (in press)

59. Pitt B. Diseases of the aorta. In: *The Principles and Practice of Medicine*, ed. by MA Harvey, RJ Johns, AH Owens, and RS Ross, New York, Appleton-Century-Crofts, 1976

60. Zerhouni EA, Barth KW, Siegelman SS. Detection of venous thrombosis by computed tomography. *Am J Roentgenol* 134:753–758, 1980

61. Goldstein G, Mackey IR. *The Human Thymus*. St. Louis, Warren H. Green, 1969

62. Dixon AK, Hilton CJ, Williams GT. Computed tomography and histological correlation of the thymic remnant. *Clin Radiol* 32:255–257, 1981

63. Perlo VP, Arnason B, Castleman B. The thymus gland in elderly patients with myasthenia gravis. *Neurology* 25:294–295, 1975

64. Baron RL, Lee JKT, Sagel SS, Peterson RR. Computed tomography of the normal thymus. *Radiology* 142:121–125, 1982

65. Gelfand DW, Goldman AS, Law EJ, MacMillan BG, Larson D, Abston S, Schreiber JT. Thymic hyperplasia in children recovering from thermal burns. *J Trauma* 12:813–817, 1972

66. Castleman B, Norris EH. The pathology of the thymus in myasthenia gravis. A study of 35 cases. *Medicine* 28:27–58, 1949

67. LeGolvan DP, Abell MR. Thymomas. *Cancer* 39:2142–2157, 1977

68. Bergh N, Gatzinsky P, Larson S, Ludin P, Ridell B. Tumors of the thymus and thymic region: 1. Clinicopathological studies on thymomas. *Ann Thorac Surg* 25:91–98, 1978

69. Zerhouni EA, Scott WW, Baker RR, Wharam MO, Siegelman SS. Invasive thymomas: Diagnosis and evaluation by computed tomography. *J Comput Assist Tomogr* 6:92–100, 1982

70. Blalock H, Harvey AM, Ford FR, Lilienthal JL Jr. The treatment of myasthenia gravis by removal of the thymus gland: Preliminary report. *JAMA* 117:1529–1533, 1941

71. Brown LR, Muhm JR, Sheepy PF, Unni KK, Bermatz PE, Hermann RC. The value of computed tomography in myasthenia gravis. *Am J Roentgenol* 140:31–35, 1983

72. Suzuki M, Takashima T, Itoh H, Choutoh S, Kawamura I, Watanabe Y. Computed tomography of mediastinal teratomas. *J Comput Assist Tomogr* 7:74–76, 1983

73. Glazer GM, Axel L, Moss AA. CT diagnosis of mediastinal thyroid. *Am J Roentgenol* 138:495–498, 1982

74. Pilla TJ, Wolverson MK, Sundaram M, Heiberg E, Shields JB. CT evaluation of cystic lymphangiomas of the mediastinum. *Radiology* 144:841–842, 1982

75. Mencini RA, Proto AV. The high left and main pulmonary arteries: A CT pitfall. *J Comput Assist Tomogr* 6:452–459, 1982

76. Norris EH. The parathyroid adenoma: A study of 322 cases. *Int Abst Surg* 84:1–41, 1947

77. Kruddy AG, Doppman JL, Brennan MF, et al. The detection of mediastinal parathyroid glands by computed tomography, selective arteriography, and venous sampling. *Radiology* 140:739–744, 1981

78. Whitley NO, Bohlman M, Connor TB, McCrea ES, Mason GR, Whitley JE. Computed tomography for localization of parathyroid adenomas. *J Comput Assist Tomogr* 5:812–817, 1981

79. Doppman JL, Kruddy AG, Brennan MF, Schneider P, Lasker RD, Marx SJ. CT appearance of enlarged parathyroid glands in the posterior-superior mediastinum. *J Comput Assist Tomogr* 6:1099–1102, 1982

80. Nakata H, Nakayama C, Kimoto T, et al. Computed tomography of mediastinal bronchogenic cysts. *J Comput Assist Tomogr* 6:733–738, 1982

81. Halber MD, Daffner RH, Thompson WM. CT of the esophagus: Normal appearance. *Am J Roentgenol* 133:1047–1050, 1979

82. Daffner RH, Halber MD, Posthlewait RW, Korobkin M, Thompson WM. CT of the esophagus: II. Carcinoma, *Am J Roentgenol* 133:1051–1055, 1982

83. Picus D, Balfe DM, Koehler RE, Roper CL, Owen JW. Computed tomography in the staging of esophageal carcinoma. *Radiology* 146:433–438, 1983

84. Kumar AJ, Kuhajda FP, Martinez CR, et al. CT of extracranial nerve sheath tumors. *J Comput Assist Tomogr* 7:857–865, 1983

Airways

The central airways include the trachea, the carina, the main-stem bronchi, and the lobar and segmental bronchi. Because of the clarity of anatomic detail that can be obtained with cross-sectional imaging, these structures are easily definable with CT (1,2). Evaluation of the central airways is important for the following reasons. (a) The bronchi are important sites of disease, both neoplastic and inflammatory. The ability to detect and potentially differentiate between various forms of bronchial pathology is of obvious clinical significance. (b) The bronchi, as seen in cross section, provide a roadmap into the pulmonary parenchyma. This is important for both localization and characterization of pulmonary parenchymal disease. (c) The bronchi serve as a lattice on which the pulmonary arteries and veins are draped in characteristic fashion. The bronchi, therefore, serve as the point of orientation for interpreting the pulmonary hila (3–6).

The purpose of this chapter will be, first, to review in detail the normal cross-sectional appearance of the central airways, with special emphasis on the lobar and segmental bronchi, and, second, to illustrate how this knowledge can be applied to the interpretation of bronchial abnormalities. The role of bronchial anatomy as it applies to evaluation of pulmonary collapse will be reviewed in Chapter 5: applications of bronchial anatomy as it relates to the pulmonary hila will be discussed in Chapter 6.

GENERAL PRINCIPLES AND METHODOLOGY

There is no standardized technique for evaluating the bronchi with CT. As shown by Osborne et al. (7), simply imaging the thorax with 10-mm-thick sec-

tions at 10-mm intervals is unsatisfactory. In their series of 50 patients imaged in this way, only 70% of the segmental bronchi were visualized.

To properly visualize and analyze the bronchi, scans must be monitored while the CT examination is in progress. Depending on which bronchial segment must be visualized, a few extra sections through the area of interest are almost always mandatory. In general, if scans have been obtained initially at 10-mm increments, then only two or three additional scans are necessary. Either sequential 5-mm-thick sections or overlapping 10-mm sections are usually satisfactory. Ordinarily, this technique adds only a few minutes to the overall time of examination.

If such an approach is taken, virtually all segmental bronchi can be visualized in all cases. Even more important, careful evaluation of segmental bronchi with thin and/or overlapping sections will prevent misinterpretation in a significant proportion of cases. This is because bronchi are small structures; unless sections are obtained through the center of the bronchi it is relatively easy to "distort" their appearance, rendering the interpretation invalid. An example of this important principle is illustrated in Fig. 1. Figure 1 is a 10-mm-thick section through the right upper lobe bronchus, which is normal in appearance. Figure 1b is a 10-mm-thick section obtained 10 mm below that shown in Fig. 1a. At this level, the right upper lobe bronchus is "abnormal," and if this section alone were interpreted, the configuration of the distal portion of the right upper lobe bronchus might be misinterpreted as showing narrowing from tumor.

In principle, cross-sectional images should not be viewed in isolation; any given section should be

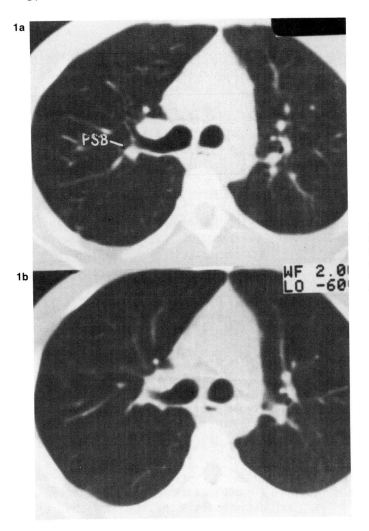

FIG. 1. Normal variant. **a,b:** Sections through the center of the right upper lobe bronchus and 10 mm below the center of the right upper lobe bronchus, respectively. It is easy to simulate bronchial pathology by scanning below or above the center of the right upper lobe bronchus. The appearance could be misinterpreted as showing narrowing from tumor (see Fig. 6b). PSB, posterior segmental bronchus.

viewed in relation to the anatomy imaged immediately above and below it to create proper perspective. In this manner, a composite picture can be created in three dimensions.

Of course, in any given case, not all bronchi need to be evaluated with such care. Correlation with appropriate radiographs should be routine prior to the CT exam to localize as carefully as possible the precise area to be studied.

BRONCHIAL ANATOMY

The ability to visualize a given bronchus on CT depends on the size and orientation of that bronchus. The origin and proximal portion of every major bronchus that courses horizontally can be identified regularly on CT, provided meticulous scanning technique is employed (see General Principles and Methodology above). These include the right upper lobe bronchus (including both the anterior and posterior segmental bronchi), the left upper lobe bronchus (including the anterior segmental bronchus), the middle lobe bronchus (generally including some portion of both the medial and lateral segmental bronchi), and the superior segmental bronchi of both lower lobes.

Bronchi having a vertical course will be seen only in cross section, and will then appear as circular lucencies. These include the apical segmental bronchus of the right upper lobe, the apical-posterior segmental bronchus of the left upper lobe, the bronchus intermedius, and the proximal portions of both lower lobe bronchi (below the takeoff of the superior segmental bronchi).

The most difficult bronchi to visualize are those that run obliquely. This is especially true of the lingular bronchus, including the superior and inferior lingular divisions, as well as the basilar segmental bronchi. On occasion, the lateral and medial segmental bronchi of the middle lobe course with a shallow obliquity. Such bronchi appear oval or elliptical when viewed in cross section.

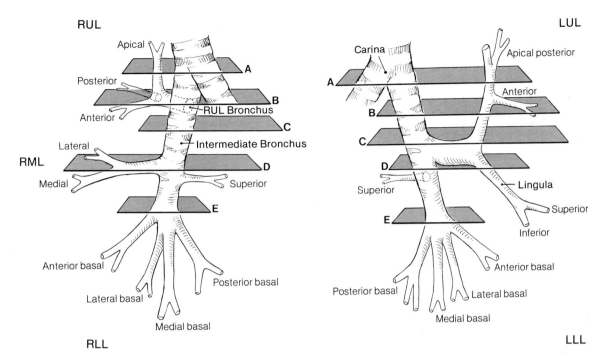

FIG. 2.a: Diagrammatic representation of the right bronchial tree in a steep oblique projection. Levels A–E represent key levels and correspond to the same levels shown in Fig. 1b. RUL; right upper lobe; RML, right middle lobe; RLL, right lower lobe. **b:** Diagrammatic representation of the left bronchial tree in 45° oblique projection. LUL, left upper lobe; LLL, left lower lobe.

Only the proximal portions of the bronchial tree, specifically the proximal portions of the segmental bronchi, can be visualized and identified on CT. Reduced size as well as variable anatomic course limit interpretation distal to segmental bronchi. As will be discussed later in the section on bronchiectasis, visualization of bronchi in the periphery of the lung on 10-mm-thick sections is itself abnormal, suggesting either thickening of the bronchial walls and/or parenchymal abnormality.

The right and left bronchial trees will be considered independently. Emphasis will be placed on recognition of characteristic sections, as illustrated in Figs. 2a and b.

SEGMENTAL ANATOMY

Right Lung

As shown in Fig. 2a, the right bronchial tree may be viewed as a sequence of five characteristic sections: the distal trachea–carina, the right upper lobe bronchus, the bronchus intermedius, the middle lobe bronchus, and the lower lobe bronchus.

Figure 3 is a CT section through the distal trachea (corresponding to level A, Fig. 2a). At this level, the apical segmental bronchus of the right upper lobe can be seen in cross section, appearing as a circular lucency immediately lateral to a main branch of the

right upper lobe pulmonary artery and immediately medial to a branch of the right superior pulmonary vein. These relationships are characteristic (3,5).

Figure 4 is a section through the right upper lobe bronchus (corresponding to level B, Fig. 2a). This bronchus is always found at or just below the carina. In Fig. 4, the carina is easily identified; a thin septum separates the right from the left main bron-

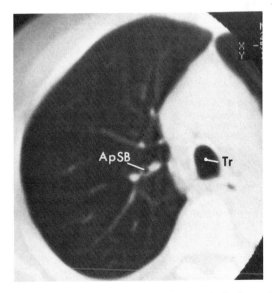

FIG. 3. Level A (per Fig. 2a): Section through the lower trachea. ApSB, apical segmental bronchus of the right upper lobe; TR, trachea.

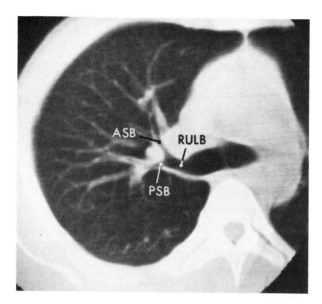

FIG. 4. Level B (per Fig. 2a): Right upper lobe bronchus. RULB, right upper lobe bronchus; ASB, anterior segmental bronchus; PSB, posterior segmental bronchus. Although the major fissure is not visualized as a line, its presence may be detected by noting a hypovascular zone which represents the junction of the posterior portion of the posterior segment of the right upper lobe and the anterior portion of the superior segment of the right lower lobe. Thus, a portion of the superior segment of the right lower lobe marginates the right main bronchus.

chi. The right upper lobe bronchus originates more cephalad than the left upper lobe bronchus, above the level of the right main pulmonary artery. The right upper lobe bronchus courses horizontally; the origins and proximal portions of the anterior and posterior segmental bronchi are visualized routinely. Note that the posterior wall of the right upper lobe bronchus is in direct contact with air in the posterior segment of the right upper lobe. Medially,

a small quantity of air in the superior segment of the right lower lobe can be defined marginating the most medial portion of the right upper lobe bronchus and the right main-stem bronchus. Differentiation between the posterior segment of the right upper lobe and the superior segment of the right lower lobe is facilitated by identification of the upper portion of the oblique fissure (see Fig. 4).

The origin of the apical segment of the right upper lobe bronchus can be visualized routinely with careful scanning technique. The origin appears as a rounded area of decreased density "superimposed" on the distal portion of the right upper lobe bronchus. This is illustrated in Fig. 5.

The overall anatomy of the right upper lobe bronchus and its relationship to both the carina and the bronchus intermedius are easy to visualize with coronal reconstructions, as illustrated in Fig. 6. This reconstruction was obtained with contiguous 10-mm-thick sections.

Any discussion of bronchial anatomy invariably raises questions concerning anatomic variants. In our experience, the greatest variable encountered in cross-sectional imaging stems from scanning technique. As has already been discussed (see General Principles and Methodology), accurate visualization of bronchi requires meticulous scanning technique. As shown in Fig. 1, it is easy to "distort" the normal appearance of a bronchus if sections are not obtained through the center of the bronchus. Another common "scan abnormality" is illustrated in Fig. 7. In this case, the right upper lobe bronchus and the anterior segmental bronchus are seen while the posterior segmental bronchus appears to be missing. In fact, the posterior segmental bronchus is normal in this case (not shown); the reason it is

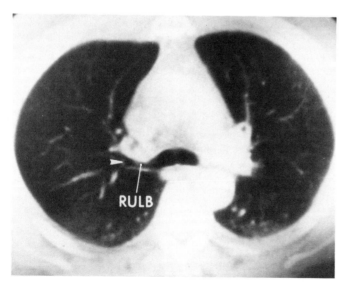

FIG. 5. Section through the right upper lobe bronchus (RULB). The origin of the apical segmental bronchus (arrowhead) can be seen as a circular lucency superimposed on the distal end of the right upper lobe bronchus.

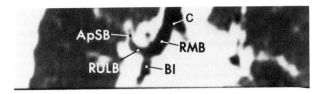

FIG. 6. Coronal reconstruction. C, carina; RMB, right mainstem bronchus; RULB, right upper lobe bronchus; ApSB, apical segmental bronchus; BI, bronchus intermedius.

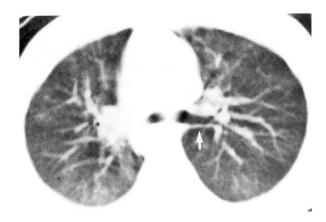

FIG. 8. Situs inversus: Kartagener's syndrome. Section through the right upper lobe bronchus *(arrow)* and both the anterior and posterior segmental bronchi. The appearance is a mirror image of normal.

not visualized is because its course is slightly oblique, and is therefore not seen in the plane of this CT section.

While minor variations in the bronchi are commonplace (and generally easy to recognize and define with CT), true anomalies of the bronchial tree are rare. An example of situs inversus in a patient with Kartagener's syndrome is shown in Fig. 8. The usual appearance of the right upper lobe bronchus, with anterior and posterior segmental bronchi, is easily recognizable on the left side.

The posterior wall of the right upper lobe bronchus is an important anatomic landmark. In general, this stripe is uniform in caliber. In our experience, there is some variability in the overall thickness of this stripe; the upper limits of normal should be less than 0.5 cm, as illustrated in Fig. 9a. As noted, this posterior stripe should have a uniform configura-

tion; nodularity or irregularity is abnormal, generally signifying tumor infiltration and/or adenopathy. One significant exception is the finding of a prominent azygos vein (8) (Fig. 9b; compare with Fig. 4). This appearance should not cause confusion; analysis of sections just above and below should establish the presence of a prominent azygos vein. If doubt persists, scans taken following a Valsalva maneuver should show marked decrease in the size of the azygos vein.

Figure 10 is a section through the bronchus intermedius (corresponding to level C, Fig. 2a). The bronchus intermedius extends from the point at which the right upper lobe bronchus originates to the point of origin of the middle lobe bronchus. The bronchus intermedius lies directly posterior to the right main pulmonary artery and, at a slightly lower level (Fig. 10), just medial to the right interlobar pulmonary artery. The entire posterior wall of this bronchus is in contact with air in the superior segment of the right lower lobe. Additionally, pulmonary parenchyma lies posteromedial to the bronchus intermedius. This represents lung in the azygoesophageal recess, the medial border of which is formed by the azygos vein. Except for the pediatric population, lung in this recess is normally convex medially. This convexity is obliterated when there are enlarged subcarinal lymph nodes. The region of the minor fissure separating the right upper and middle lobes is generally manifested as a hypovascular zone lateral to the right interlobar pulmonary artery frequently seen at this level (Fig. 10).

Figs. 11a and b are sequential 5-mm-thick sections through the origin of the middle lobe bronchus and just below it, respectively. This corresponds to level D in Fig. 2a. The middle lobe bronchus ex-

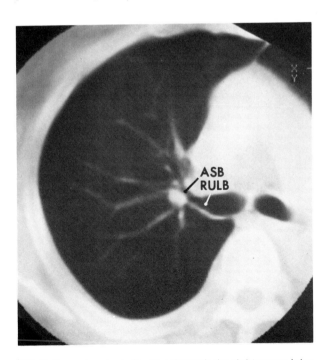

FIG. 7. Normal variant. Section through the right upper lobe bronchus (RULB). The anterior segmental bronchus (ASB) is clearly visible. The posterior segmental bronchus appears to be missing because it is not coursing in the plane of the CT scan.

9a,b

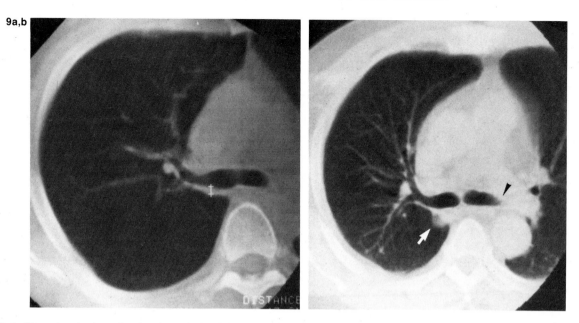

FIG. 9. Normal variants. **a:** Section through the right upper lobe bronchus. The posterior wall is top normal in size (0.5 cm). Notice that the posterior wall is extremely smooth. **b:** Prominent azygos vein *(arrow)*. This appearance may simulate adenopathy. Note also that the left upper lobe bronchus has a tapered appearance where it is crossed by the left pulmonary artery *(arrowhead)*. This should not be confused with an endobronchial lesion.

tends anteriorly at a slightly oblique angle. The origin of the middle lobe bronchus also marks the point of origin of the right lower lobe bronchus. In Fig. 11a, the middle lobe spur can be seen separating the middle and lower lobe bronchus. A thin septum of tissue can be identified; more frequently, only the lateral aspect of the spur can be seen. This can be identified as a triangular wedge of tissue just lateral to the bronchial bifurcation.

In 60% of cases, the middle lobe bronchus divides

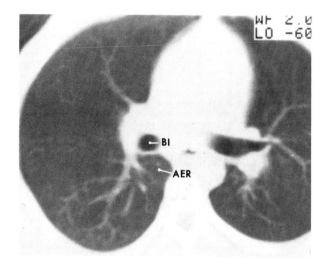

FIG. 10. Level C (per Fig. 2a): Bronchus intermedius (BI). The bronchus intermedius lies immediately posterior and medial to the right main and interlobar pulmonary arteries. The extensive hypovascular region on the right represents the region of the minor fissure. AER, azygo-esophageal recess.

into equally prominent medial and lateral segmental bronchi (9). The medial segmental bronchus has a more oblique orientation than does the lateral segmental bronchus, which courses horizontally. This is shown in Fig. 11b. In a small percentage of cases, a large medial segmental bronchus is associated with a small lateral segmental bronchus. Even more rarely, the two segmental bronchi appear to arise independently from a very truncated middle lobe bronchus (Fig. 12). None of these variations should cause confusion.

As one may note in Fig. 2a, the middle lobe bronchus courses inferiorly as well as anteriorly. If the origin of the middle bronchus is visualized, the medial and lateral segmental bronchi may be located in a slightly inferior plane.

The superior segmental bronchus of the right lower lobe may arise at the same level as the point of origin of the middle lobe bronchus, or, frequently, at a slightly lower level. The superior segmental bronchus courses posteriorly and runs in a horizontal plane (Fig. 13).

Figure 14 is a section through the proximal portions of both lower lobe bronchi, just inferior to the origin of the superior segmental bronchi (corresponding to level E, Fig. 2a). The lower lobe bronchi, at this level, are vertically oriented, and hence are visualized as circular lucencies. The lower lobe bronchi always lie medial and anterior to the corresponding lower lobe pulmonary arteries, which also course vertically. The lower lobe bronchi charac-

11a

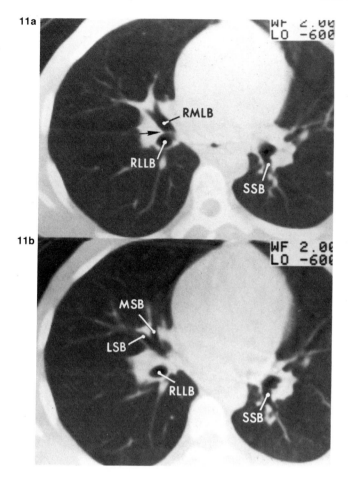

11b

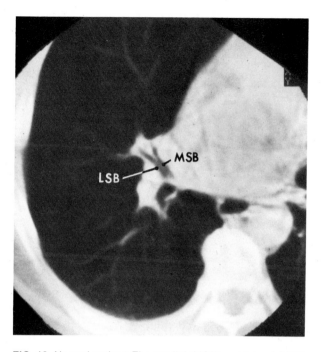

FIG. 12. Normal variant. The medial (MSB) and lateral (LSB) segmental bronchi of the middle lobe appear to arise independently.

FIG. 11. a: Level D (per Fig. 2a): Right middle lobe bronchus (RMLB). This section shows the origin of the middle lobe bronchus coursing anteriorly on an oblique angle. There is a thin line, or septum, separating the middle lobe bronchus anteriorly from the right lower lobe bronchus (RLLB); this represents the middle lobe spur *(arrow)*. SSB, superior segmental bronchus of the left lower lobe. **b:** Section just caudal to that shown in a, through the medial (MSB) and lateral (LSB) segmental bronchi of the middle lobe.

tions relative to one another, and because of their general configuration coursing toward the anticipated positions of their respective pulmonary segments.

More peripherally, the same relationships hold, allowing for accurate identification (Fig. 16). This

teristically appear "suspended" in the lung by the superior portions of the inferior pulmonary ligaments.

The basilar segmental bronchi are easiest to identify when all four are imaged in the same plane (Fig. 15). There is considerable variability in the cross-sectional appearance of the basilar segmental bronchi. The following characteristics may be noted in Fig. 15. First, the medial basilar segmental bronchus characteristically lies just anterior to the inferior pulmonary vein. This is a constant relationship. Second, while variable in appearance, the basilar segmental bronchi always course in the direction of their respective basilar pulmonary segments. This is the key to their identification. The anterior, lateral, and posterior basilar bronchi may all be identified individually because of their posi-

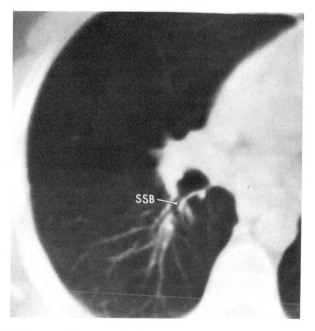

FIG. 13. Section through the superior segmental bronchus (SSB) of the right lower lobe. This bronchus courses posteriorly and runs in a horizontal plane.

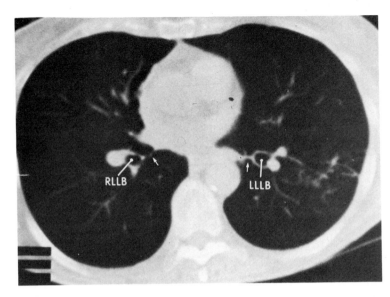

FIG. 14. Level E (per Fig. 2a): Lower lobe bronchi. Proximal portions of the right (RLLB) and left (LLLB) lower lobe bronchi. *Arrows* point to the superior portions of the inferior pulmonary ligaments.

level is the most inferior one at which the basilar bronchi should be identifiable.

A common, normal variant is shown in Fig. 17. In this case, the lateral and posterior basilar segmental bronchi of both the right and left lower lobes originate from a common trunk.

Left Lung

Figures 18a and b are sections through the lower trachea and carina, respectively, and correspond to levels A and B in Fig. 2b. These two levels are grouped together because both are sections through the apical-posterior segmental bronchus of the left upper lobe. The left upper lobe bronchus originates at a level lower than the right upper lobe bronchus and forms a "sling" over which the main left pulmonary artery passes. In Fig. 18a the apical-posterior segmental bronchus is seen as a circular lucency surrounded medially and laterally by main branches of the left upper lobe pulmonary artery and vein. In Fig. 18b, the apical-posterior segmental bronchus is

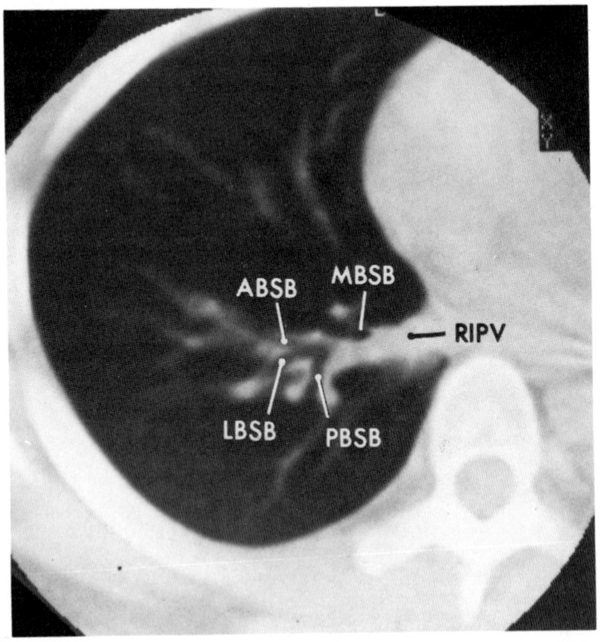

FIG. 15. Section through the basilar segmental bronchi. The medial basilar bronchus always lies anterior to the inferior pulmonary vein. MBSB, medial basilar segmental bronchus; ABSB, anterior basilar segmental bronchus; LBSB, lateral basilar segmental bronchus; PBSB; posterior basilar segmental bronchus; RIPV, right inferior pulmonary vein.

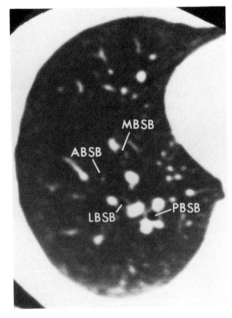

FIG. 16. Section through the basilar segmental bronchi. The key to the identification of the basilar segmental bronchi is that they subtend the expected location of the various basilar lung segments. MBSB, medial basilar segmental bronchus; ABSB, anterior basilar segmental bronchus; LBSB, lateral basilar segmental bronchus; PBSB, posterior basilar segmental bronchus.

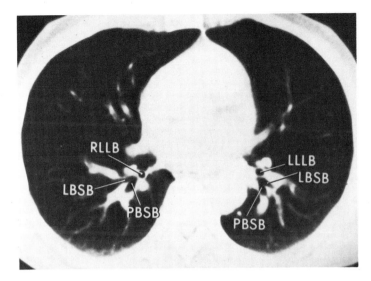

FIG. 17. Normal variant. Posterior basilar segmental bronchus (PBSB) and lateral basilar segmental bronchus (LBSB). These two basilar segmental bronchi frequently originate from a common trunk. RLLB, right lower lobe bronchus; LLLB, left lower lobe bronchus.

separated from the left main bronchus by the left main pulmonary artery as it courses posteriorly.

The key to understanding the anatomy of the left upper lobe bronchus and its branches is to realize that the left upper lobe bronchus is large, and it is therefore possible to obtain sections through both the upper and lower portions of this bronchus. Each has a characteristic appearance.

Figure 19 is a section through the "upper" portion of the left upper lobe bronchus (corresponding to level C, Fig. 2b). At this level, the posterior wall of the left upper lobe bronchus is slightly concave; this concavity is caused by the left pulmonary artery as it passes above and then posterior to the left upper lobe bronchus. The origin of the apical-posterior segmental bronchus can be recognized as a rounded

area of increased lucency "superimposed" on the distal portion of the left upper lobe bronchus (Fig. 19). Just posterior to the medial portion of the left upper lobe bronchus air in the superior segment of the left lower lobe abuts the posteromedial wall of the bronchus. Webb and Gamsu (10) have referred to this invagination of lung between the descending aorta and the left interlobar pulmonary artery as the left "retrobronchial stripe." Adenopathy and/or a hilar mass will efface this segment of lung, similar to the effacement of the azygo-esophageal recess on the right side caused by subcarinal adenopathy.

The anatomy of the left upper lobe bronchus and the apical posterior segment bronchus of the left upper lobe may be seen clearly using parasagittal reconstructions. Figures 20a and b are coronal

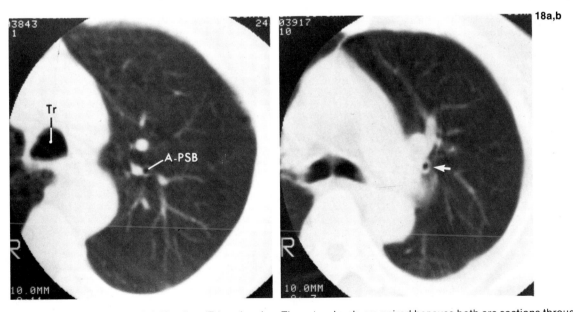

FIG. 18. a,b: Levels A and B (per Fig 2a): Trachea (Tr) and carina. These two levels are paired because both are sections through the apical-posterior segmental bronchus (A-PSB) of the left upper lobe (see *arrow* in **b**).

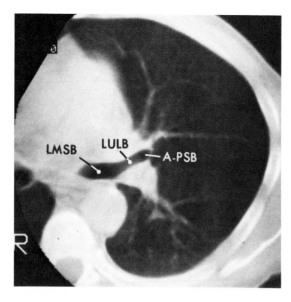

FIG. 19. Level C (per Fig. 2a): Upper portion of the left upper lobe bronchus (LULB). The posterior wall of the left upper lobe bronchus is slightly concave. The origin of the apical-posterior segmental bronchus (A-PSB) can be identified as a circular lucency superimposed in the distal portion of the left upper lobe bronchus. LMSB, left main-stem bronchus.

views, respectively, of the left main-stem bronchus and the proximal portion of the left upper lobe bronchus, and the apical-posterior segmental bronchus (which can be seen originating from the upper surface of the left upper lobe bronchus; compare with Fig. 2b).

Figure 21 is a section through the lower portion of the left upper lobe bronchus (corresponding to level D, Fig. 2b). The most important anatomic landmark in this section is the left upper lobe spur. This spur marks the point of origin of the left lower lobe bronchus. The spur can be recognized as a triangular density separating the lower portion of the left upper from the left lower lobe bronchus, and is exactly analagous to the middle lobe spur on the right side (compare with Fig. 11a).

The lingular bronchus arises from the undersurface of the distal portion of the left upper lobe bronchus and has an oblique course inferiorly. The origin of the lingular bronchus can be identified as a circular area of increased lucency "superimposed" on the distal portion of the left upper lobe bronchus, in much the same manner in which the origin of the apical-posterior segmental bronchus can be identified (compare Figs. 19 and 21). The key to differentiating the origin of the apical-posterior segmental bronchus from the origin of the lingular bronchus is identification of the left upper lobe spur (Fig. 21) and confirming that the section showing the origin of the lingular bronchus is through the lower portion of the left upper lobe bronchus.

The lingular bronchus runs inferiorly on an oblique path. In cross section, the lingular bronchus has an oval or elliptical shape. If sections are obtained just below the left upper lobe bronchus, the lingular bronchus will appear as a discrete oval lucency separated spatially from the left lower lobe bronchus (Fig. 22). Sequential sections obtained below the origin of the lingular bronchus will show progressively wider separation between the lingular bronchus anteriorly and the left lower lobe bronchus posteriorly.

The superior and especially the inferior divisions of the lingular bronchus are seen on CT only infrequently. These segmental bronchi tend to originate at a considerable distance from the origin of the lingular bronchus and are generally too small and peripheral to be visualized. The proximal portion of the superior division of the lingular bronchus can be seen in Fig. 23.

The anterior segmental bronchus of the left upper lobe has been omitted from discussion so far because it is highly variable. In approximately 75% of individuals, the left upper lobe bronchus divides into superior and lingular divisions (11). In this instance, the anterior segmental bronchus originates

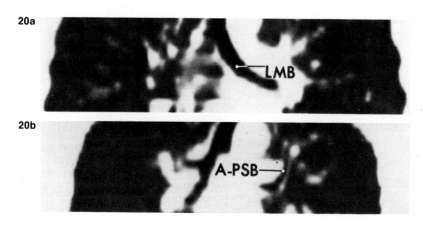

FIG. 20. a,b: Coronal reconstructions through the left main-stem bronchus (LMB) and the lateral portion of the left upper lobe bronchus, respectively. A-PSB, apical-posterior segmental bronchus (arising from the upper portion of the left upper lobe bronchus).

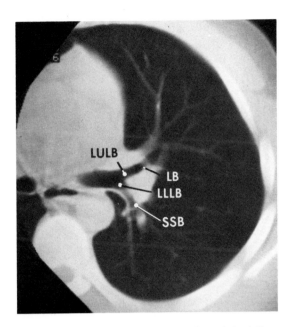

FIG. 21. Level (per Fig. 2a): Lower portion of the left upper lobe bronchus (LULB). The left upper and lower lobe bronchi are separated by the left upper lobe spur, which can be identified as a triangular wedge of tissue. The lingular bronchus (LB) arises from the lower portion of the left upper lobe bronchus. LLLB, origin of the left lower lobe bronchus; SSB, superior segmental bronchus.

as a branch of the apical-posterior segmental bronchus (Figs. 2b and 24).

In 25% of cases, the left upper lobe trifurcates. The anterior segmental bronchus then arises between a modified superior division bronchus (api-

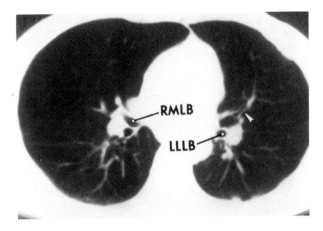

FIG. 23. Section through the proximal portion of the superior division of the lingular bronchus (arrowheads). LLLB, left lower lobe bronchus; RMLB, right middle lobe bronchus.

cal-posterior segmental bronchus) superiorly and the lingular bronchus inferiorly. When the left upper lobe bronchus trifurcates in this manner, the anterior segmental bronchus will arise in close proximity to the apical-posterior segmental bronchus (Fig. 25), or, occasionally, close to the origin of the lingular bronchus.

Identification of the anterior segmental bronchus is facilitated by recognizing that it is the only bronchus arising from the left upper lobe bronchus that courses anteriorly in a horizontal plane.

The superior segmental bronchus of the left lower

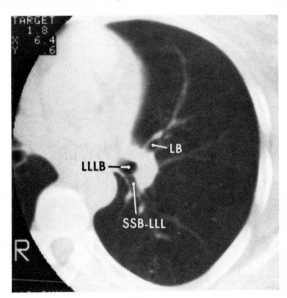

FIG. 22. Section below the left upper lobe bronchus. Sequential sections below the left upper lobe bronchus will show progressively wider separation between the lingular and lower lobe bronchi. LB, lingular bronchus; LLLB, left lower lobe bronchus; SSB-LLL, superior segmental bronchus of the left lower lobe.

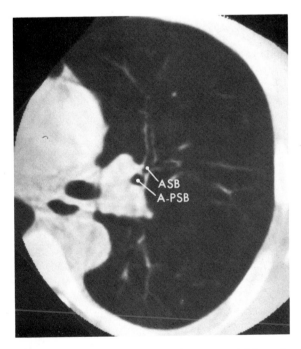

FIG. 24. Section through the anterior segmental bronchus (ASB), in this case arising from the proximal portion of the apical-posterior segmental bronchus (A-PSB).

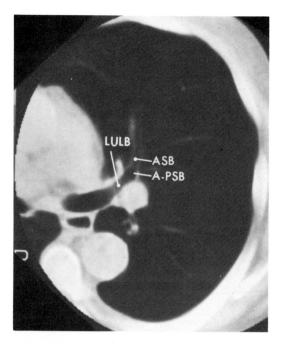

FIG. 25. Section through the anterior segmental bronchus (ASB) arising at the distal end of the left upper lobe bronchus (LULB), alongside the origin of the apical-posterior segmental bronchus (A-PSB).

lobe is analagous in shape and configuration to the same bronchus on the right side. The superior segmental bronchus of the left lower lobe is seen in Figs. 21 and 22.

The left lower lobe bronchus usually conforms to the same pattern as the right lower lobe bronchus. The proximal portion of the left lower bronchus, below the origin of the superior segmental bronchus, is shown in Fig. 14 and corresponds to level E in Fig. 2b. The proximal portion of the left lower lobe bronchus at this level appears suspended in the lung by the upper portion of the left inferior pulmonary ligament.

The basilar segmental bronchi are essentially mirror images of the patterns shown for the right lower lobe basilar bronchi. Again, the key to identification is to note the general configuration and position of these bronchi as they course to their corresponding basilar lung segments (see Fig. 17).

In this section, the right and left bronchial trees have been considered and illustrated separately. By way of comparison, right to left, it should be noted that levels A to E are the same (i.e., they correspond) in both Figs. 2a and b. This is true only as long as the patient being examined is in perfect alignment. Unfortunately, even minor degrees of tilt will distort the correspondence of the right and left bronchial trees—hence the emphasis on learning right- and left-sided bronchial anatomy independently.

BRONCHIAL NEOPLASIA

In the evaluation of bronchial neoplasia, CT is efficacious in localizing the presence and/or confirming the absence of bronchial malignancy, as well as in determining the true extent of disease. Recognition of pathology rests on thorough knowledge of normal bronchial anatomy, as well as mediastinal and hilar anatomy (see Chapters 2 and 6). CT is less useful in differentiating among the various types of bronchial malignancy, although certain features of particular tumors tend to be characteristic, as will be discussed. On occasion, CT can be useful in differentiating benign from malignant disease.

The most important role of CT in evaluating patients with bronchial neoplasia is in planning the best diagnostic approach for accurate staging. In this chapter, the role of CT in detecting bronchial neoplasia will be stressed. A detailed discussion of the value of CT in the diagnostic evaluation of the mediastinum, especially of the significance of mediastinal adenopathy, is presented in Chapter 3.

Bronchial Adenomas

Evaluation of the appearance on CT of bronchial adenomas serves as a useful model for all bronchial neoplasia. The neoplasms grouped under this heading include bronchial carcinoids, adenoid-cystic carcinomas, and mucoepidermoid carcinomas. The term "bronchial adenoma" is a misnomer; these tumors, while slow growing, invade locally and have a marked tendency to recur after they have been excised (12). Less frequently, they metastasize to distal, extrathoracic sites. For these reasons, they should all be considered to be low-grade malignancies (13,14).

Bronchial adenomas have a common tendency to arise centrally, either in the trachea or proximal bronchial tree. They are, therefore, ideally situated for evaluation by CT.

An important principle in the evaluation of bronchial neoplasms, and in particular in the evaluation of bronchial adenomas, is definition of the true extent of disease. Bronchial adenomas show variable growth patterns. They may grow primarily intraluminally, or, alternatively, they may have a small intraluminal component and extend deeply into the adjacent peribronchial soft tissues. While routine radiography, including tomography and bronchography, can define the presence of disease, and endoscopic biopsy can reliably establish the diagnosis, proper preoperative evaluation requires accurate definition of both the intra- and extraluminal components of these tumors (15,16) (see Figs. 26 and 27).

Endobronchial lesions may be manifested in a va-

26a,b

26c,d

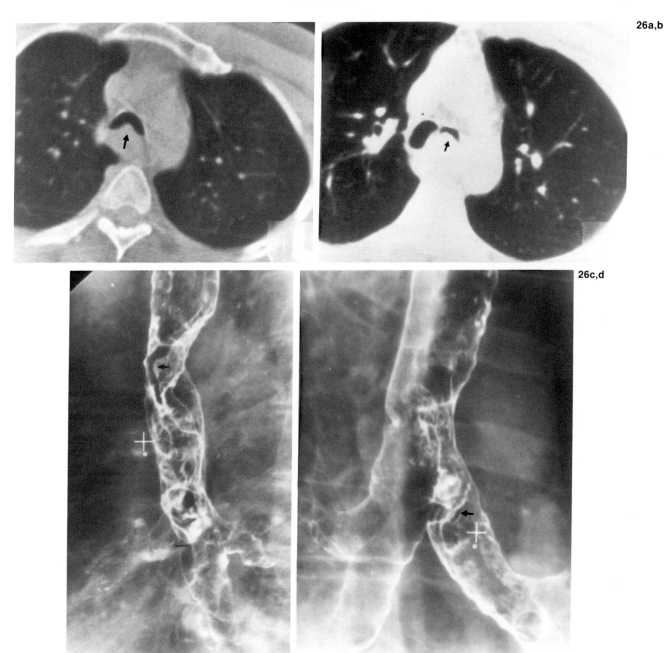

FIG. 26. Adenoid cystic carcinoma (carina). **a:** Section through lower trachea at the level of the aortic arch. The trachea is displaced anteriorly; the posterior wall of the trachea is deformed by tumor mass *(arrow)*. **b:** Section at the level of the carina. The left main-stem bronchus is narrowed and deformed posteriorly by tumor mass *(arrow)*, which also encroaches on the medial aspect of the right main-stem bronchus. **c,d:** Lateral and AP views from an inhalational tantalum tracheogram. A large mass deforms the posterior wall of the lower trachea. The *arrow* in (c) is at the same level as the scan illustrated in (a). The *arrow* in (d) is at the same level as the scan illustrated in (b). Note that, in the AP tracheogram, there is no evidence that the mass involves the right main-stem bronchus.

riety of ways. If a lesion is primarily endobronchial, tumor may partially occlude the bronchial lumen and act as a ball valve, trapping air in the subtended lung, with resultant emphysema (Fig. 28).

More frequently, endobronchial obstruction causes pneumonitis and atelectasis in the subtended lung. This may be lobar or segmental, depending on

the location and size of the lesion. This pattern of presentation is illustrated in Figs. 29 and 30. It should be noted that when there is no evidence of extension outside the bronchial wall, local resection of the tumor with plastic repair of the bronchi may be feasible (16). The value of CT in preoperative staging is illustrated in Fig. 29.

27,a,b

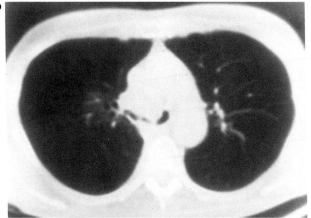

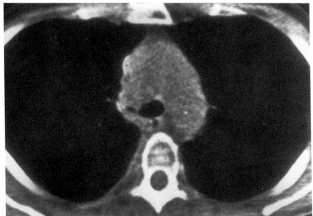

27c

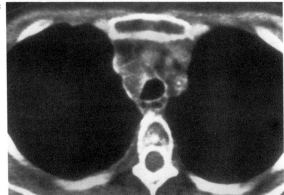

FIG. 27. Adenoid-cystic carcinoma (carina). **a:** Section at the level of the carina. An irregular tumor mass arises anteriorly and partially occludes both the right and left main bronchi. **b:** Section obtained slightly higher than that shown in (a). The fascial planes of the mediastinum have been obliterated by tumor. **c:** Section at the level of the great vessels. Tumor extends along the right lateral tracheal wall, minimally deforming the tracheal configuration.

Computed tomography also is of value in follow-up examinations in patients whose tumors have been excised. Bronchial adenomas tend to recur, either as metastases or as primary tumors, and, as a consequence, repeat bronchoscopy at regular intervals is frequently necessary, especially if the patient becomes symptomatic. CT obviates the need for follow-up bronchoscopy, as illustrated in Fig. 31.

Although adenomas usually arise centrally in relation to either the trachea, carina, or lobar and/or proximal segmental bronchi, they occasionally present as pulmonary nodules. As a rule, adenomas are well-marginated, sharply defined lesions; they are almost always in close proximity to an adjacent bronchus, which may be deformed, and they frequently show stippled areas of peripheral calcification. This is illustrated in Fig. 32. (A detailed discussion of the use of CT in the evaluation of pulmonary nodules can be found in Chapter 7.) While not pathognomonic, this triad of findings is sufficiently characteristic to suggest the diagnosis. This is important, since adenomas are very vascular lesions that may bleed extensively if they are not biopsied carefully.

Bronchogenic Carcinoma

As noted previously, bronchial adenomas serve as a useful model of bronchial neoplasia. The appearance on CT of bronchogenic carcinoma may be indistinguishable from that of a bronchial adenoma (Fig. 33; compare with Fig. 26).

Certain features of bronchogenic carcinomas, however, are distinctive. Centrally, bronchogenic carcinoma may arise in a central airway and infiltrate circumferentially for a considerable length. This appearance, as illustrated in Fig. 34, may be exceedingly subtle (see also Figs. 29 and 30 in Chapter 6).

Peripherally, bronchogenic carcinomas frequently have lobulated or spiculated margins, although perfectly smooth lesions may still be malignant (Figs. 35a and b). More important, bronchogenic carcinoma frequently arises at points of bronchial bifurcation. In these cases, the only apparent bronchial abnormality may be widening of the spur (Fig. 36; compare with the normal appearance of the first bifurcation of the superior segmental bronchus of the right lower lobe in Fig. 13).

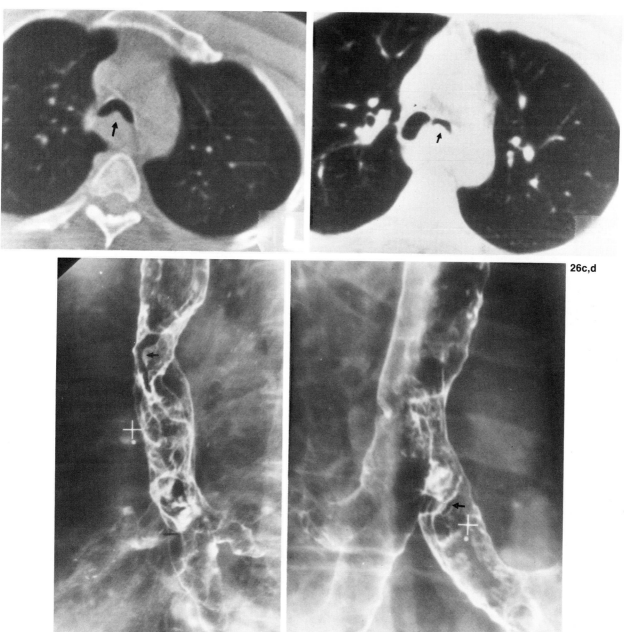

26a,b

26c,d

FIG. 26. Adenoid cystic carcinoma (carina). **a:** Section through lower trachea at the level of the aortic arch. The trachea is displaced anteriorly; the posterior wall of the trachea is deformed by tumor mass *(arrow).* **b:** Section at the level of the carina. The left main-stem bronchus is narrowed and deformed posteriorly by tumor mass *(arrow),* which also encroaches on the medial aspect of the right main-stem bronchus. **c,d:** Lateral and AP views from an inhalational tantalum tracheogram. A large mass deforms the posterior wall of the lower trachea. The *arrow* in (c) is at the same level as the scan illustrated in (a). The *arrow* in (d) is at the same level as the scan illustrated in (b). Note that, in the AP tracheogram, there is no evidence that the mass involves the right main-stem bronchus.

riety of ways. If a lesion is primarily endobronchial, tumor may partially occlude the bronchial lumen and act as a ball valve, trapping air in the subtended lung, with resultant emphysema (Fig. 28).

More frequently, endobronchial obstruction causes pneumonitis and atelectasis in the subtended lung. This may be lobar or segmental, depending on

the location and size of the lesion. This pattern of presentation is illustrated in Figs. 29 and 30. It should be noted that when there is no evidence of extension outside the bronchial wall, local resection of the tumor with plastic repair of the bronchi may be feasible (16). The value of CT in preoperative staging is illustrated in Fig. 29.

27,a,b

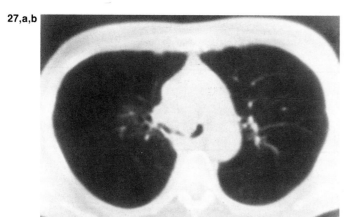

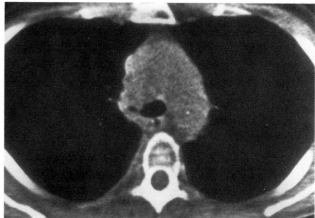

27c

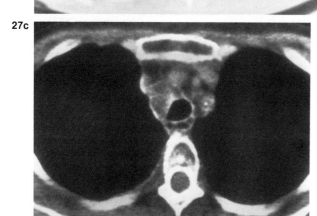

FIG. 27. Adenoid-cystic carcinoma (carina). **a:** Section at the level of the carina. An irregular tumor mass arises anteriorly and partially occludes both the right and left main bronchi. **b:** Section obtained slightly higher than that shown in (a). The fascial planes of the mediastinum have been obliterated by tumor. **c:** Section at the level of the great vessels. Tumor extends along the right lateral tracheal wall, minimally deforming the tracheal configuration.

Computed tomography also is of value in follow-up examinations in patients whose tumors have been excised. Bronchial adenomas tend to recur, either as metastases or as primary tumors, and, as a consequence, repeat bronchoscopy at regular intervals is frequently necessary, especially if the patient becomes symptomatic. CT obviates the need for follow-up bronchoscopy, as illustrated in Fig. 31.

Although adenomas usually arise centrally in relation to either the trachea, carina, or lobar and/or proximal segmental bronchi, they occasionally present as pulmonary nodules. As a rule, adenomas are well-marginated, sharply defined lesions; they are almost always in close proximity to an adjacent bronchus, which may be deformed, and they frequently show stippled areas of peripheral calcification. This is illustrated in Fig. 32. (A detailed discussion of the use of CT in the evaluation of pulmonary nodules can be found in Chapter 7.) While not pathognomonic, this triad of findings is sufficiently characteristic to suggest the diagnosis. This is important, since adenomas are very vascular lesions that may bleed extensively if they are not biopsied carefully.

Bronchogenic Carcinoma

As noted previously, bronchial adenomas serve as a useful model of bronchial neoplasia. The appearance on CT of bronchogenic carcinoma may be indistinguishable from that of a bronchial adenoma (Fig. 33; compare with Fig. 26).

Certain features of bronchogenic carcinomas, however, are distinctive. Centrally, bronchogenic carcinoma may arise in a central airway and infiltrate circumferentially for a considerable length. This appearance, as illustrated in Fig. 34, may be exceedingly subtle (see also Figs. 29 and 30 in Chapter 6).

Peripherally, bronchogenic carcinomas frequently have lobulated or spiculated margins, although perfectly smooth lesions may still be malignant (Figs. 35a and b). More important, bronchogenic carcinoma frequently arises at points of bronchial bifurcation. In these cases, the only apparent bronchial abnormality may be widening of the spur (Fig. 36; compare with the normal appearance of the first bifurcation of the superior segmental bronchus of the right lower lobe in Fig. 13).

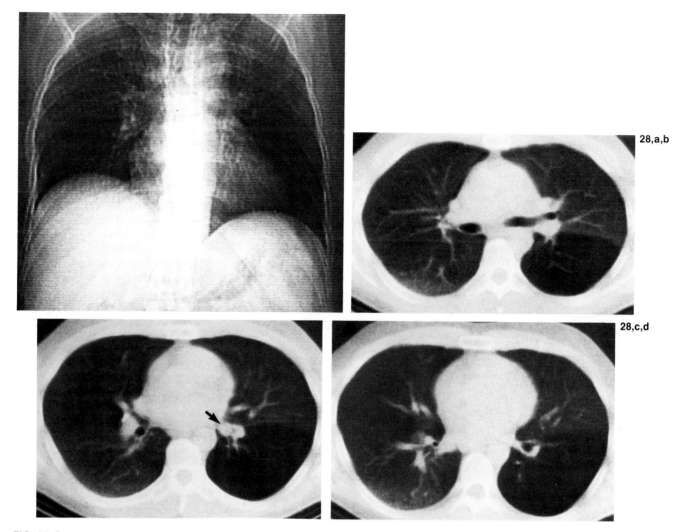

FIG. 28. Bronchial adenoma (left lower lobe bronchus). **a:** Scanogram shows hyperlucency of the left lower lobe and minimal depression of the left hemidiaphragm. **b–d:** Sequential sections through the left upper lobe and left lower lobe bronchi. There is hyperlucency and slight expansion of the left lower lobe in all sections. A 3-mm tumor mass partially occludes the left lower lobe bronchus (*arrow in* **(c)**), acting as a ball valve. This appearance is accentuated by scanning at end expiration.

Because of the precision with which lesions may be visualized with CT, this modality may be used to facilitate diagnostic evaluation. In certain patients, CT may help differentiate benign from malignant disease, obviating the need for further workup (Fig. 37).

In those cases in which bronchial neoplasia cannot be excluded, CT is most helpful in determining whether parenchymal lesions should be approached bronchoscopically or by percutaneous, transthoracic needle biopsy. As already illustrated throughout this chapter, in select cases, CT may serve as an accurate roadmap for the bronchoscopist. This principle is illustrated in Figs. 38–40. While localization is easiest when a lesion is adjacent to bronchi that course in a horizontal plane, it is still possible to determine the location of a lesion even when the adjacent bronchi have a vertical or oblique course (Fig. 40); as important, even when a lesion does not lie adjacent to a bronchus, the particular segment of lung in which a lesion is located can be determined in nearly all cases. This knowledge is helpful in assessing the best route for biopsy.

If it has been determined that a lesion is most easily approached transthoracically, CT can also have several potentially useful roles. First, CT can be used to plan the best approach for percutaneous biopsy (CT-assisted, transthoracic needle biopsy). For example, in our experience, small subpleural blebs are frequently seen with CT that were unsuspected on plain films; their presence frequently necessitates a change in the direction of biopsy.

29,a,b

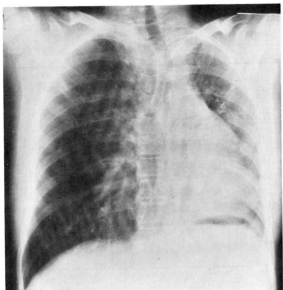

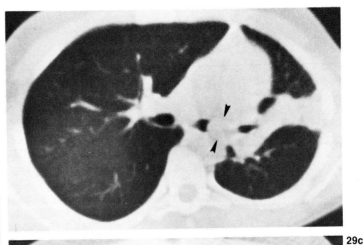

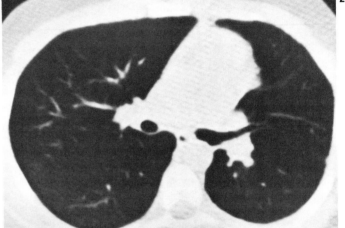

29c

FIG. 29. Carcinoid tumor. **a:** PA radiograph. There is volume loss in the left upper lobe. **b:** Section at the level of the left upper lobe bronchus. There is a sharply defined mass in the midportion of the left upper lobe bronchus *(arrowheads).* There is infiltrate in the posterior portion of the left upper lobe, sharply demarcated posteriorly by the oblique fissure. Hyperinflation of the right lung is apparent. **c:** Section through the left upper lobe bronchus following surgical resection of the tumor and plastic repair of the left upper lobe bronchus. There is no evidence of residual tumor.

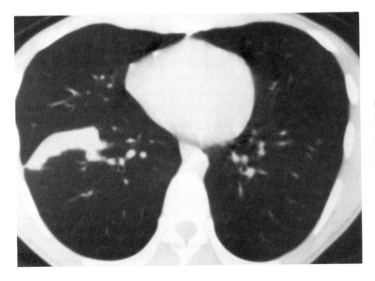

FIG. 30. Bronchial adenoma. Section through the lower lobes. There is a sharply defined area of parenchymal consolidation in the anterior basal segment of the right lower lobe, demarcated anteriorly by the oblique fissure. At bronchoscopy, a small tumor mass occluded the anterior basilar segmental bronchus.

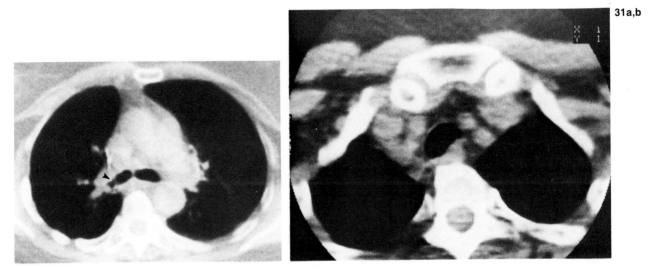

FIG. 31. Recurrent adenoid-cystic carcinoma. **a:** Section at the level of anastomosis between the right main-stem bronchus and the bronchus intermedius *(arrowhead)*. Adenoid-cystic carcinoma within the right upper lobe bronchus had been resected several years previously. **b:** Section through the great vessels. There is a mass deforming the posterolateral wall of the trachea, infiltrating adjacent soft tissues. (Biopsy proven.)

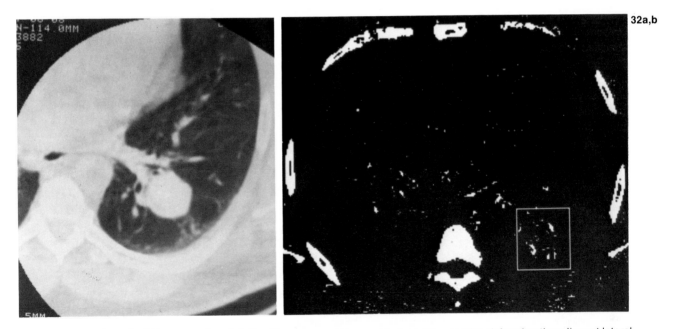

FIG. 32. Peripheral carcinoid tumor. **a:** A well-defined tumor mass is present in the left lower lobe, deforming the adjacent lateral basilar segmental bronchus. **b:** Same section shown in (a), imaged with a window width of 4. The area of the tumor is contained within the rectangle; peripheral areas of calcification can be seen. This constellation of findings should suggest a diagnosis of bronchial adenoma.

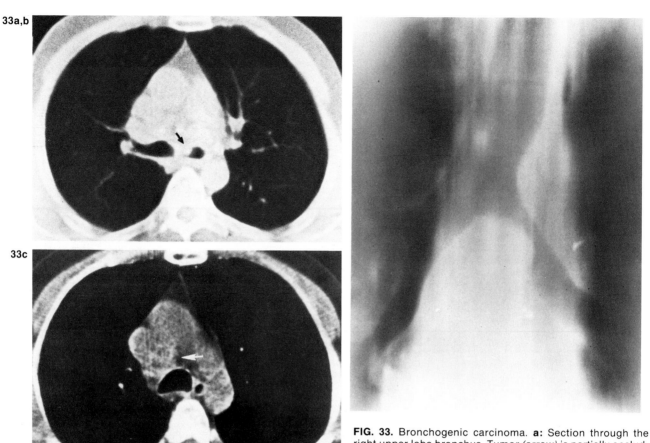

FIG. 33. Bronchogenic carcinoma. **a:** Section through the right upper lobe bronchus. Tumor *(arrow)* is partially occluding the left main bronchus. Extension outside the bronchial lumen can be identified even in this section imaged with wide windows. **b:** AP tomogram shows the mass partially occluding the left main bronchus. Tomography fails to define the true extent of tumor. **c:** Section obtained just above the level of the carina. The extraluminal component of this tumor extends superiorly in front of the trachea *(arrow)*.

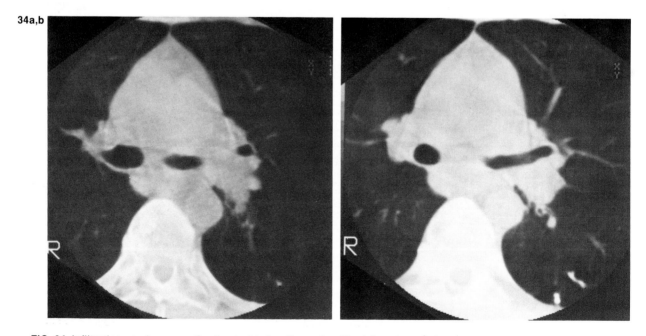

FIG. 34. Infiltrating carcinoma. **a:** Section just below the carina. The left main-stem bronchus is circumferentially narrowed and slightly irregular in contour. Subcarinal adenopathy deforms the azygo-esophageal recess. **b:** Section through the left upper lobe bronchus. Tumor infiltrates the entire length of the left upper lobe bronchus (compare the caliber of the left upper lobe bronchus with that of the bronchus intermedius).

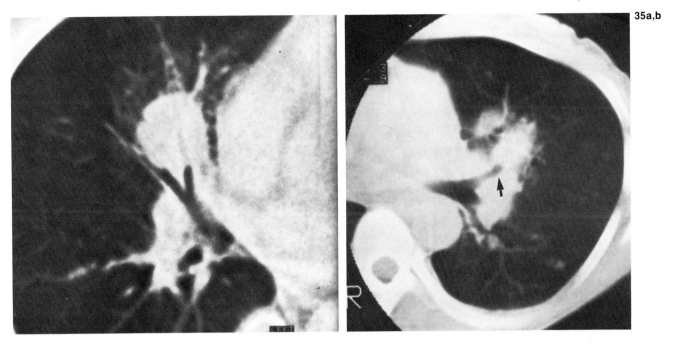

FIG. 35. Peripheral bronchogenic carcinoma. **a:** A large, irregular and spiculated mass is present in the middle lobe, deforming the medial border of the lateral segmental bronchus and displacing inferiorly the medial segmental bronchus. Endoscopic biosy showed adenocarcinoma. **b:** Section through the origin of the lingular bronchus *(arrow)* A lobulated tumor mass is present just beyond the lingular origin. Biopsy showed small cell carcinoma.

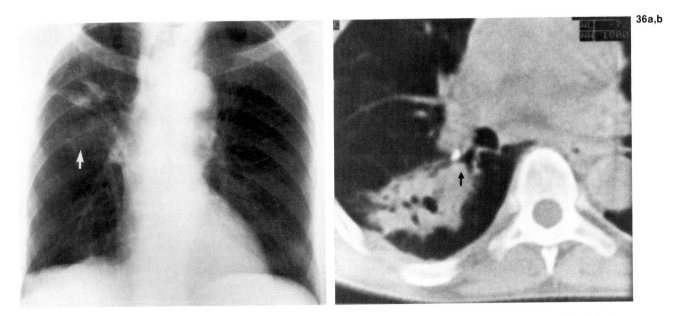

FIG. 36. Bronchogenic carcinoma. **a:** PA radiograph shows ill-defined mass–infiltrate in the superior segment of the right lower lobe *(arrow)*. **b:** Scan at the level of the origin of the superior segmental bronchus. Tumor involves and widens the spur at the first major bifurcation of the superior segmental bronchus *(arrow)*. Although patent, the subsegmental bronchi are splayed by tumor. Biopsy at this site showed squamous cell carcinoma.

37a,b

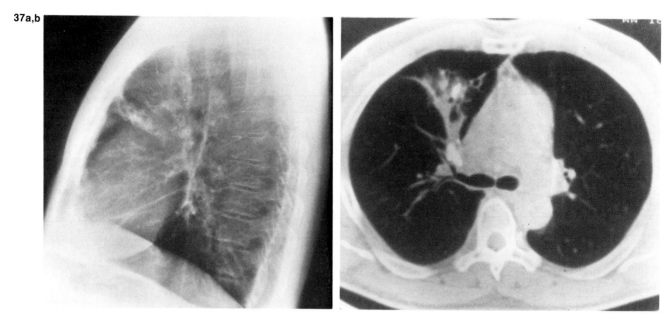

FIG. 37. Tuberculosis (calcified broncholith). **a:** Lateral radiograph shows an ill-defined infiltrate in the anterior segment of the right upper lobe, within which are ill-defined calcifications. Tumor cannot be excluded. **b:** Section at the level of the right upper lobe bronchus. The anterior segmental bronchus is patent. At the level of first bifurcation, the medial subsegmental bronchus is obliterated by an adjacent calcified lymph node. At bronchoscopy, this had eroded into the bronchus, causing obstruction.

38a,b

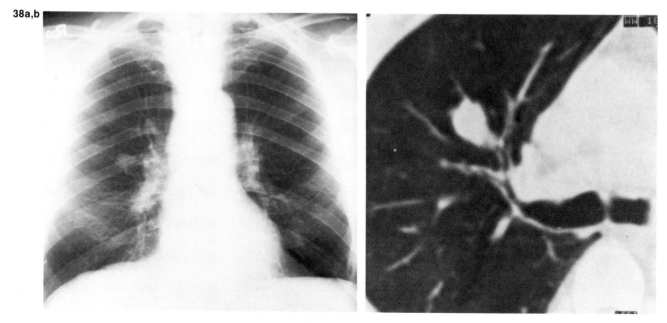

FIG. 38. Bronchogenic carcinoma (localization). **a:** PA radiograph. Mass is present in the right upper lobe. **b:** Section through the right upper lobe bronchus. Tumor mass can be seen adjacent to a fourth-order division of the right upper lobe bronchus. In this case, CT provided a roadmap for the bronchoscopist. Biopsy showed adenocarcinoma.

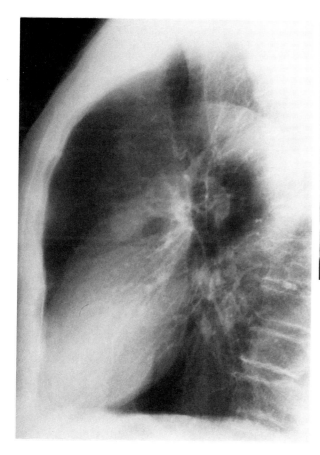

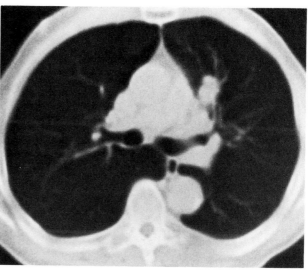

39a,b

FIG. 39. Bronchogenic carcinoma (localization). **a:** Lateral radiograph. A mass is present in the left upper lobe. This could not be accurately localized on the PA radiograph. **b:** Section through the left upper lobe bronchus. An irregular tumor mass is present in the medial portion of the left upper lobe in close proximity to the anterior segmental bronchus. Biopsy showed large cell undifferentiated carcinoma. It is apparent why this lesion was difficult to localize on the PA radiograph.

Alternatively, Fink et al. (17) have shown that in cases in which peripheral lesions are difficult to identify accurately with biplanar fluoroscopy, biopsy can be performed under CT guidance. Even in those cases in which the lesion is easily seen and localized fluoroscopically, CT may be useful in determining the exact site at which a biopsy should be performed. This is most significant in larger lesions in which considerable necrosis may be present. As shown by Pinstein et al. (18), contrast enhancement can disclose areas of viable tumor tissue distinct from areas of necrosis, thus establishing the best location for biopsy.

BRONCHIECTASIS

In addition to the evaluation of bronchial neoplasia, CT may be useful in defining inflammatory diseases of the bronchial wall, especially bronchiectasis.

Bronchiectasis is defined as generally localized, irreversible dilatation of the bronchial tree. The radiographic manifestations of bronchiectasis have been described (19). Typically, there is crowding and loss of definition of vascular markings in specif-

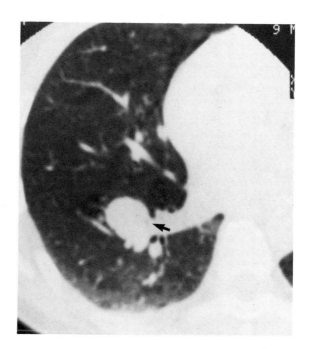

FIG. 40. Hamartoma (localization). Section through a well-defined tumor mass that at biopsy proved to be a hamartoma. The lesion lies behind the oblique fissure (confirming that it is in the lower lobe). The tumor is adjacent to and deforms the anterior basilar segmental bronchus (*arrow*).

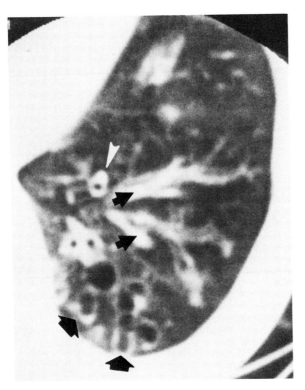

FIG. 41. Cylindrical and cystic bronchiectasis. Cylindrical bronchiectasis will appear as a "tramline" if the involved bronchi course horizontally in the plane of the CT scan *(narrow black arrows)*, and will appear to resemble a "signet ring" if the involved bronchus courses vertically *(white arrowhead)*. The signet-ring sign is caused by a pulmonary artery that runs alongside the bronchus. Cystic bronchiectasis can be identified in this section by its "string of pearls" appearance *(wide black arrows)*. This results when a bronchus with discrete foci of cystic bronchiectasis is sectioned along its length.

ic segments of lung, changes reflecting peribronchial fibrosis, and loss of volume. With more extensive disease, discrete cystic spaces can be defined, occasionally containing air–fluid levels. In its most severe form, bronchiectasis causes a "honeycomb" pattern. The honeycombing is caused by fibrosis and resultant emphysema, not by dilated bronchi.

Bronchiectasis has been classified by Reid (20) into three groups, depending on the severity of bronchial dilatation: cylindrical, in which the bronchi are dilated but retain regular outlines; varicose, in which the bronchi show a greater degree of dilatation and have irregular contours, and cystic, in which the bronchi have "ballooned" and are progressively more dilated toward the periphery.

Each type of bronchiectasis has a characteristic appearance on CT; however, the differentiation between various forms of bronchiectasis is less important than the simple identification of the disease process *per se* (21). Dilated bronchi with thickened walls and air-filled distended lumens are distinguishable in cross section from normal lung parenchyma. The key to the CT diagnosis of bronchiectasis is the recognition of distinct and characteristic patterns of abnormalities within the pulmonary parenchyma.

Cylindrical Bronchiectasis

Cylindrical bronchiectasis may be recognized by the finding of dilated, thick-walled bronchi extending toward the lung periphery. Using 10-mm-thick sections, bronchi are normally visualized only in the medial or proximal portions of the lung parenchyma. Peribronchial fibrosis, with resultant thickening of the bronchial wall and dilatation of the bronchial lumen, allows visualization of bronchi in more peripheral locations.

The appearance of cylindrically dilated bronchi will vary depending on whether the bronchi have a horizontal or vertical course. When horizontal, the bronchi are visualized along their length; they are recognizable as "tramlines." This pattern is illustrated in Fig. 41.

When cylindrically dilated bronchi course in a vertical direction, they are cut in cross section and appear as thick-walled, circular lucencies. Dis-

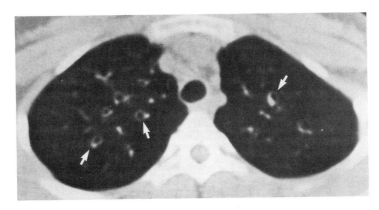

FIG. 42. Cylindrical bronchiectasis (cystic fibrosis). Cylindrical bronchiectasis involving a vertically oriented bronchus results in the "signet-ring" sign *(arrows)*.

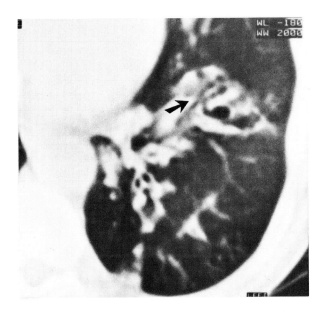

FIG. 43. Varicose bronchiectasis. Varicose bronchiectasis results in the involved bronchus having a beaded appearance. This can be identified for certain only if the involved bronchus has a horizontal course *(arrow)*.

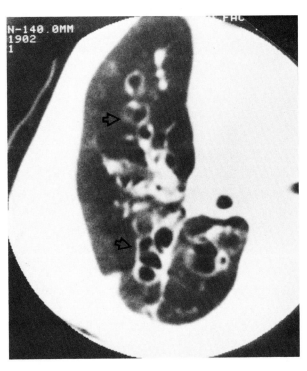

FIG. 45. Cystic bronchiectasis. Several dilated bronchi can be identified in both the middle and lower lobes, aligned in a linear fashion and resembling a string of pearls *(arrows)*.

tended bronchi can be differentiated from emphysematous blebs in two ways. First, blebs generally have no definable wall thickness. Second, and more characteristically, bronchi, even in the lung periphery, are accompanied by branches of the pulmonary artery. When cut in cross section, the result is a "signet ring" pattern. Examples of this pattern are illustrated in Figs. 41 and 42.

Varicose Bronchiectasis

Varicose bronchiectasis is essentially similar in appearance to cylindrical bronchiectasis, the chief difference being that with varicose bronchiectasis the walls of the bronchi assume a beaded appear-

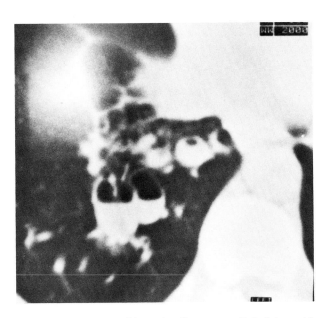

FIG. 44. Cystic bronchiectasis. Numerous dilated bronchi with air–fluid levels can be identified in the right lower lobe. Normally, bronchi cannot be seen this far peripherally.

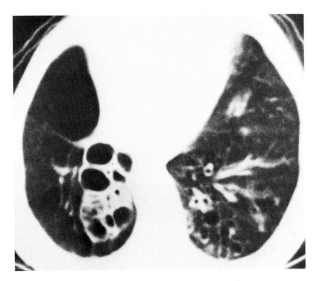

FIG. 46. Cystic bronchiectasis. Section through the right lower lobe. (Note: Fig. 41 is an enlargement of the left lower lobe shown in this section.) Numerous, dilated bronchi are grouped together in the right lower lobe; the appearance resembles a "cluster of grapes."

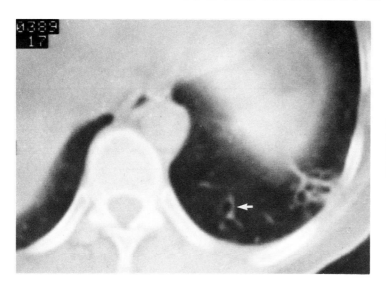

FIG. 47. Cystic bronchiectasis. Subtle, focal bronchiectatic changes can be seen in the peripheral portions of the left lower lobe. Notice the juxtaposition of one isolated, cystically dilated bronchus and its accompanying vessel *(arrow)*.

ance. Varicose bronchiectasis is easiest to identify when the involved bronchi course horizontally, as illustrated in Fig. 43.

Cystic Bronchiectasis

Cystic bronchiectasis may be most reliably recognized by the following patterns:

(a) Air–fluid levels. Retained secretions in the dependent portions of dilated bronchi are a very specific sign of cystic bronchiectasis. An example is illustrated in Fig. 44.

(b) Strings of cysts. The presence of a patent bronchus with consecutive areas of cystic dilatation leads to the production of a linear array or string of cysts if the bronchus courses horizontally within the scanning plane. The greater the length of bron-

chus visualized on one section, the longer is the string of cysts. Strings, however, need not be lengthy to be diagnostic of cystic bronchiectasis (Figs. 41 and 45).

(c) Clusters of cysts. In more severe cases, dilated bronchi can be found grouped together. The appearance suggests a cluster of grapes, as shown in Fig. 46. Recognition of some combination of dilated bronchi, air–fluid levels, and strings and clusters of cysts should be diagnostic of cystic bronchiectasis. More than one pattern may be present, often on a single section (Fig. 41). Varicose and cylindrical bronchiectasis may be present as well. It should be emphasized that the findings on CT of bronchiectasis may be quite focal and exceedingly subtle. Reliance on the patterns described above should lead to accurate diagnosis (Fig. 47).

48a,b

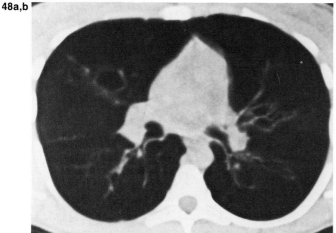 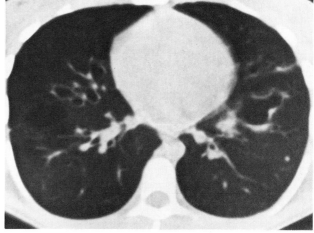

FIG. 48. Allergic bronchopulmonary aspergillosis. **a,b:** Sections through the mid- and lower thorax, respectively, show central bronchiectasis typical of this disease.

Certain patterns of bronchiectasis are sufficiently characteristic to suggest a specific diagnosis. For example, central bronchiectasis is a frequent finding in patients with allergic bronchopulmonary aspergillosis (Fig. 48).

There are other patterns of bronchiectasis that warrant special mention so that errors in diagnosis can be avoided. While retained secretions give rise to characteristic air–fluid levels, occasionally the entire bronchial lumen may become filled with fluid. This may resemble superficially intrapulmonary nodules (Fig. 49). The key to accurate diagnosis in these cases is recognition of the unusual, frequently linear distribution of these "pseudo-masses," as well as recognition in other parts of the lung of characteristic patterns of bronchiectasis.

A more important caveat in the diagnosis of bronchiectasis is illustrated in Fig. 50, which is an enlargement of a section through the left lower lobe in a patient with pneumonia. Numerous dilated bronchi can be identified, similar in appearance to the dilated bronchi shown in Figs. 41 and 45. The diagnosis of bronchiectasis implies irreversible dilatation. Bronchi will become dilated when there is airspace consolidation, yet, unlike true bronchiectasis, once this consolidation has cleared, the bronchi return to normal size. This appearance has been termed "reversible bronchiectasis." It overemphasizes that bronchiectasis cannot be diagnosed accurately in the face of parenchymal consolidation. In specific cases in which the diagnosis is questioned, repeat scans should be obtained after treatment. In the case illustrated in Fig. 50, a follow-up scan after therapy showed no evidence of residual bronchial dilatation.

SUMMARY

The bronchi serve as constant anatomic landmarks. Air within the bronchial lumen serves as a perfect contrast agent, allowing visualization of the central airways in virtually every case. Additionally, as seen in cross section, each bronchus has a typical and unique configuration, further aiding identification. Our approach has been to stress characteristic levels. In fact, once these are learned, any section through any portion of the bronchial tree should be immediately identifiable.

If CT is primarily an anatomic imaging modality, then anatomic orientation in three dimensions is one of the most important goals in learning to interpret abnormalities. This is most easily achieved by reference to the bronchial tree. Traditionally, anatomic orientation has centered around mediastinal structures. This is unsatisfactory because the appearance and relationships of the aortic arch and great vessels provide little, if any, orientation to the remainder of the thorax.

Conceptually and anatomically, the bronchi and pulmonary vessels are the nexus between the mediastinum, the hila, and the pulmonary parenchyma. Of these, the bronchi are easiest to visualize and identify, having the most characteristic configurations. The notion that the airways are the central or core structures of the thorax is easiest to appreciate visually (22). As shown in Fig. 51 (an example of a patient with extensive neurofibromatosis), anatomically, the airways represent a major "pathway" between the mediastinum, the hila, and the pulmonary

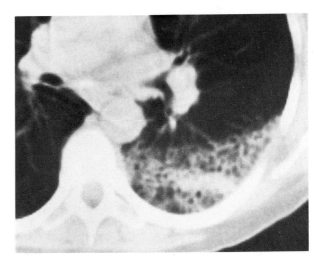

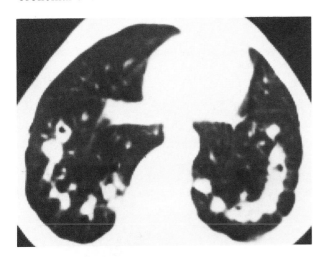

FIG. 49. Cystic bronchiectasis. Innumerable "nodular" densities can be identified in both lower lobes, superficially resembling pulmonary nodules. This may occur if cystically dilated bronchi are entirely filled with fluid.

FIG. 50. Reversible bronchiectasis. Section through the left lower lobe shows numerous dilated bronchi in an area of parenchymal consolidation. Following appropriate antibiotic therapy, a repeat scan was entirely normal. Bronchiectasis cannot be diagnosed with certainty in the presence of parenchymal consolidation.

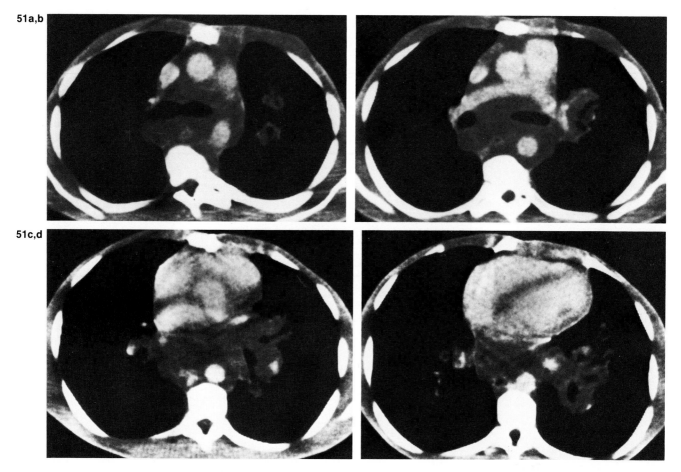

FIG. 51. Neurofibromatosis. **a–d:** Sequential images in a patient with diffuse neurofibromatosis that has infiltrated and distorted the mediastinum. Note that tumor extends in a continuous sheet from the mediastinum to involve the hila (especially on the left side) and then the pulmonary parenchyma in the vicinity of the lobar bronchi. In this case, the airways can be conceptualized as unifying structures, serving as a pathway from the mediastinum to the pulmonary parenchyma.

parenchyma, serving to unite these otherwise disparate anatomic units.

Because of the critical role the airways play in conceptually unifying the thorax, emphasis has been placed in this chapter on the normal cross-sectional appearance of the airways, as well as on characteristic patterns of abnormalities.

The protean significance of the airways in interpreting thoracic pathology is best illustrated by analysis of bronchial neoplasia. Lung cancer directly or indirectly affects the airways of the mediastinum, hila, and the pulmonary parenchyma, and thus serves to conceptually unify the entire thorax. Endobronchial and peribronchial lesions are easily identified because they distort the bronchial tree. Such lesions can be identified peripherally (Figs. 32, 35, 36, 38, 39, and 40) or centrally (Figs. 26, 27, 29, 31, 33, and 34). They may appear as areas of pulmonary consolidation and/or collapse (Figs. 29 and 30) or they may cause focal emphysema (Fig.

28). Occasionally, endobronchial obstruction may cause no appreciable parenchymal changes at all, even when obstruction is total (see Fig. 1 in Chapter 5). Despite this wide variability of presentation, involving pathology in the mediastinum, hila, and pulmonary parenchyma, the airways (including the trachea and carina) serve as the point of departure for accurate interpretation.

This unifying principle of the airways also has therapeutic applications. As previously discussed, CT may be used to determine the best diagnostic approach to parenchymal lesions (Figs. 30, 32, 35, and 36–40). Central endobronchial lesions may also be defined, even when not apparent or unsuspected on plain radiographs (Figs. 26, 27, 29, 31, 33, and 34).

Recent attention has focused on the use of transtracheal and transbronchial needle aspiration biopsy using a standard bronchoscope and a retractable needle in a catheter to assess patients with mediasti-

52a,b

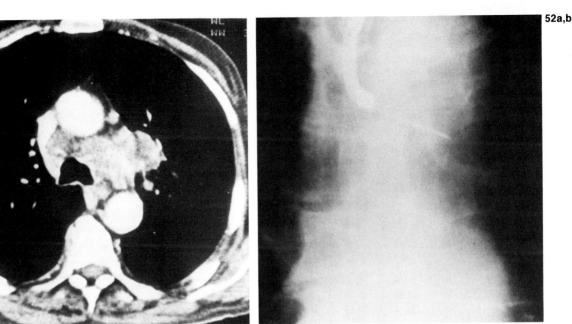

FIG. 52. CT-guided transbronchial needle aspiration and biopsy. **a:** CT section shows extensive adenopathy in the aorticopulmonary window. No endobronchial tumor is present. **b:** PA radiograph obtained at bronchoscopy. The bronchoscope is present in the left main-stem bronchus. The exact position of the transbronchial aspirating needle can be seen, with the tip in the region of the aorticopulmonary window. The exact position for this biopsy was determined by the CT scan. Aspiration yielded small cell carcinoma.

nal disease. There is a significant number of patients with bronchogenic carcinoma in whom the main or only finding is mediastinal disease, frequently paratracheal and/or peribronchial in location. Wang et al. (23) have shown that pre- and paratracheal masses, including nodes in the aorticopulmonary window, and subcarinal nodes and masses may be accurately biopsied with this technique. Even in the absence of an endobronchial component to these lesions, the airways still serve as points of anatomic orientation. Other lesions within the mediastinum and hilum are also accessible with this technique, including mediastinal abscesses. An example of the role of CT in determining accessibility of disease for transtracheal and transbronchial needle aspiration is shown in Fig. 52.

The full potential of CT for evaluating the airways has not yet been realized. While a large variety of disease processes affecting the airways in all compartments of the thorax may be identified, as illustrated throughout this chapter, much work remains to be done in determining the limits to which bronchial and peribronchial disease may be defined. Most significant for future developments is the use of CT in the early diagnosis of bronchogenic carcinoma. In this regard, the development of some type of inhalational contrast medium to detect peripheral airway disease would be most useful.

REFERENCES

1. Naidich DP, Terry, PB, Stitik, FP, and Siegelman SS. Computed tomography of the bronchi. 1. Normal anatomy. *J. Comput Assist Tomogr* 4:746–753, 1980
2. Naidich DP, Stitik FP, Khouri NF, Terry PB, Siegelman SS. Computed tomography of the bronchi. 2. Pathology. *J Comput Assist Tomogr* 4:754–762, 1980
3. Naidich DP, Khouri NF, Scott WW, Wang KP, Siegelman SS. Computed tomography of the pulmonary hila. 1. Normal anatomy. *J Comput Assist Tomogr* 5:459–467, 1981
4. Naidich DP, Khouri NF, Stitik FP, McCauley DI, Siegelman SS. Computed tomography of the pulmonary hila. 2. Abnormal anatomy. *J Comput Assist Tomogr* 5:468–475, 1981
5. Webb WR, Glazer G, Gamsu G. Computed tomography of the normal pulmonary hilum. *J Comput Assist Tomogr* 5:476–484, 1981
6. Webb WR, Gamsu G, Glazer G. Computed tomography of the abnormal pulmonary hilum. *J Comput Assist Tomogr* 5:485–490, 1981
7. Osbourne D, Vock P, Godwin D, Korobkin M. Computed tomographic evaluation of the normal lung. Paper presented at the 68th Scientific Assembly and Annual Meeting of the Radiological Society of North America, November 28–December 3, 1982
8. Landay M. Azygos vein abutting the posterior wall of the right main and upper lobe bronchi: A normal CT variant. *AJR* 140:461–462, 1983
9. Felson B. *Chest Roentgenology*. Philadelphia, W.B. Saunders, 1973
10. Webb WR, Gamsu G. Computed tomography of the left retrobronchial stripe. *J Comput Assist Tomogr* 7:65–69, 1983
11. Borman N. Broncho-pulmonary segmental anatomy and bronchography. *Minn Med* 41:820–830, 1958
12. Spencer H. *Pathology of the Lung, Excluding Pulmonary Tuberculosis* 2nd ed. Oxford, Pergamon Press, 1968

13. Turnbull AD, Huvos AG, Goodner JT, Beattie EJ. The malignant potential of bronchial adenoma. *Ann Thorac Surg* 14:453–464, 1972

14. Naidich DP, McCauley DI, Siegelman SS. Computed tomography of bronchial adenoma. *J Comput Assist Tomogr* 6:725–782, 1982

15. Boyd AD, Spencer FC, Lind AL. Why has bronchial resection and anastomosis been reported infrequently for treatment of bronchial adenoma? *J Thorac Cardiovasc Surg* 59:359–365, 1970

16. Jensik RJ, Faber LP, Brown CM, Kittle CF. Bronchial adenoma. *J Thorac Cardiovasc Surg* 68:556–565, 1974

17. Fink I, Gamsu G, Harter L. CT-guided aspiration biopsy of the thorax. *J Comput Assist Tomogr* 6:958–962, 1982

18. Pinstein ML, Scott RL, Salazaar J. Avoidance of negative percutaneous lung biopsy using contrast-enhanced CT. *AJR* 140: 265–267, 1983

19. Gudbjerg CE. Roentgenologic diagnosis of bronchiectasis. An analysis of 112 cases. *Acta Radiol (Stockh)* 43:209, 1955

20. Reid LM. Reduction in bronchial subdivision in bronchiectasis. *Thorax* 5:233–236, 1950

21. Naidich DP, McCauley DI, Khouri NF, Stitik FP, Siegelman SS. Computed tomography of bronchiectasis. *J Comput Assist Tomogr* 6:437–444, 1982

22. Ross CR, McCauley DI, Naidich DP. Clinical images: Intrathoracic neurofibroma of the vagus nerve associated with bronchial obstruction. *J Comput Assist Tomogr* 6:406–412, 1982

23. Wang KP, Terry P, Marsh B. Bronchoscopic needle aspiration biopsy of paratracheal tumors. *Am Rev Resp Dis* 118:17–21, 1978

Chapter 5

Lobar Collapse

The radiographic patterns of lobar collapse have been extensively reviewed (1–9). A wide range of abnormalities has been described, characterizing the appearance of the collapsed lobe as well as secondary, compensatory changes, including shifts or changes of position of mediastinal structures, the hila, the hemidiaphragms, and the fissures.

Computed tomography is a useful adjunct to routine radiography in the evaluation of lobar collapse (10–13). This is because CT allows unobstructed cross-sectional visualization of thoracic anatomy. Not only can the affected lobe and involved airways be evaluated, but changes involving the mediastinum, chest wall, hilum, pleura, and adjacent lung can be appreciated as well.

The purpose of this chapter will be to review the basic patterns of lobar collapse, with specific emphasis on the underlying pathophysiology. It is only through an understanding of the mechanics of collapse that cross-sectional images can be interpreted properly.

GENERAL PRINCIPLES AND METHODOLOGY

Obviously, accurate interpretation of the cross-sectional appearance of lobar collapse necessitates thorough knowledge of normal CT anatomy, especially bronchial anatomy. CT can accurately identify and localize the presence of an obstructing bronchial lesion. Even in the absence of bronchial obstruction, alterations in the normal appearance of the bronchi are to be expected consequent to volume loss in the affected lobe and resultant change in the position of normal bronchi. While these changes

may be appreciated on routine radiographs, they are far more apparent with CT.

Proper technique for evaluating the airways has been described in detail in Chapter 4. Correlation with appropriate radiographs is mandatory to define which bronchi need to be closely evaluated. Initially, 10-mm sections every 10 mm are obtained and should be reviewed while the CT exam is in progress. Additional, thinly collimated sections (5-mm-thick sections are generally adequate) should then be obtained through the regions of greatest interest, i.e., the pertinent lobar and/or segmental bronchi. This ensures accurate delineation of the presence or confirmation of the absence of pathology.

Use of intravenous contrast medium is reserved for those cases in which further anatomic detail is required. This is especially important in evaluating the presence and extent of central tumor masses, and occasionally is helpful in evaluating pleural disease. Additionally, intravenous contrast medium is of value in analyzing the mediastinum, although in a surprising number of cases adequate delineation of mediastinal disease is possible without the use of contrast agents.

Lobar collapse may be caused by one of four mechanisms: endobronchial obstruction; passive atelectasis (collapse caused by extrinsic pressure, either from air, fluid, or both in the pleural space); cicatrization; and more rarely, adhesions, such as may be caused by radiation with resultant loss of surfactant (14). Each of these mechanisms results in a distinctive radiographic pattern, and is easily assessed with CT.

111

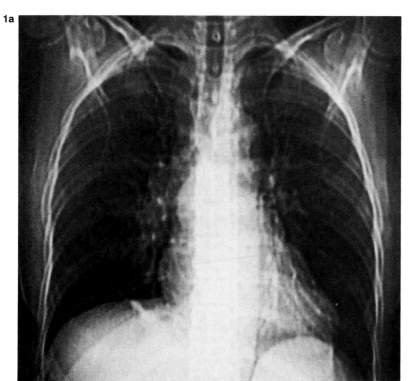

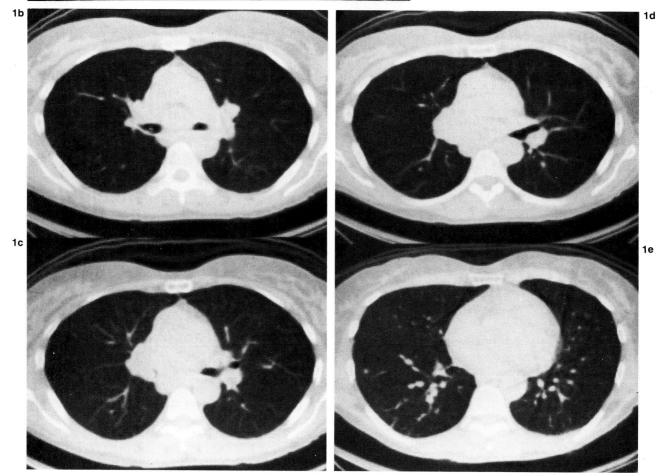

FIG. 1. Endobronchial obstruction: Metastatic renal cell carcinoma. **a:** Scanogram. A nodular density is present in the right lower lobe. A subcarinal mass is present as well. There is no evidence of volume loss on the right side. **b–e:** Sequential images through the right upper lobe bronchus, bronchus intermedius, right lower lobe bronchus and right lower lobe. A small density can be seen within the lumen of the right upper lobe bronchus. The bronchus intermedius is obliterated. Despite this, there is normal aeration of the middle and right lower lobes. Total obstruction was confirmed bronchoscopically.

ENDOBRONCHIAL OBSTRUCTION

Endobronchial obstruction causes a spectrum of radiographic changes, reflecting both the nature and extent of the disease process within the affected lobe, as well as compensatory changes involving the adjacent lung, the mediastinum, the diaphragm, and the chest wall. Lobar collapse due to endo-bronchial occlusion should thus be viewed as a dynamic process accounting for a wide variability of radiographic appearances.

Bronchial obstruction usually causes increased density within the affected lobe, secondary to the presence of intra-alveolar fluid. How much fluid is present within the obstructed lung is generally a function of both the degree of obstruction and time.

Occasionally, in the presence of endobronchial obstruction, the affected lobe may contain air and appear relatively normal in density. In this situation, obstruction may be difficult to detect (Fig. 1). In the presence of total bronchial obstruction, distal lung may appear normally aerated if there is sufficient collateral air-drift. This may occur between various portions of a single lobe, or, as illustrated in Fig. 1, between lobes, presumably as a function of incompletely formed fissures.

Despite great variability, lobar collapse secondary to endobronchial obstruction forms a discrete and easily definable subset, the characteristic appearance of which will be described (see Table 1).

Right Upper Lobe Collapse

The right upper lobe is bordered medially by the mediastinum, superiorly by the chest wall, inferiorly by the minor fissure, and posteroinferiorly by the superior portion of the oblique fissure. When collapsed, the right upper lobe progressively pancakes against the mediastinum, maintaining its connection to the hilum by a tongue of tissue that has been referred to as the mediastinal wedge (Fig. 2).

The lower and middle lobes both become hyper-aerated in compensation; this results in upward displacement of the minor fissure and anterior displacement of the upper portion of the oblique fissure. As the right upper lobe collapses toward the midline, the middle lobe (especially the lateral segment) insinuates itself laterally between the chest wall and the lateral portion of the collapsing right upper lobe. With hyperaeration and expansion, the pulmonary vessels within the middle and lower lobes will appear abnormally spaced. Ancillary

TABLE 1. *CT of lobar collapse: primary changes*

Segmental bronchi are variable in appearance. Endobronchial tumor causes irregular narrowing and/or occlusion; patent bronchi may be established with other forms of lobar collapse.

With collapse, the involved lobe becomes pie-shaped rather than hemispherical in cross section.

The proximal portion of the lobe assumes a V-shape, with the apex situated at the origin of the affected bronchus.

There is an overall increase in the density of the lobe. Endobronchial obstruction, over time, produces an airless lobe with soft-tissue density. Lucency within collapsed lobes is generally secondary to extensive bronchiectasis, such as is seen with cicatrization atelectasis.

Large tumor masses produce a bulge in the contour of the collapsed lobe (S-sign of Golden), and may be identified separately from the remainder of the collapsed lobe following a bolus of i.v. contrast medium.

Loss of volume results in a reduced zone of contact between the pleural surface of the lobe and the chest wall.

Partial fixation of the lobe by prior pleural adhesions may affect the pattern of collapse, as will fluid and/or air in the pleural space, in which case the affected lobe may be displaced from the chest wall or mediastinum.

An entire lobe may be replaced by tumor; this gives a lobular rather than wedge-shaped appearance to the collapsed lobe in the absence of endobronchial occlusion.

changes, such as shift to the right of the trachea and mediastinum and elevation of the right hemi-diaphragm, may occur, but are more variable.

This sequence of events is readily identifiable with CT. As illustrated in Fig. 2, the collapsed right upper lobe appears as a wedge of soft-tissue density extending alongside the mediastinum to the anterior chest wall. Hyperaerated middle and lower lobes can be differentiated by identification of the oblique fissure, which marginates the posterior border of the collapsed right upper lobe. Separation of vessels within the hyperaerated middle and lower lobes is easy to appreciate by comparison with the normal, contralateral lung. As the right upper lobe retracts from the lateral chest wall, the apex of the lobe remains affixed to the hilum.

Endobronchial obstruction is readily identifiable with CT. In the case illustrated in Fig. 2, a polypoid mass occludes the origin of the right upper lobe bronchus and prolapses into the right main-stem bonchus and proximal portion of the bronchus intermedius, causing partial occlusion. Unfortunately, there is little specificity in the appearance of most endobronchial lesions. Primary bronchogenic carcinoma, bronchial adenomas, endobronchial metastases, and even lymphoma may be indistinguishable. Accurate histologic diagnosis requires biopsy.

2a,b

2c,d

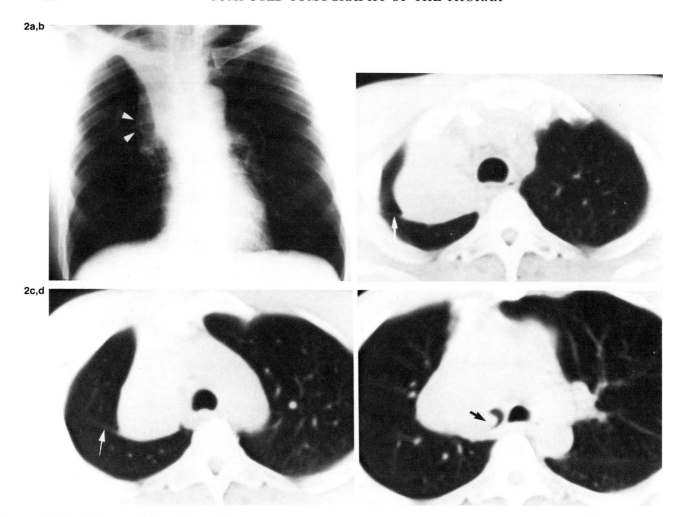

FIG. 2. Right upper lobe collapse: Adenocarcinoma. **a:** PA radiograph shows right upper lobe collapse. The line that is convex medially represents the elevated middle lobe fissure; the line that is convex laterally represents tumor mass (*arrowheads*). **b–d:** Sequential images through the mid- and lower trachea and the right upper lobe bronchus. The collapsed right upper lobe can be identified as a wedge of uniform density extending along the mediastinum to the anterior chest wall. There is hyperinflation of the middle and lower lobes, which can be clearly separated by identification of the lateral margin of the oblique fissure (*arrows* in (b) and (c)). The middle lobe is insinuated between the collapsed upper lobe medially and the lateral chest wall. A large polypoid lesion obstructs the origin of the right upper lobe bronchus (*arrows* in (d)). Notice that there is convex bulging of the contour of the collapsed upper lobe laterally, which becomes more pronounced as sections are taken closer to the right upper lobe bronchus. This bulge is caused by central tumor mass and accounts for the S-shaped configuration of the collapsed right upper lobe scan on the PA radiograph.

In the absence of a large, proximally obstructing lesion, the collapsed right upper lobe should taper relatively smoothly into the hilum. When central tumor mass is present, the lateral border of the collapsed lobe widens centrally, having a convex border directed laterally, as shown in Fig. 2. This is the CT counterpart of the radiologic "S-sign of Golden," and may be seen on CT with collapse of any lobe that is caused by central tumor (15). With right upper lobe collapse, the concave line seen on PA films is caused by upward displacement of the minor fissure; the convex line is caused by tumor (Fig. 3). Identification of central tumor mass is facilitated by use of a bolus of i.v. contrast medium. As

shown in Fig. 3, following contrast medium administration, the borders of a central tumor can be distinguished from the remainder of the collapsed lobe, as well as from the mediastinum.

In addition to the changes already mentioned, right upper lobe collapse may result in a rearrangement of bronchial anatomy (Fig. 4). Such changes may be difficult to detect with routine films. Rotation of the carina, such as may occur in right upper lobe collapse, probably reflects the fact that, unlike the left upper lobe bronchus which is anchored superiorly by the left main pulmonary artery, the right upper lobe bronchus is more freely able to change position.

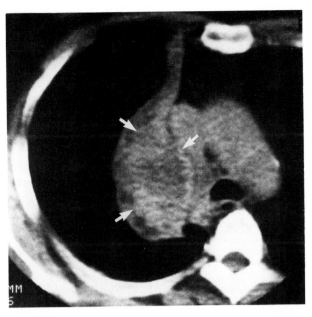

FIG. 3. Right upper lobe collapse: Adenocarcinoma. Section through a collapsed right upper lobe following an i.v. bolus of contrast medium. Tumor mass can be defined separate from the remainder of the collapsed lobe as well as from the mediastinum *(arrows)*. This pattern of central convexity may be seen with collapse of any lobe if it is caused by a central tumor.

The findings on CT in right upper lobe collapse are summarized in Tables 1 and 2.

Left Upper Lobe Collapse

The left upper lobe is bounded medially by the mediastinum and more inferiorly by the left heart border, superiorly and laterally by the chest wall,

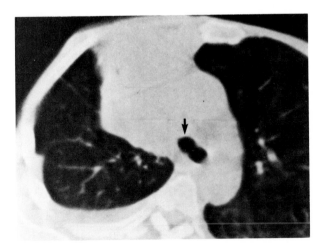

FIG. 4. Right upper lobe collapse: Squamous cell carcinoma. Section at the level of the carina shows that the right mainstem bronchus has rotated anteriorly *(arrow)*. Right upper lobe collapse is apparent (compare with Fig. 2).

TABLE 2. *CT of lobar collapse: specific findings*

Right upper lobe
  Posterior margin of the collapsed lobe (the major fissure) is displaced anteromedially.
  Medial margin of collapsed lobe abuts the mediastinum.
  Anterior margin of collapsed lobe consists of a reduced zone of pleural contact.

Left upper lobe
  Posterior margin of collapsed lobe (the major fissure) is displaced anteromedially.
  Medial margin of collapsed lobe approaches the mediastinum, but frequently makes incomplete contact because of intrusion of overexpanded superior segment of left lower lobe.

Middle lobe collapse
  Medial margin of lobe abuts the right heart border.
  Posterior margin of collapsed lobe is displaced anteromedially.
  Compensatory changes are less marked because of small volume of middle lobe.

Lower lobe collapse
  Medial margin makes contact with the mediastinum inferiorly.
  The anterior margin (the major fissure) is displaced posteromedially.
  Contact between the collapsed lobe and the medial portion of the diaphragm is maintained, probably as a result of the inferior pulmonary ligament.

and posteriorly by the major fissure. With collapse, the left upper lobe moves anterosuperiorly. Unlike the right upper lobe, which collapses against the mediastinun along its entire length, the left upper lobe generally retains more contact with the anterior and lateral chest wall as it collapses. Superiorly, the left upper lobe may be displaced from the mediastinum by the hyperaerated left lower lobe. This accounts for the frequent finding of peri-aortic lucency on PA radiographs following left upper lobe collapse (Fig. 5). Inferiorly, the left upper lobe, like the right upper lobe, marginates the mediastinum and is connected to the left hilum by a wedge of collapsed tissue.

Superiorly, the collapsed upper lobe has a wedge-shaped, triangular configuration, with the apex pointing posteriorly. This configuration is caused by the general anterosuperior direction of collapse; the broad base of the triangular collapsed lobe retains its connection to the anterior chest wall. Hyperinflation of the left lower lobe and right lung (which crosses the midline) is somewhat greater than that seen in right upper lobe collapse, probably because the left upper lobe has a much greater volume. Superiorly, hyperaerated left lower lobe insinuates between the aorta and mediastinum medially and the collapsed upper lobe laterally.

Depending on the degree of collapse, the left hilum will become elevated. The degree of elevation of the left hilum, and subsequent rotation of the left bronchial tree, is of less magnitude on the left side,

5a,b

5c,d

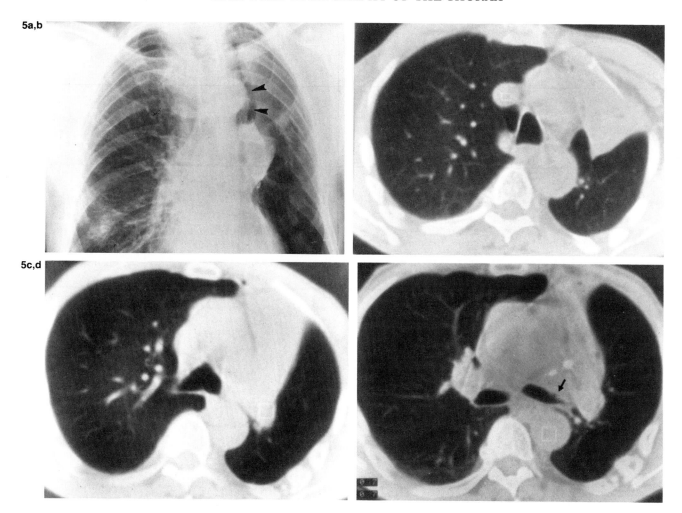

FIG. 5. Left upper lobe collapse: Squamous cell carcinoma. **a:** PA radiograph. There is a mass in the left hilum. Peri-aortic lucency can be seen (*arrows*). **b:** Section at the level of the great vessels shows the classic appearance of left upper lobe atelectasis. The collapsed left upper lobe forms a sharply defined triangular density, with the apex pointing posteriorly. The hyperinflated left lower lobe lies between the collapsed upper lobe and the aorta. **c:** Section through the carina. The atelectatic left upper lobe forms a sharply defined soft-tissue wedge adjacent to the ascending aorta and left main pulmonary artery. **d:** Section through the left upper lobe bronchus. The left upper lobe bronchus tapers to a point (*arrow*) laterally, due to a squamous cell carcinoma that has infiltrated submucosally.

compared with changes accompanying right upper lobe collapse, because the left upper lobe bronchus is "anchored" by the left pulmonary artery superiorly. As shown in Fig. 5, despite considerable volume loss in the left upper lobe, the left upper lobe bronchus has undergone little elevation or rotation.

Endobronchial obstruction is easily defined with CT (Fig. 5d). Tumor infiltration frequently results in irregular tapering of the distal portion of the left upper lobe bronchus. Care must be taken to confirm this appearance as abnormal with sequential, thin sections. The left upper lobe bronchus normally may have a tapered appearance if sections are obtained at the level at which the left main pulmonary artery courses over the left upper lobe bronchus (see Fig. 9b in Chapter 4).

The triangular, wedge-shaped configuration of

the collapsed left upper lobe is generally a result of considerable volume loss. Acutely, the degree of volume loss within the left upper lobe may be minimal, in which case the posterior margin of the collapsed lobe may appear convex posteriorly (Fig. 6). Such an appearance of an expanded lobe following endobronchial obstruction has been referred to as "drowned lung."

Collapse may be associated with a large hilar mass, as well as with extensive mediastinal disease. The separation of these components may be possible with CT (Fig. 7). Differentiation between the collapsed lung and masses in the hilum and mediastinum depends on identification of the characteristic triangular configuration of the collapsed left upper lobe.

While lesions involving the left upper lobe bron-

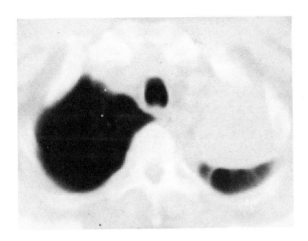

FIG. 6. Left upper lobe collapse: Drowned lung. Section through the left lung apex. The posterior aspect of the left upper lobe has a convex margin directed posteriorly (compare with Fig. 5b; in this case, the left upper lobe is expanded by intralobar fluid).

chus generally cause collapse of the whole lobe, occasionally, collapse is more pronounced in one of the segments of the left upper lobe. As illustrated in Fig. 8, despite total occlusion of the left upper lobe bronchus, volume loss is most marked in the lingula. This portion of the left upper lobe collapses against the left heart border, causing marked anteromedial displacement of the major fissure. Presumably, volume differential to this degree between different segments of a lobe implies prior segmental obstruction.

The findings on CT in left upper lobe collapse are reviewed in Tables 1 and 2.

Middle Lobe Collapse

The middle lobe is bounded medially by the right heart border, anteriorly and laterally by the chest wall, posteriorly by the major fissure, and superiorly by the minor fissure. As the middle lobe collapses, the two fissures begin to approximate one another; that is, there is downward shift of the minor fissure and forward displacement of the oblique fissure. The major fissure is clearly seen with CT because the axis of this fissure is perpendicular to the plane of the scan (see Chapter 9). The minor fissure, parallel to the plane of the scan, is never as sharply defined. As the middle lobe loses volume, it collapses medially against the right heart border. This accounts for the silhouette sign on PA radiographs. The middle lobe normally has a triangular or wedge-shaped configuration; this becomes accentuated as the lobe collapses, with the apex of the triangle directed toward the hilum. Because of the relatively smaller volume of the middle lobe, compared with the other lobes, compensatory changes, such as shift of the mediastinum and hyperaeration of the remainder of the lung, tend to be less pronounced (Fig. 9).

Bronchial obstruction may be caused by endobronchial tumor; alternatively, peribronchial tumor and/or enlarged nodes may compress and obstruct bronchi. In both cases, the result is lobar collapse. These conditions may be difficult to differentiate by CT (Fig. 9).

The typical configuration of middle lobe collapse, as in any other form of lobar collapse, will be altered if adhesions form between the pleural surfaces. This may cause confusion, especially when seen on radiographs. CT may prove valuable in this circumstance, as illustrated in Fig. 10. As with other forms of collapse, the presence of central tumor will deform the contour of the collapsed lobe, causing an S-shaped configuration. Use of i.v. con-

7a,b

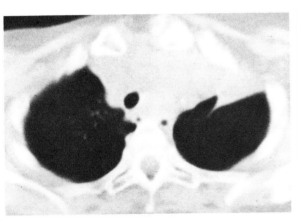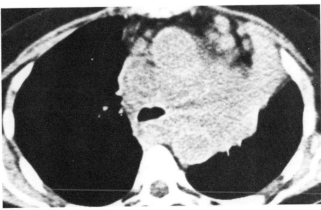

FIG. 7. Left upper lobe collapse: Small cell carcinoma. **a,b:** Sections through the mid-trachea and carina, imaged with wide and narrow windows, respectively. The collapsed left upper lobe can be identified by its characteristic wedge-shaped triangular configuration. Additionally, extensive mediastinal tumor is present, effacing the normal mediastinal fascial planes. Differentiation between collapse and tumor is facilitated by transverse imaging.

8a

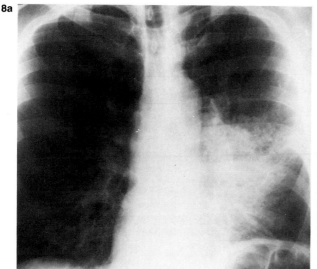

8b

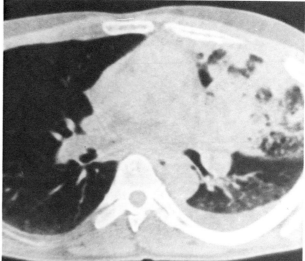

8c

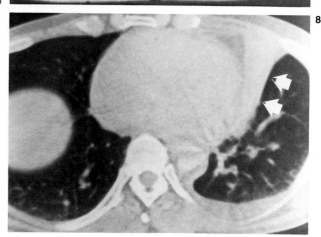

FIG. 8. Left upper lobe collapse: Large cell carcinoma. **a:** PA radiograph shows left upper lobe collapse. Increased density in the left lung is more apparent inferiorly. **b:** Section at the level of the left upper lobe spur. The left upper lobe bronchus is obliterated by tumor. Mass and infiltrate are present in the left upper lobe, sharply marginated posteriorly by the major fissure. At this level, volume loss is slight. **c:** Section through the lower thorax. The lingula is totally collapsed, identifiable as a wedge of uniformly increased density, marginating the left heart border and extending to the anterior chest wall. The major fissure has rotated anteromedially (*arrow*). In this case, obstruction of the lingular bronchus must have antedated obstruction of the left upper lobe bronchus.

trast medium may disclose the true extent of tumor (Fig. 10).

The findings on CT of middle lobe collapse are summarized in Tables 1 and 2.

Lower Lobe Collapse

The lower lobes should be considered together, since anatomically they appear identical in the collapsed state. The lower lobes are bordered inferiorly by the hemidiaphragms, posteriorly and laterally by the chest wall, medially by the heart and mediastinum, and anteriorly by the major fissure. The lower lobes collapse medially toward the mediastinum, generally maintaining contact with the hemidiaphragms. These changes reflect the attachments of the inferior pulmonary ligaments. Occasionally, the attachments between the lower lobes and the pulmonary ligaments are incomplete. In this case, collapse of the lower lobes may assume an unusual or rounded configuration. The major fis-

sure, especially the lateral portion, moves posteriorly. This accounts for the usually sharp line of the lateral portion of the collapsed lobe on PA radiographs (Fig. 11).

Figures 11a–d are sequential sections from a patient with left lower lobe collapse. The left upper lobe bronchus is narrowed and irregular; the left lower lobe bronchus is obliterated at the spur by tumor. The collapsed, airless lower lobe can be identified, displaced medially against the descending aorta and posterior mediastinum. The major fissure is displaced posteromedially, and there is hyperinflation of the left upper lobe. The lateral contour of the collapsed left lower lobe is convex (best seen in Figs. 11c and d).

Right lower lobe collapse mimics the appearance of left lower lobe collapse (Fig. 12). Collapse is generally posteromedial against the posterior mediastinum and spine. The lateral contour of the collapsed lobe is convex laterally when collapse is secondary to central tumor. Use of i.v. contrast medium accentuates this appearance by defining areas

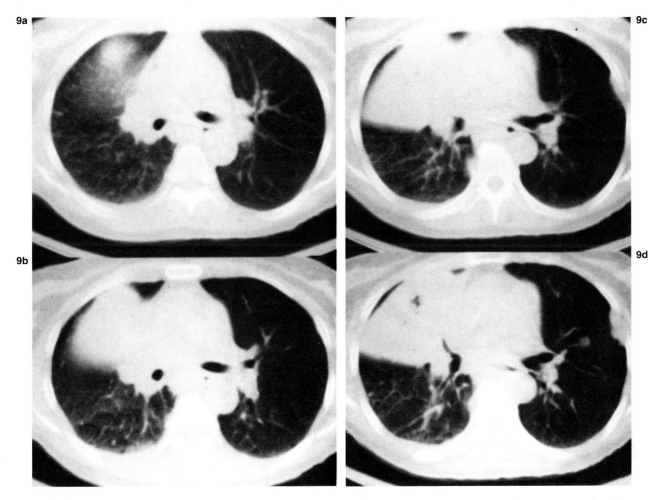

FIG. 9. Middle lobe collapse: Lymphoma. **a–d:** Sequential images through the bronchus intermedius and middle lobe bronchus. The origin and proximal portions of the middle lobe bronchus are patent. The middle lobe bronchus is narrowed extrinsically in a pattern suggestive of adenopathy (confirmed bronchoscopically). The middle lobe has a roughly triangular configuration, with the apex pointing toward the hilum. The posterior margin of the middle lobe is sharply demarcated because the major fissure lies perpendicular to the plane of the CT scan. The minor fissure, roughly parallel to the plane of the CT scan, is not so well-defined.

of tumor necrosis (Fig. 13). Occasionally, air-bronchograms may be identified within a collapsed lobe, even when not apparent on routine radiographs (Fig. 14). Their presence should not be assumed to be evidence of bronchial patency, either because central obstruction may be of recent onset or because endobronchial obstruction may not be complete. It is for this reason that careful scanning with thin sections through the origin and proximal portions of potentially abnormal bronchi is mandatory.

The findings on CT of lower lobe collapse are reviewed in Tables 1 and 2.

BENIGN VERSUS MALIGNANT BRONCHIAL OCCLUSION

Bronchial obstruction with resultant collapse may be caused by a variety of benign conditions, including bronchostenosis, congenital bronchial atresia, and trauma with bronchial laceration, among others. The findings on CT of obstruction secondary to an aspirated foreign body, as well as a broncholith, have been reported (16–18). It has recently been shown that CT can be used to differentiate between benign and malignant causes of bronchial obstruction (1,2). Occasional false positives will be encountered, although in our experience, this has been the exception (Fig. 15).

Perhaps the most important and most common benign cause of endobronchial obstruction is mucous plugs. These most frequently form when there is some interruption in the normal mechanism for clearing bronchial secretions, such as, for example, in the immediate postoperative period. Potentially, a mucus-filled bronchus can mimic an endobronchial lesion; in fact, the diagnosis of a mucous plug

10a

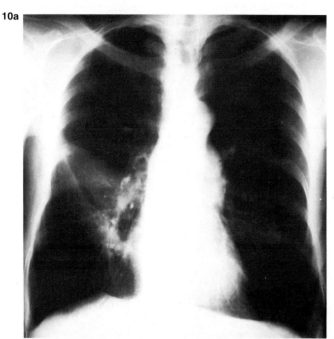

FIG. 10. Middle lobe collapse: Squamous cell carcinoma. **a:** PA radiograph showing unusual configuration of the middle lobe. **b:** Section through the origin of the middle and right lower lobe bronchi. The middle lobe bronchus is obstructed just past its origin. The middle lobe can be defined as an airless wedge extending from the hilum to the lateral chest wall, defined posteriorly by the right lower lobe and anteriorly by the hyper-inflated upper lobe. In this case, the unusual configuration of the middle lobe is due to lateral pleural adhesions causing fixation. **c:** Same section as in b, following administration of i.v. contrast medium, and imaged with a narrow window. The posterior bulge or convexity seen along the posteromedial aspect of the collapsed middle lobe is caused by a central tumor mass with necrosis.

10b,c

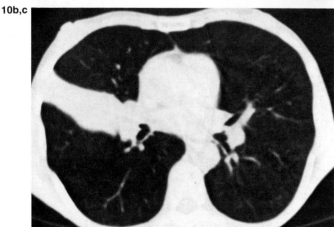
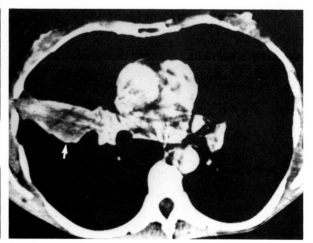

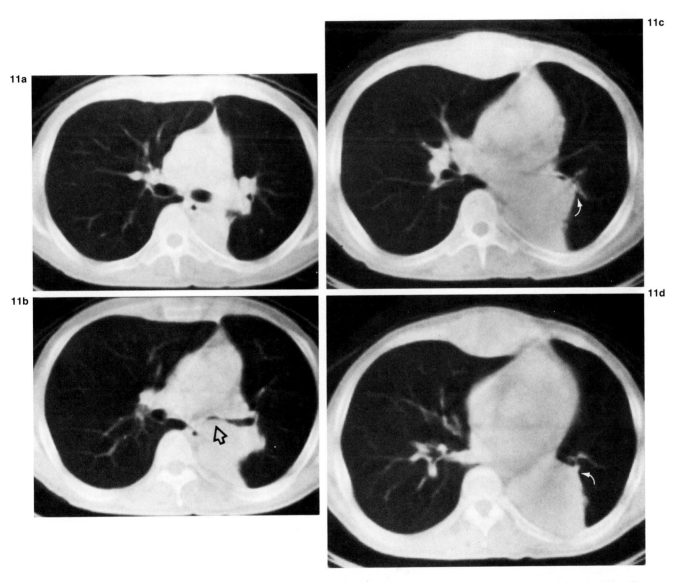

FIG. 11. Left lower lobe collapse: Squamous cell carcinoma. **a–d:** Sequential images through the collapsed left lower lobe. The left upper lobe bronchus is narrowed; there is occlusion of the left lower lobe bronchus at the level of the spur (*arrow* in b). The left lower lobe is airless and collapsed against the posterior mediastinum. The left upper lobe is hyperinflated, as is the right lung which crosses the midline anteriorly. There is a pronounced convexity in the lateral margin of the collapsed left lower lobe, caused by presence of central tumor (*arrows* in c and d). (Incidentally, note that the lower half of the sternum is destroyed (c and d). This was not initially appreciated on the routine radiographs. On biopsy, this proved to be a metastasis from a primary squamous carcinoma of the left lower lobe bronchus.)

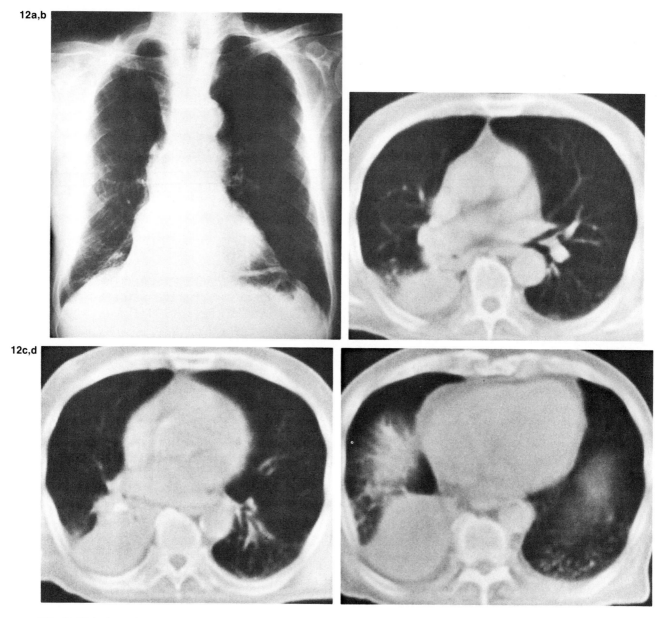

FIG. 12. Right lower lobe collapse: Squamous cell carcinoma. **a:** PA radiograph. **b–d:** Sequential sections from the lower portion of the bronchus intermedius to the lower thorax. The bronchus intermedius is circumferentially narrowed by infiltrating tumor. The right lower lobe is collapsed posteromedially against the mediastinum and spine in a manner analogous to the pattern seen in left lower lobe collapse (compare with Fig. 11).

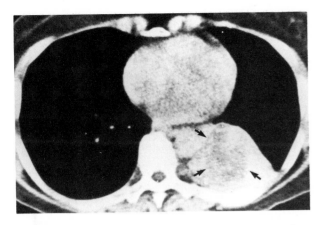

FIG. 13. Left lower lobe collapse: Large cell carcinoma. Section through the lower thorax. There is heterogeneous density in the left lower lobe following administration of i.v. contrast medium; a distinct tumor mass is defined (*arrows*), causing a bulge in the contour of the collapsed lower lobe, which is convex laterally.

can be made because mucous plugs conform to the branching pattern of the involved bronchus and have heterogeneous density. Additionally, unlike occluding tumor, visualization of the entire length of the bronchial wall is possible, distinct from the mucous plug (Fig. 16).

Mucous plugs may also form in bronchi distal to an occluding tumor. Presumably, most cases of lobar collapse due to endobronchial obstruction, if examined pathologically, would demonstrate this routinely, visualization of mucous plugs distal to central occluding tumors is not possible. Occasionally, however, when a follow-up CT scan is obtained, after radiation therapy, in patients with endobronchial tumor causing lobar collapse, evidence of bronchiectasis in the distal lobar bronchi can be defined (Fig. 17).

PASSIVE ATELECTASIS

Passive atelectasis denotes loss of volume within a lobe or lobes secondary to interference with the normal balance that exists between the lung, which tends to retract toward the hilum, and the chest wall, which tends to expand the lung and keep it aerated. This most frequently occurs because of pleural disease, i.e., the presence of air, fluid, or both within the pleural space. Of all forms of collapse, in our experience, this is the most common. Fluid within the pleural space is easily defined, even when the underlying lung is collapsed. This differentiation may be made simpler by use of i.v. contrast medium, because of the difference in density between pleural fluid and consolidated, col-

lapsed pulmonary parenchyma (Fig. 18). Pleural fluid, when sufficiently massive, will distort the "usual" configuration of collapsed lobes. The configuration of collapse caused by endobronchial obstruction is typified by characteristic relationships between the collapsed lobes and the chest wall; these are distorted in the presence of fluid (Fig. 19).

Once a lobe has collapsed, it is frequently difficult to exclude the presence of tumor. If the lobar bronchi are patent, and air-bronchograms can be defined in every portion of the collapsed lobe, tumor is unlikely. Unfortunately, this is not often the case. However, if tumor within the collapsed lobe is difficult to exclude, the presence of tumor within the pleural space is generally easy to recognize. If collapse is passive, secondary to a large accumulation of fluid in the pleural space, characterization of the nature of the pleural disease process is clearly of primary concern. (For a full discussion of pleural malignancy and differentiation from benign pleural disease, see Chapter 9.) The value of CT in differentiating benign from malignant pleural effusions is illustrated in Fig. 20. The diagnosis of malignant pleural disease is dependent on recognition of the presence of soft tissue densities within the pleural space. These will appear either as nodular foci of soft-tissue density or as an enveloping rind of thickened nodular pleura, usually in association with loculated areas of pleural fluid. In a recent report, 22 of 23 cases of malignant pleural effusions causing lobar collapse were accurately diagnosed with CT (11). In the exceptional case, malignant pleural disease may be nondescript in appearance (Fig. 18).

As already noted, unusual configurations of collapse may result when fluid or air is present in the pleural space. The magnitude of pressure exerted on lung by adjacent pleural fluid, or especially by air, may be great; the result may be confusing at first. As illustrated in Fig. 21, CT may be helpful in evaluating such cases.

CICATRIZATION ATELECTASIS

Cicatrization atelectasis is lobar collapse consequent to scarring and fibrosis from inflammatory disease. This form of collapse is a frequent sequela of tuberculosis, and is best typified by the chronic middle lobe syndrome (Fig. 22). Cicatrization atelectasis may be differentiated from other forms of lobar collapse by the following criteria.

(a) Endobronchial obstruction is absent. With careful scan technique, patency of the bronchial

14a,b

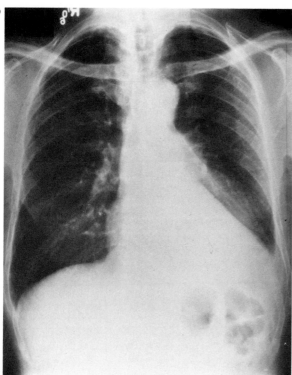

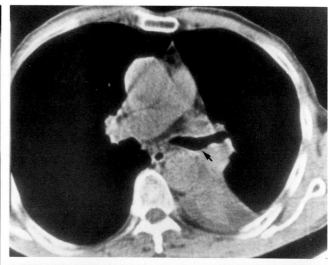

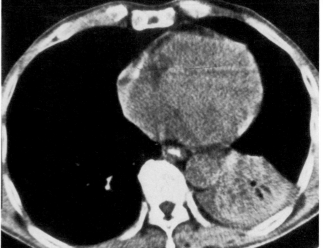

14c

FIG. 14. Left lower lobe collapse: Squamous cell carcinoma. **a:** PA radiograph. The left lower lobe appears to be airless. **b,c:** Sections through the left upper lobe spur and the left lower lobe, respectively. Air-bronchograms can be defined within the collapsed lower lobe, despite total occlusion of the origin of the left lower lobe bronchus (*arrow* in (b)). A small quantity of pleural fluid surrounds the collapsed lower lobe, easily distinguishable from the airless pulmonary parenchyma.

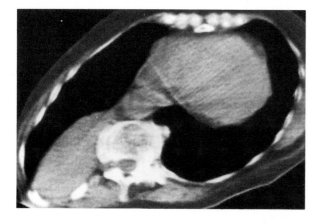

FIG. 15. Bronchostenosis. Section through the right lower lobe in a patient with marked scoliosis. The right lower lobe bronchus was obliterated at its origin (not shown). The right lower lobe has collapsed against the mediastinum posteriorly. An erroneous diagnosis of carcinoma was made (i.v. contrast was not used). At surgery, there was bronchostenosis of the right lower lobe. Additionally, there was evidence of extensive bronchiectasis throughout the resected specimen. This is inapparent on CT because all bronchi were filled with fluid.

tree subtending the involved lobe can be confirmed (Fig. 23).

(b) The degree of volume loss, in general, is more marked in cicatrization atelectasis than in other forms of collapse, particularly collapse from endobronchial obstruction. Any question of central obstruction, of course, is easily resolved by scanning through the appropriate lobar bronchus.

(c) Collapse is frequently accompanied by bronchiectatic changes within the involved lobe.

(d) Collapse is present in the absence of demonstrable pleural or chest wall pathology.

There has been some controversy about whether the chronic middle lobe syndrome is due to bronchostenosis or to cicatrization from inflammatory parenchymal disease. In our and others' experience, in all cases of chronic middle lobe syndrome examined with CT, the middle lobe bronchus has been patent, excluding bronchostenosis (i.e., fibrous narrowing of the middle lobe bronchus) as etiologic (19).

16a,b

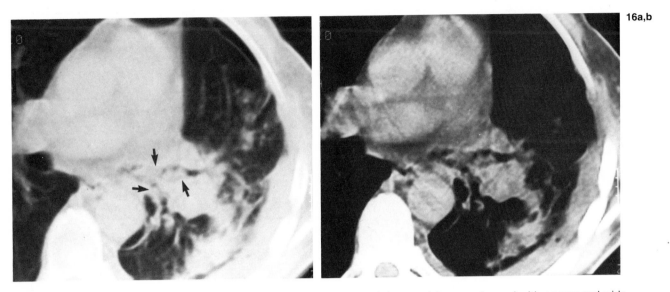

FIG. 16. Left lower lobe collapse: Mucous plug. **a,b:** Sections through the left upper lobe spur, imaged with narrow and wide windows, respectively. Irregular density fills the left upper and lower lobe bronchi (*arrows*). Despite this, the walls of the bronchi are clearly delineated. Follow-up scan after physical therapy showed normal left upper and lower lobe bronchi.

17a,b

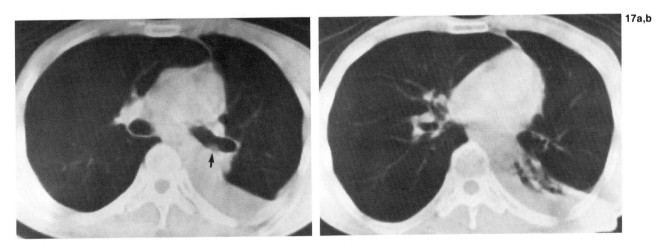

FIG. 17. Left lobe collapse: Bronchiectasis. **a:** Section through the left upper lobe spur. There is a tumor mass occluding the origin of the left lower lobe bronchus, a portion of which prolapses into the left upper lobe bronchus *(arrow)*. The left lower lobe is collapsed. **b:** Section through the left lower lobe following radiation therapy. The left lower lobe is still collapsed; however, there is aeration of the distal bronchi, which are beaded and irregular in contour (changes are compatible with bronchiectasis).

18a

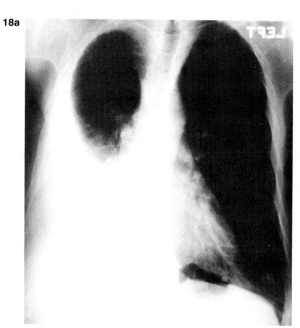

FIG. 18. Passive atelectasis: Right pleural effusion. **a:** PA radiograph shows large right-sided pleural fluid collection. **b,c:** Sequential images through the middle and lower lobes. Fluid fills the right pleural space (air within the pleural space is secondary to a previous thoracentesis). The middle and lower lobes are collapsed. The pattern of collapse is different from that seen in endobronchial occlusion, in that the collapsed lobes have been displaced away from the chest wall by the pleural fluid. Patent bronchi within both lobes can be defined.

18b,c

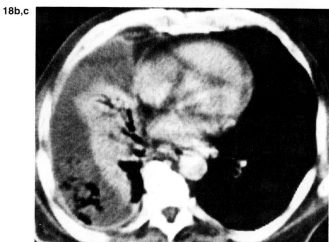
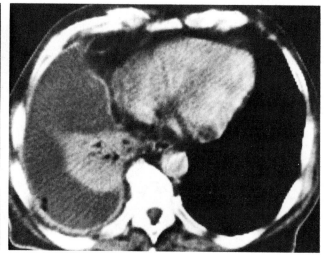

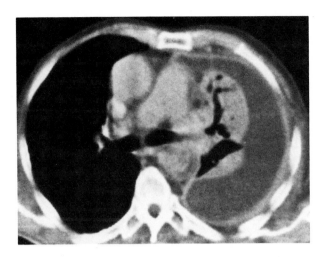

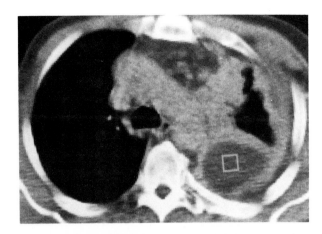

FIG. 19. Passive atelectasis (left upper and lower lobes). **a:** Large pleural fluid collection has collapsed the left lung. Air-bronchograms can be defined in both the left upper and lower lobes. The configuration of the collapsed lobes is "uncharacteristic" because pleural fluid is interposed between the collapsed lobes and the chest wall. Note that the pleural margins are slightly thickened in a uniform manner. Despite the nondescript appearance of the pleural space, pleural biopsy was compatible with metastatic pleural disease.

FIG. 20. Passive atelectasis: Malignant pleural disease (left upper lobe). Section through the aortic arch shows considerable volume loss in the left upper lobe, within which discrete air-bronchograms can be defined (better seen with wide windows). A loculated pleural fluid collection is present posteriorly (*cursor*). Note that the pleural surface is markedly irregular and that anterior mediastinal adenopathy is present. These changes are characteristic of malignant pleural disease. Biopsy revealed poorly differentiated adenocarcinoma.

21a,b

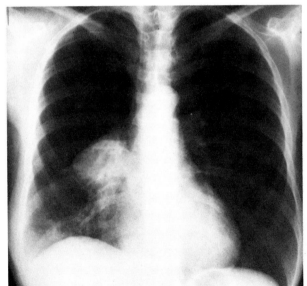

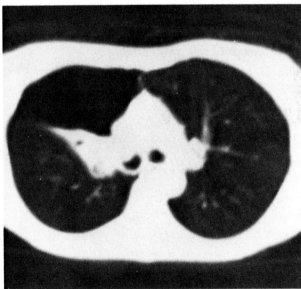

FIG. 21. Passive atelectasis (right upper lobe). **a:** PA radiograph shows a right apical pneumothorax. The right upper lobe is collapsed and displaced inferiorly. **b:** Section through the right upper lobe bronchus. The right upper lobe is collapsed, identifiable as a triangular wedge of uniform density, with the apex pointing toward the hilum. A focal anterior pneumothorax can be seen. The right upper lobe bronchus appears to be obstructed. In fact, there has been torsion around the right upper lobe bronchus secondary to the pneumothorax. Following chest tube placement and re-expansion of the right upper lobe, bronchoscopy was negative.

22a

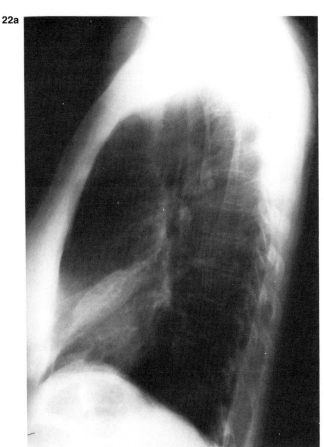

FIG. 22. Cicatrization atelectasis: Chronic middle lobe syndrome. **a:** Lateral radiograph shows marked volume loss in the middle lobe. **b:** Section through the middle lobe bronchus. The middle lobe bronchus is patent. Adjacent to the origins of the medial and lateral segmental bronchi, punctate calcification can be identified (*arrows*). **c:** Section through the middle lobe. The middle lobe is totally collapsed. Dilated, irregular bronchi can be identified within the collapsed lobe. The lateral border of the collapsed middle lobe is sharply defined by the major fissure, which is displaced anteromedially (*arrowheads*). The anterior border of the collapsed middle lobe is less well-defined. This is because the minor fissure is roughly parallel to the plane of the CT scan. Despite the appearance of retraction of the middle lobe from the anterior chest wall, some contact is generally maintained, usually at a more inferior level (not shown).

22b,c

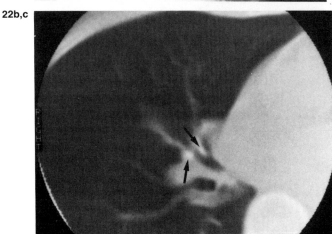 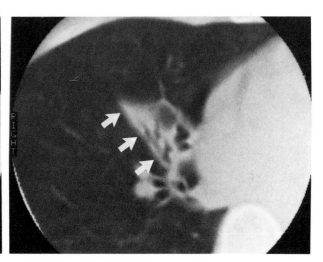

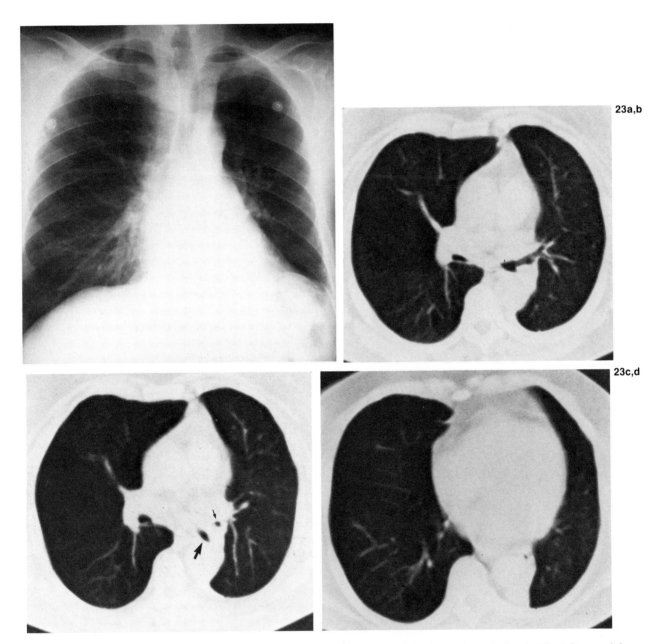

FIG. 23. Cicatrization atelectasis (left lower lobe). **a:** PA radiograph. **b–d:** Sequential images from the level of the left upper lobe spur to the lower thorax. The left lower lobe is markedly atelectatic. The bronchi are displaced posteromedially, but are otherwise patent (*large arrow* points to the left lower lobe bronchus and *small arrow* points to lingular bronchus in (c)). The left lower lobe has collapsed against the posterior mediastinum. Note that the lateral contour of the collapsed lobe is smooth, with no evidence of convexity (i.e., there is no central tumor mass).

24a,b

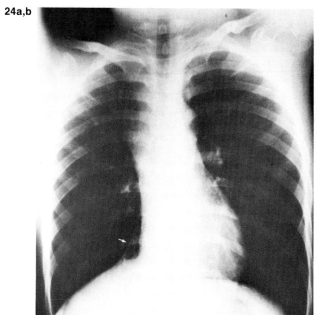

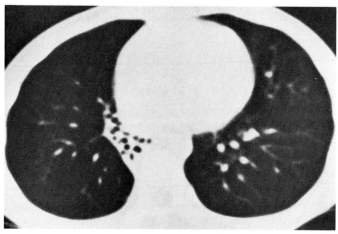

24c

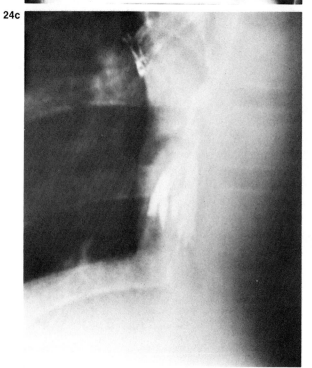

FIG. 24. Cicatrization atelectasis (right lower lobe). **a:** PA radiograph shows poorly defined border of the superior mediastinum on the right, subsequently proven to be due to a prominent thymus. A faintly definable oblique line can be seen inferiorly *(arrow)*, initially thought to represent an accessory fissure. **b:** Section through the lower thorax. The right lower lobe is collapsed. Dilated, irregular bronchi can be defined within it. This degree of collapse is usually secondary to extensive fibrosis within the involved lobe. **c:** Cone-down view from a selective right lower lobe bronchogram shows total collapse of the right lower lobe and bronchiectasis.

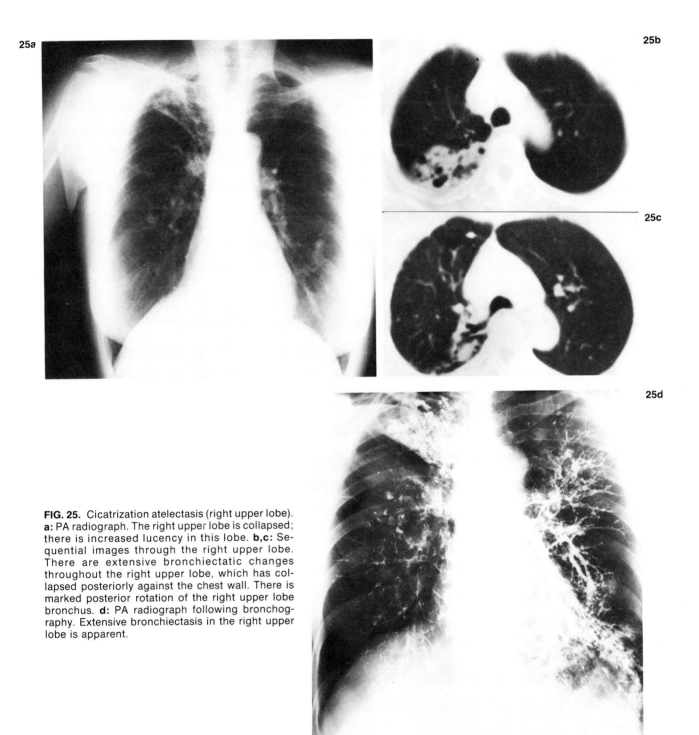

FIG. 25. Cicatrization atelectasis (right upper lobe). **a:** PA radiograph. The right upper lobe is collapsed; there is increased lucency in this lobe. **b,c:** Sequential images through the right upper lobe. There are extensive bronchiectatic changes throughout the right upper lobe, which has collapsed posteriorly against the chest wall. There is marked posterior rotation of the right upper lobe bronchus. **d:** PA radiograph following bronchography. Extensive bronchiectasis in the right upper lobe is apparent.

26a

26b

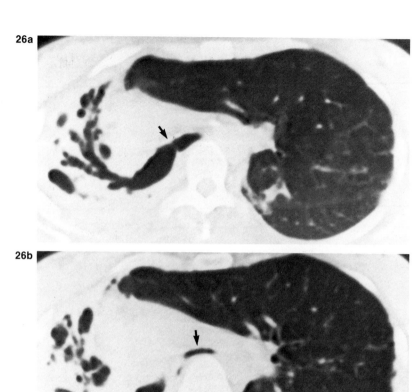

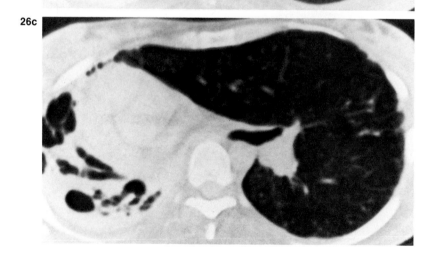

26c

FIG. 26. Cicatrization atelectasis: Bronchiectasis (right upper lobe). **a–c:** Sequential images show right upper lobe collapse, with evidence of extensive bronchiectasis. The carina (*arrow* in (a)) is displaced to the right. The left main-stem bronchus is stretched across the spine (*arrow* in (b)), with resultant narrowing. The left upper lobe bronchus (in (c)) is of normal caliber. In this case, respiratory distress resulted not from pathology in the right upper lobe but was secondary to compression of the left main-stem bronchus, caused by its displacement.

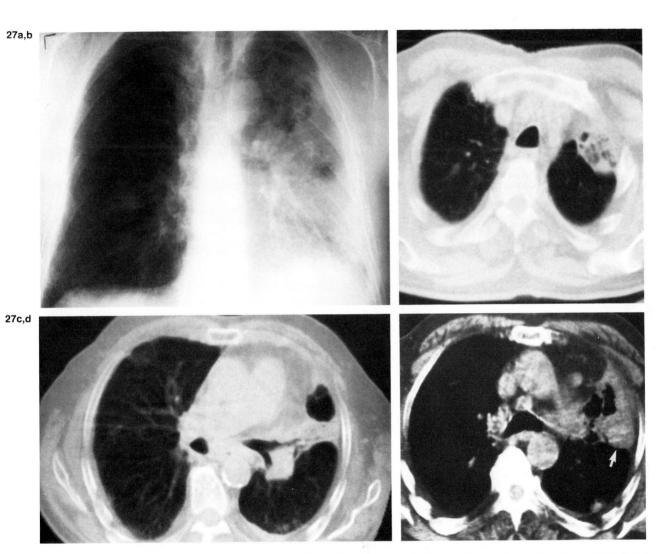

FIG. 27. Cicatrization atelectasis: Adenocarcinoma. **a:** PA radiograph shows left upper lobe collapse. **b,c:** Sequential images through the left lung apex and left upper lobe bronchus, respectively. The characteristic triangular shape of a collapsed left upper lobe is apparent, within which there are extensive bronchiectatic changes. The left upper lobe bronchus is patent. **d:** Section through the carina imaged with narrow windows. In addition to left upper lobe collapse, a rounded left upper lobe density can be seen (*arrow*). A nodule is adjacent to the pleura posteriorly, and both anterior and pretracheal adenopathy are present as well. At surgery, the left upper lobe was fibrosed and extensive bronchiectasis could be seen. The left upper lobe bronchus was irregular, but otherwise normal. A 3 × 3 cm tumor mass was present in the same location as shown in D. This proved to be adenocarcinoma with pulmonary and mediastinal metastases.

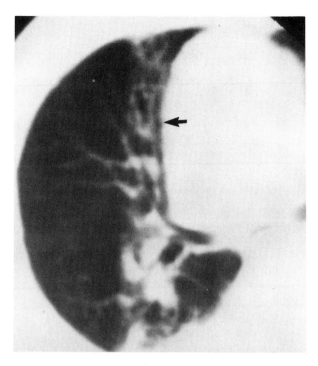

FIG. 28. Adhesive atelectasis: Radiation. A sharp line demarcates normal pulmonary parenchyma laterally from irradiated parenchyma medially. The middle lobe bronchus, as well as the medial and lateral segmental bronchi, is irregular. The medial segmental bronchus can be traced to the chest wall (arrows).

Bronchiectasis within scarred and shrunken lobes is common. This may occur even in the absence of bronchial occlusion. Although the pathogenesis of this form of bronchiectasis is disputed, it probably results from stasis of secretions with subsequent infection (20–22). In the absence of endobronchial occlusion, bronchi within a collapsed lobe may appear dilated on CT. If the degree of collapse is marked, and bronchiectasis is extensive, the overall result may be hyperlucency of a shrunken lobe on routine radiography (Figs. 24 and 25).

Occasionally, cicatrization atelectasis may result in the compromise of respiratory function as a result of compensatory spatial rearrangements affecting otherwise uninvolved portions of the lung. This detrimental effect on other portions of the airways and lung may not be apparent on routine radiographs (Fig. 26).

When collapse is as marked as that shown in Figs. 22–26, the etiology can safely be considered to be inflammatory, provided a central endobronchial lesion has been ruled out. Care must be taken, however, as previously suggested, to define dilated, bronchiectatic airways in each portion of the collapsed lung in order to survey for a peripheral rather than a central malignancy in the involved lobe. This

potential problem is illustrated in Fig. 27. Such lesions are apt to be scar carcinomas.

ADHESIVE ATELECTASIS

Adhesive atelectasis is a somewhat controversial subject. Presumably, this form of atelectasis occurs as a result of an absence or lack of production of surfactant, and may be thought of as a form of resorption atelectasis occurring without bronchial obstruction. The prototype for this form of collapse is radiation pneumonitis. The spectrum of changes seen in the thorax consequent to radiation have been described (23). The hallmark of this type of atelectasis is that involved lung is sharply demarcated from normal lung, usually conforming to known radiation ports (Fig. 28).

REPLACEMENT ATELECTASIS

Volume loss may occur as a consequence of obliteration of pulmonary parenchyma by unchecked tumor growth. Endobronchial obstruction is generally absent. We have termed this "replacement atelectasis" (Fig. 29). The key to identifying this type of collapse is to note that the margins of the "collapsed" lobe do not conform to lobar or segmental anatomy. In the case illustrated in Fig. 29, there is uniform density throughout the right upper lobe. Superficially, this mimics parenchymal consolidation. However, the contours of this density do not conform to the shape of the right upper lobe. Unchecked tumor growth has resulted in replacement of the right upper lobe, with extension into the chest wall. More frequently, tumor is restricted to the involved lobe; in this setting, the diagnosis can be made by noting that the margins of the collapsed lobe are exceedingly nodular and irregular (Fig. 30).

CONCLUSIONS

Lobar collapse is a significant indicator of a variety of pulmonary abnormalities. Commonly associated with central endobronchial tumor, collapse may also denote, among other disease processes, long-standing infection, pleural disease (both benign and malignant), or evidence of radiation. The sorting out of these various etiologies is a frequently difficult and perplexing problem encountered by all radiologists.

In the preceding sections, representative examples of "typical" forms and patterns of collapse have been reviewed. As has been stressed repeatedly, collapse, in all its forms, represents a pathophysiologic spectrum; images obtained at any given time, therefore, represent only one point on a continuum of changes. Nonetheless, certain patterns

29a

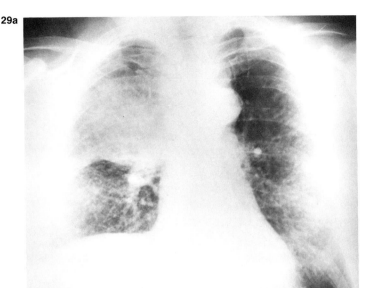

9b,c

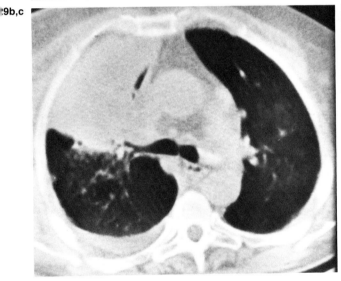

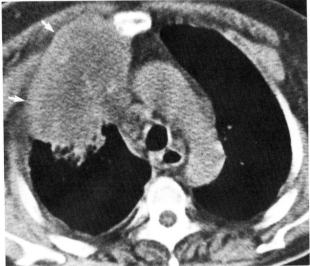

FIG. 29. Replacement atelectasis: Small cell carcinoma. **a:** PA radiograph shows uniform density in the right upper lobe. There is slight elevation of the middle lobe fissure and the right hemidiaphragm. **b:** Section through the right upper lobe bronchus. The proximal portion of the bronchus is patent. There is uniform density throughout the right upper lobe, which superficially mimics consolidation. **c:** Section through the right upper lobe. Uniform density is present; however, this does not conform to the shape of the right upper lobe. Tumor has replaced the lobe and infiltrated into the chest wall anteriorly *(arrows)*.

are characteristic and are important models. It is in this sense that the examples illustrated have been chosen to be representative.

It is clear that CT can complement routine radiographs in the evaluation of patients with lobar collapse. CT provides previously unavailable information concerning the mechanics of lobar collapse. Most important, CT is an effective means for differentiating among the various etiologies of collapse.

Endobronchial obstruction may be differentiated from other forms of collapse by detailed evaluation of the bronchial tree. The hallmark of tumorous bronchial occlusion is the presence of an endobronchial lesion associated with a central tumor mass, causing a bulging or convexity in the margin of the collapsed lobe.

Passive lobar collapse caused by pleural effusions is equally characteristic. Most important, although histologic diagnosis is difficult, the presence of pleural malignancy can be accurately diagnosed in a majority of cases. The hallmarks of pleural malignancy are thickened, irregular, nodular pleural surfaces associated with loculated fluid. CT represents a marked improvement over plain radiographs in the assessment of pleural malignancy because of its ability to differentiate more precisely among various tissue densities. Differentiation between pleural fluid and collapsed lung is usually possible, and, furthermore, endobronchial obstruction can be excluded with confidence in these cases, obviating the need for bronchoscopy.

Cicatrization atelectasis is a discrete subdivision

30a

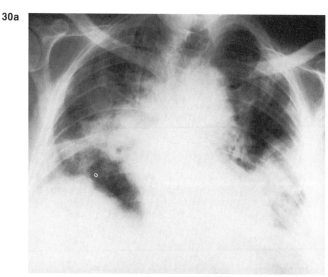

FIG. 30. Pulmonary parenchymal lymphoma. **a:** PA radiograph. **b,c:** Section through the carina imaged with wide and narrow windows, respectively. Massively enlarged pretracheal nodes can be identified. The right upper lobe is partially collapsed, and there are extensive air-bronchograms throughout. A small pleural fluid collection on the left side and a pleural nodule can be seen as well. **d,e:** Section through the middle lobe bronchus imaged with wide and narrow windows, respectively. There is volume loss in both lower lobes; air-bronchograms can be defined in both lobes as well. Despite this, the contour of the lower lobe is nodular (*arrow* on right), suggesting that a diffuse infiltrative process is present. Additionally, a large mass is present in the left upper lobe, in which air-bronchograms can be defined. It is apparent why parenchymal lymphoma may superficially mimic more routine causes of lobar collapse. Differentiation is based on recognition of the unusual contours of areas of involved parenchyma.

30b,c

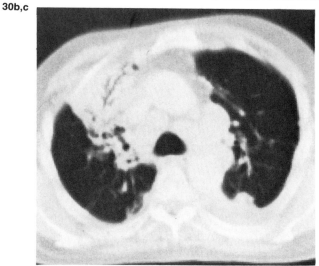

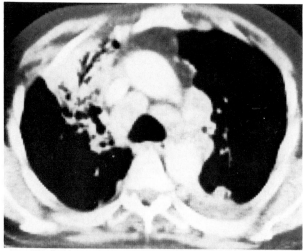

30d,e

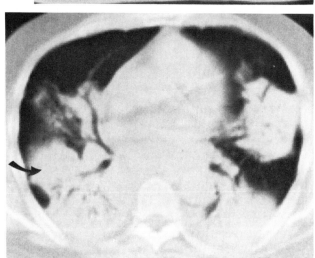

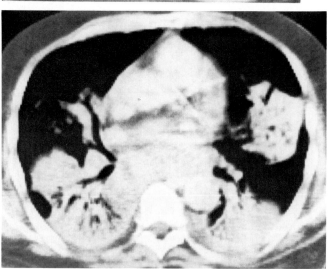

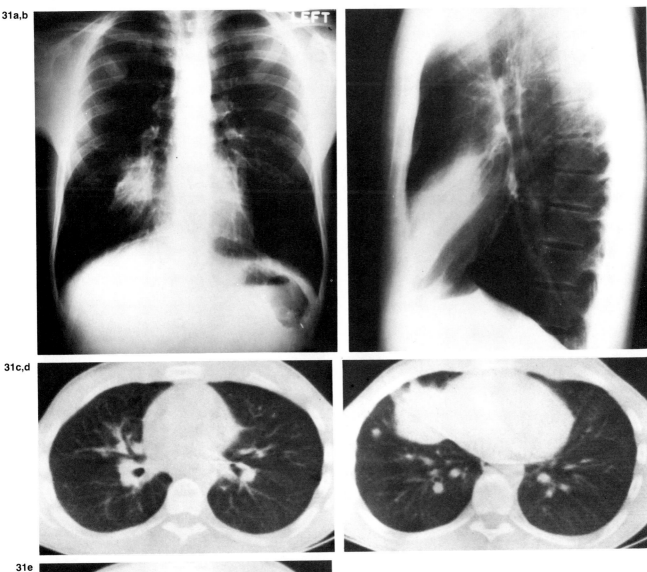

FIG. 31. Lymphoma. **a,b:** PA and lateral radiographs in a patient previously treated with mediastinal radiation for lymphoma. Recurrent pleural masses are present superiorly. The middle lobe is collapsed. **c:** Section through the middle lobe bronchus, confirming patency. **d,e:** Sequential sections through the middle and lower portions of the middle lobe. A large parenchymal mass of lymphomatous tissue (biopsy-proven) occupies the peripheral portion of the middle lobe in (d). At a lower level, the peripheral portion of the middle lobe is collapsed in a characteristic fashion.

of lobar collapse, and has a characteristic appearance on CT. In these cases, endobronchial obstruction is absent; the lobes tend to be markedly shrunken; and there is frequent evidence of diffuse bronchiectasis. CT is especially efficacious for this group of patients because collapse so frequently tends to be "atypical." In our experience, the appearance of cicatrization atelectasis may be sufficiently characteristic to obviate the need for further workup. This is especially true of those patients with chronic middle lobe syndrome. Tumor may be superimposed on chronically inflamed, fibrotic lobes; identification of this complication is possible if care is taken to examine each part of the collapsed lobe. Clearly, recognition of tumor is dependent on the size of the lesion; it may be anticipated that small lesions will be overlooked.

Other forms of collapse are equally characteristic, including collapse secondary to radiation and collapse caused by unchecked tumor growth. CT is efficacious in differentiating these different forms of collapse from more typical forms, such as endobronchial obstruction.

With the increasing availability and use of CT, it is probable that variations of lobar collapse will be encountered. Clarification of the characteristic patterns of collapse on CT, therefore, must be understood in order to avoid potential confusion and misdiagnoses.

Additionally, it is to be hoped that, with continued study, the mechanics of plain-film findings with lobar collapse will be further clarified. In this regard, Fram et al. (24) have recently developed a method of three-dimensional reconstructions that would be ideally suited to the characterization of the patterns and mechanisms of lobar collapse.

Computed tomography may play an important role in the treatment of patients with unresectable carcinoma. The usefulness of CT in planning radiation ports in patients with bronchogenic neoplasia has been documented (25–28). Babcock (29) has compared the efficacy of CT to that of routine radiographs in determining tumor location, volume, and expected radiation doses in 59 patients with primary unresectable bronchial tumors. Fifty-nine percent of the patients required alterations in their radiation treatment plans because of additional information supplied by CT. While the usefulness of CT in evaluating patients with central tumors and lobar collapse has not been specifically addressed, it is anticipated that CT will have an important impact on the therapy for this subset of patients.

Invariably, any discussion of lobar collapse will lead to the diagnostic dilemma posed by alveolar cell carcinoma and pulmonary parenchymal lymphoma. In these cases, there may be radiographic evidence of collapse associated with patent bronchi. Although our experience is limited, cross-sectional imaging has proven to be valuable, especially in clarifying the patterns of parenchymal involvement in patients with pulmonary lymphoma (Figs. 30 and 31). In these cases, parenchymal masses frequently appear to have a lobar configuration, and, further, are frequently associated with air-bronchograms. CT clarifies the pattern of lymphomatous infiltration that is only partially lobar in distribution.

In conclusion, CT represents an important advance in our ability to evaluate patients with lobar collapse of all types; it is indicated in those cases in which plain radiographic findings are equivocal or when further clarification of the mechanism of collapse is required.

REFERENCES

1. Robbins LL, Hale EH, Merril OE. The roentgen appearance of lobar and segmental collapse of the lung. I. Technique of examination. *Radiology* 44:471–476, 1945
2. Robbins LL, Hale CH. The roentgen appearance of lobar and segmental collapse of the lung. II. The normal chest as it pertains to collapse. *Radiology* 44:543–547, 1945
3. Robbins LL, Hale CH. The roentgen appearance of lobar and segmental collapse of the lung. III. Collapse of an entire lung or the major part thereof. *Radiology* 45:23–26, 1945
4. Robbins LL, Hale CH. The roentgen appearance of lobar and segmental collapse of the lung. IV. Collapse of the lower lobes. *Radiology* 45:120–127, 1945
5. Robbins LL, Hale CH. The roentgen appearance of lobar and segmental collapse of the lung. V. Collapse of the right middle lobe. *Radiology* 45:260–266, 1945
6. Robbins LL, Hale CH. The roentgen appearance of lobar and segmental collapse of the lung. VI. Collapse of the upper lobes. *Radiology* 45:347–355, 1945
7. Lubert M, Krause GR. Patterns of lobar collapse as observed radiologically. *Radiology* 56:165–182, 1951
8. Krause GR, Lubert M. Gross anatomic spatial changes occurring in lobar collapse: A demonstration by means of three-dimensional plastic models. *Am J Roentgenol Radium Ther Nucl Med* 79:258–268, 1958
9. Proto AV, Tocino I. Radiographic manifestations of lobar collapse. *Semin Roentgenol* 15:117–173, 1980
10. Naidich DP, Khouri NF, McCauley DI, Leitman BS, Hulnick D, Siegelman SS. Computed tomography of lobar collapse: Part I. Endobronchial obstruction. *J Comput Assist Tomogr* 7:745–757, 1983
11. Naidich DP, Khouri NF, McCauley DI, Leitman BS, Hulnick D, Siegelman SS. Computed tomography of lobar collapse: Part II. Collapse in the absence of endobronchial obstruction. *J Comput Assist Tomogr* 7:758–767, 1983
12. Raasch BN, Heitzman ER, Carsky EW, Lane EJ, Berlow ME, Witwer G. A computed tomographic study of bronchopulmonary collapse. Exhibit presented at the 68th Scientific Assembly and Annual Meeting of the Radiological Society of North America, November 28–December 3, 1982
13. Glazer HS, Aronberg DJ, Van Dyke JA, Seigel SS. Computed tomographic manifestation of pulmonary collapse. *Contemporary Issues in CT* vol. 4 1984 (in press)

14. Fraser RG, Pare JA. *Diagnosis of Diseases of the Chest*, 2nd ed. Philadelphia, W.B. Saunders, 1979

15. Golden R. The effect of bronchostenosis upon the roentgen ray shadows in carcinoma of the bronchus. *Am J Roentgenol Radium Ther Nucl Med* 13:21–30, 1925

16. Cohen AM, Solomon EH, Alfidi RJ. Computed tomography in bronchial atresia. *AJR* 135:1097–1099, 1980

17. Kowal LE, Goodman LR, Zarro VJ, Haskin ME. Case report: CT diagnosis of broncholithiasis. *J Comput Assist Tomogr* 7:321–323, 1983

18. Berger PE, Kuhn JP, Kuhns LR. Computed tomography and the occult tracheobronchial foreign body. *Radiology* 134:133–135, 1980

19. Putnam CE, Rosenbloom SA, Vock P, Godwin D, Chen JT, Hedlung LW, Effman EL, Bober EL, Rowin CE. Peripheral middle lobe syndrome. Exhibit displayed at the 68th Scientific Assembly and Annual Meeting of the Radiological Society of North America, November 28–December 3, 1982

20. Tannenberg J, Pinner M. Atelectasis and bronchiectasis. *J Thorac Surg* 11:571–616, 1942

21. Croxatto OC, Lanari A. Pathogenesis of bronchiectasis. Experimental study and anatomic findings. *J Thorac Surg* 27:514–528, 1954

22. Spencer H. *Pathology of the Lung*. Oxford, Pergamon Press, 1968

23. Nabawi P, Mantrauaot R, Breyer D, Capek V. Case report: Computed tomography of radiation-induced lung injuries. *J Comput Assist Tomogr* 5:568–570, 1981

24. Fram EK, Godwin JD, Putnam CE. Three-dimensional display of the heart, aorta, lungs, and airways using CT. *AJR* 139:1171–1176, 1982

25. Emami B, Melo A, Carter BL, Munzenrider JE, Piro AJ. Value of computed tomography in radiotherapy of lung cancer. *Am J Roentgenol* 131:63–67, 1978

26. Smith V, Parker DL, Stanley JH, Phillips TL, Boyd DP, Kan PT. Development of a computed tomographic scanner for radiation therapy treatment planning. *Radiology* 136:489–493, 1980

27. Barrett A, Dodds HJ, Husband JE. The value of computed tomography in radiation therapy. *CT* 5:217–218, 1981

28. Goitein M, Wittenberg J, Mondiondo M, Doucette J, Friedberg C, Ferrucci J, Gunderson L, Linggood R, Shipley W, Fineberg HJ. The value of CT scanning in radiation therapy treatment planning: A prospective study. *Int J Rad Onc Biol Phys* 5:1787–1798, 1979

29. Badcock PC. The role of computed tomography in the planning of radiotherapy fields. *Radiology* 147:214–244, 1983

Pulmonary Hila

The critical factor in accurate interpretation of computed tomographic (CT) scans of the pulmonary hila is detailed knowledge of normal cross-sectional anatomy (1–4). The purpose of this chapter will be to review pertinent anatomy; how this knowledge can be applied to the abnormal hilum will be extensively illustrated.

GENERAL PRINCIPLES AND METHODOLOGY

There is no one generally accepted method for CT evaluation of the pulmonary hila (1,3,5). A detailed guide to methodology was presented in Chapter 1. In this section, we review our approach to interpretation and methodology.

The pulmonary hila are comprised of airways, including segmental and in some cases subsegmental bronchi, and pulmonary arteries and veins. As will be discussed, there is a fairly constant relationship between these structures that allows for immediate identification at given levels. In most cases, pulmonary lymphatic vessels are not visualized, and hence they present no problems in evaluation.

Anatomically, the hila can be evaluated in two ways: with wide windows (generally window ranges of 1,800–2,000 HU are employed in this chapter and throughout the text) and narrow windows (generally 300–500 HUs depending on the individual case). The rationale for selecting these parameters was presented in Chapter 1. With wide windows, analysis centers around the bronchial tree, and the interface between the pulmonary parenchyma and the soft tissue structures of the hila. With narrow windows, attention is focused on the soft-tissue structures of the hila, the hilar vessels in particular. Both

approaches are valuable, as will be illustrated throughout this chapter.

It is our contention that each case should be individualized methodologically. Consideration must be given to the nature of the problem to be investigated, the status of the patient, and the capabilities and limitations of the particular equipment available. We begin all examinations without administration of intravenous contrast material, using 10-mm sections at 10-mm intervals. Additional unenhanced scans are obtained as needed to further clarify anatomic relationships. Depending on the indication and the appearance of the scans without contrast enhancement, either the study is deemed complete or further images are obtained following bolus injections of contrast medium. The advantages to this approach are numerous. In a considerable percentage of cases, the study may be completed noninvasively. This is of obvious value in patients who have known allergy to i.v. contrast media or renal insufficiency.

Uncooperative patients may also cause problems in interpretation. When there is significant respiratory motion, contrast enhancement is of less value; in these cases, information is generally best obtained by imaging the hila with wide windows.

If an abnormality is seen and/or suspected for which contrast is considered necessary, the precise location at which a bolus of contrast medium would be of greatest value may be selected from the nonenhanced scans. This is of critical importance when "dynamic scanning" capability is not available. In our experience, without dynamic scanning, at best only one or two images can be obtained with intense enhancement of vessels.

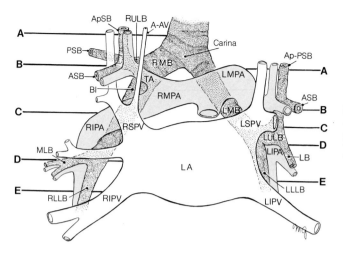

FIG. 1. Schematic representation of the pulmonary hila derived from AP hilar tomograms, as described by Yamashita (7) (see text). Characteristic sections are labeled A through E.

When dynamic scanning is available, we would concur with the methodology proposed by Glaser et al. (5) for dynamic incremental CT evaluation of the pulmonary hila. This method calls first for "priming" the patient with a slow-drip infusion and scanning through the upper thorax. Subsequent images are obtained from the level of the right upper lobe bronchus to the inferior portions of the hilum, following the injection of 50 ml of high-concentration contrast medium at 1-cm intervals.

ANATOMY

The key to cross-sectional CT anatomy of the pulmonary hila is cross-sectional bronchial anatomy (6). The bronchi form a lattice on which the pulmonary arteries and veins are draped in a characteristic fashion. The bronchi are easily recognizable, since air within the lumen of bronchi serves as a natural contrast agent (cross-sectional anatomy of the bronchi is discussed in detail in Chapter 4, and this material should be reviewed before this chapter is read).

The purpose of this review will be to present a simplified approach to the pulmonary hila, based on characteristic sections. The bronchi serve as convenient, easily identifiable reference points that allow immediate anatomic orientation. The right and left hila will be considered separately. Throughout this section, the reader should refer to Fig. 1, a schematic representation of the pulmonary hila derived from the meticulous anatomic work of Yamashita (7), and to Fig. 3, an injected anatomic specimen in which the pulmonary vessels have been opacified with colored latex (2).

Right Hilum

Figure 2a is a section through the distal portion of the trachea (compare with level A, Fig. 1). At this level, the apical segmental bronchus of the right upper lobe is cut in cross section and appears as a circular lucency. The right upper lobe pulmonary artery (segmental branch to the apical segment of the right upper lobe) and the right superior pulmonary vein (segmental branch draining the apical segment of the right upper lobe) also course vertically; the artery lies just medial to and the vein just lateral to the apical segmental bronchus. Invariably, other vessels will be imaged at this level; these generally may be recognized by their characteristic branching patterns (Figs. 3a and b). Any density larger than the pulmonary artery and vein surrounding the apical segmental bronchus is suspicious for neoplasm until it is proven vascular in origin.

Figure 2b is a section made approximately 1 cm below that shown in Fig. 2a. The pertinent anatomic relationships remain unchanged. At this level, the carina is easily identified. Comparison should be made with Fig. 3a, the corresponding injected anatomic specimen.

Figure 4a is a section through the right upper lobe bronchus, corresponding to level B in Fig. 1. Note that the border of this bronchus is in direct contact with lung parenchyma. Anterior to the right upper lobe bronchus is the truncus anterior; this is the first large branch of the right main pulmonary artery and arises within the pericardium (Fig. 4b). The right superior pulmonary vein lies within the angle formed by the bifurcation of the right upper lobe bronchus into anterior and posterior segmental bronchi.

Anterior and medial to the truncus anterior, there

2a,b

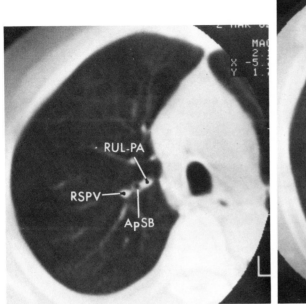
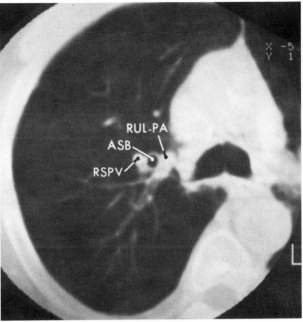

FIG. 2. a: Section through the lower trachea. ApSB, apical segmental bronchus; RUL-PA, right upper lobe pulmonary artery; RSPV, right superior pulmonary vein. Note that, at this level, the largest vascular structures surround the apical segmental bronchus. b: Section through the carina. Anatomic relationships are unchanged from those shown in (a). ASB, apical segmental bronchus; RUL-PA, right upper lobe pulmonary artery; RSPV, right superior pulmonary vein.

frequently is a small convexity (Fig. 4a). This represents another right upper lobe vein (the apical-anterior vein) which may characteristically be found in this location (Fig. 4a; compare with Figs. 1 and 3).

Figures 5a and b are sequential images through the bronchus intermedius, corresponding to level C in Fig. 1. This bronchus has a generally vertical course and is therefore seen in cross section as an oval lucency. The posterior wall of the bronchus intermedius, like the posterior wall of the right upper lobe bronchus, is in direct contact with lung parenchyma. Pulmonary parenchyma also extends posteromedially, forming the azygo-esophageal recess. The right main pulmonary artery crosses first in front and then at a slightly lower level alongside the lateral aspect of the bronchus intermedius. The right superior pulmonary vein(s) lie alongside the lateral border of the right main pulmonary artery, causing the configuration of the hila to have a slightly nodular contour at this level. This nodularity should not be mistaken for adenopathy. Comparison should be made to the corresponding injected anatomic section (Fig. 3c), as well as to the post-contrast image at the same level (Fig. 5c).

Once the right main pulmonary artery reaches the lateral border of the bronchus intermedius, it is not unusual for this artery to have a triangular and

somewhat irregular configuration (Fig. 6a). This normal variation is caused by a change in the course of the right pulmonary artery as it turns inferiorly and becomes the right interlobar pulmonary artery. Figure 6b is a lateral radiograph from a pulmonary angiogram. The sudden change in the course of the right pulmonary artery as it assumes an interlobar position is evident. When viewed in cross section, at the point at which it turns inferiorly, this artery will have a triangular configuration.

Figure 7a is a section through the origin of the middle lobe bronchus, corresponding to level D in Fig. 1. The middle lobe bronchus is separated from the lower lobe bronchus by the middle lobe spur. The interlobar pulmonary artery lies immediately lateral to the lateral borders of both the middle and lower lobe bronchi. The interlobar artery at this point is vertically oriented and is thus seen in cross section as an oval structure. The right superior pulmonary vein lies medial to the middle lobe bronchus and can be seen entering the upper portion of the left atrium (compare with the injected anatomic section in Fig. 3d).

Figure 7b is a section slightly more inferior than that shown in Fig. 7a. The middle lobe bronchus has bifurcated into lateral and medial segmental bronchi. At the point of bifurcation, the middle lobe pul-

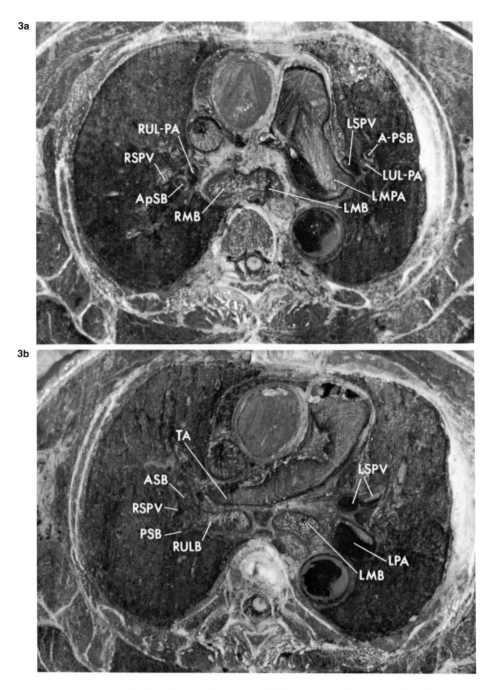

FIG. 3. Injected anatomic sections. **a:** Section through the carina. RMB, right main bronchus; RUL-PA, right upper lobe pulmonary artery; ApSB, apical segmental bronchus; RSPV, right superior pulmonary vein; LMB, left main bronchus; LMPA, left main pulmonary artery; LUL-PA, left upper lobe pulmonary artery; A-PSB, apical-posterior segmental bronchus; and LSPV, left superior pulmonary vein. **b:** Section through the right upper lobe bronchus (RULB). TA, truncus anterior; ASB, anterior segmental bronchus; PSB, posterior segmental bronchus; RSPV, right superior pulmonary vein; LMB, left main bronchus; LPA, left interlobar pulmonary artery; and LSPV, left superior pulmonary vein.

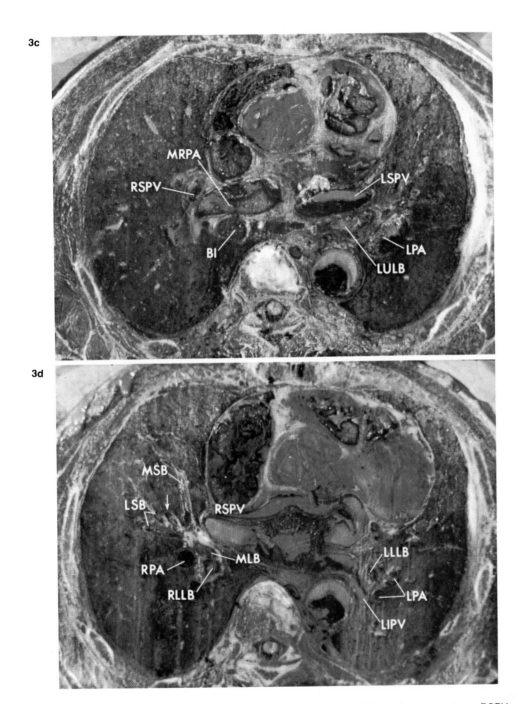

FIG 3 *(cont).*c: Section through the bronchus intermedius (BI). MRPA, main right pulmonary artery; RSPV, right superior pulmonary vein; LSPV, left superior pulmonary vein; LPA, left interlobar pulmonary artery; and LULB, left upper lobe bronchus. **d:** Section through the middle lobe bronchus (MLB). MSB, medial segmental bronchus; LSB, lateral segmental bronchi; RLLB, right lower lobe bronchus; RPA, right interlobar pulmonary artery; LLLB, left lower lobe bronchus; LPA, left lower lobe pulmonary arteries; LIPV, left inferior pulmonary vein; and RSPV, right superior pulmonary vein. The *arrow* points to branch of middle lobe pulmonary artery. (From ref. 1, with permission.)

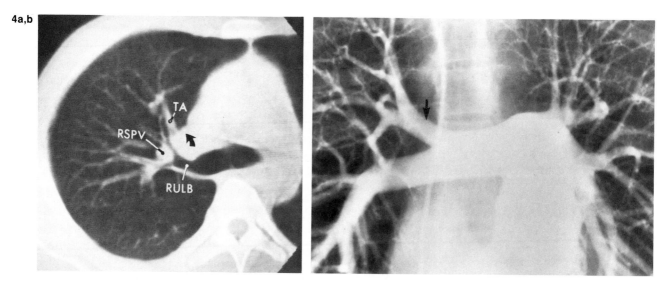

FIG. 4. a: Section through the right upper lobe bronchus (RULB). TA, right upper lobe pulmonary artery (truncus anterior); RSPV, right superior pulmonary vein. The *arrow* points to a small convexity just medial to the TA; this is the apical-anterior pulmonary vein. **b:** Posteroanterior view; normal pulmonary angiogram. The first branch of the main right pulmonary artery arises from within the pericardium, the truncus anterior *(arrow)*.

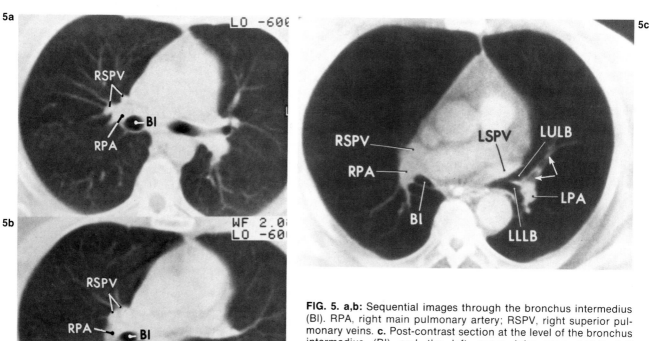

FIG. 5. a,b: Sequential images through the bronchus intermedius (BI). RPA, right main pulmonary artery; RSPV, right superior pulmonary veins. **c.** Post-contrast section at the level of the bronchus intermedius (BI) and the left upper lobe spur. LULB, left upper lobe bronchus; LLLB, left lower lobe bronchus; LPA, left interlobar pulmonary artery, LSPV, left superior pulmonary vein. The *arrows* point to the lingular pulmonary artery at its point of origin.

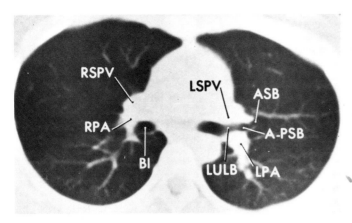

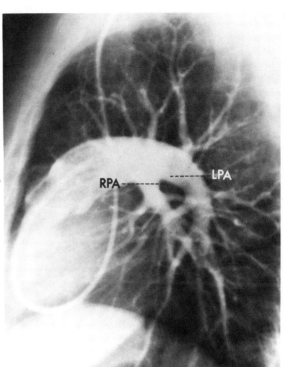

FIG. 6. a: Section at the level of the bronchus intermedius (BI) and left upper lobe bronchus (LULB). Note the triangular configuration of both the right and left pulmonaries (RPA, LPA). RSPV and LSPV, right and left superior pulmonary veins; ASB, anterior segmental bronchus; A-PSB, origin of apical-posterior segmental bronchus. **b:** Lateral radiograph from pulmonary angiogram shown in Fig. 4b. The proximal right and left interlobar pulmonary arteries (RPA, LPA) are labeled at approximately the same level shown in (a).

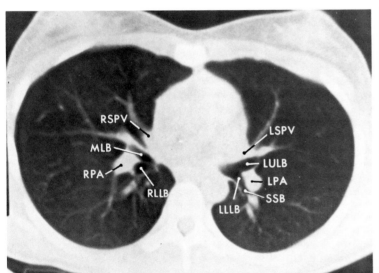

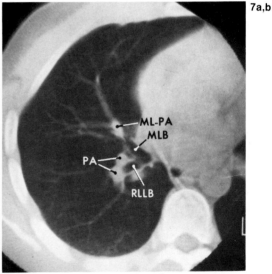

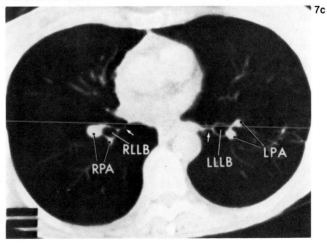

FIG. 7. a: Section through the origin of the middle lobe bronchus (MLB) and the left upper lobe spur. RLLB, right lower lobe bronchus; RPA, right interlobar pulmonary artery; RSPV, right superior pulmonary vein; LULB, left upper lobe bronchus; LLLB, left lower lobe bronchus; SSB, superior segmental bronchus, left lower lobe; LPA, left interlobar pulmonary artery; LSPV, left superior pulmonary vein. **b:** Section slightly lower than that shown in (a). MLB, middle lobe bronchus; RLLB, right lower lobe bronchus; ML-PA, middle lobe pulmonary artery; PA, pulmonary artery branches to the lower lobes. **c:** Section through the proximal portions of the lower lobe bronchi (RLLB, LLLB). The pulmonary arteries to the lower lobes (RPA, LPA) lie adjacent and posterolateral to the bronchi. The *arrows* point to the upper portions of the inferior pulmonary ligaments.

monary artery usually can be identified coursing anterolaterally. The right interlobar pulmonary artery has also bifurcated into the various basilar segmental pulmonary arteries. Note that these basilar pulmonary arteries have a characteristic, rounded configuration, lying posterolateral to the proximal portion of the right lower lobe bronchus. These relationships between the lower lobe bronchus and the lower lobe basilar pulmonary arteries remain constant even in more caudal sections (Fig. 7c).

Unlike the pulmonary arteries, the right inferior pulmonary vein is oriented horizontally. The inferior pulmonary veins can be routinely traced into the lower portion of the left atrium (Fig. 8). It should be noted that Figs. 7c and 8 are below what is formally considered part of the pulmonary hila (see level E, Fig. 1). These sections have been included to provide a sense of continuity when evaluating sequential cross-sectional images in the region of the pulmonary hila.

Left Hilum

The upper portion of the left hilum can assume various configurations. While the left superior pulmonary vein and left upper lobe pulmonary artery can always be identified, their anatomic relationships, especially to the airways, tend to be less constant on the left side, as compared with the right.

Figure 9 is section through the carina, corresponding to level A in Fig. 1. The apical-posterior segmental bronchus is cut in cross section and can be identified as a circular lucency. The apical-posterior segmental bronchus is separated from the left main bronchus by the main left pulmonary artery, which courses over the left upper lobe bronchus at

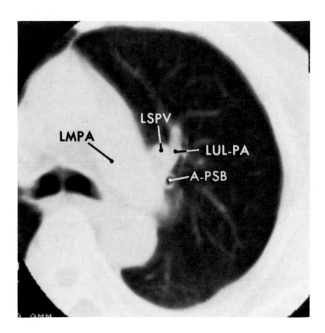

FIG. 9. Section through the carina. A-PSB, apical-posterior segmental bronchus; LMPA, left main pulmonary artery, LSPV, left superior pulmonary vein; LUL-PA, left upper lobe pulmonary artery (supplying anterior segment of the left upper lobe).

this level. The left superior pulmonary vein (the branch draining the apical-posterior segment of the left upper lobe) and the left upper lobe pulmonary artery (the main branch to the left upper lobe) can be recognized as two distinct vessels. In general, at this level the left upper lobe pulmonary artery can be traced to its origin from the main left pulmonary artery and lies posterolateral to the left superior pulmonary vein. Figure 4a is the corresponding injected anatomic section.

Figure 10 is a section at the level of the right upper lobe bronchus, corresponding to level B in Fig. 1. At this level, the anatomy on the left side is essentially the same as that shown in Fig. 9. In this specific case, note that the left upper lobe pulmonary artery courses behind the apical-posterior segmental bronchus; the pulmonary artery to the left upper lobe lies just lateral to the apical-posterior segmental bronchus (compare with Fig. 9). Minor variations of this nature are frequent at this level and should not cause confusion. Again, note the convexity caused by the left superior pulmonary vein, which in this case lies just medial to the apical-posterior segmental bronchus.

Figure 11 is a section through the upper portion of the left upper bronchus, corresponding to level C in Fig. 1. The posterior wall of the left upper lobe bronchus at this level is slightly convex because it is indented superiorly and posteriorly by the left main

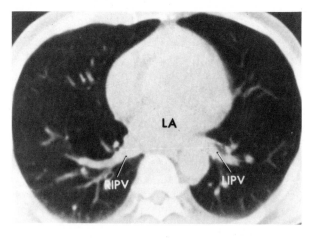

FIG. 8. Section through the inferior pulmonary veins (RIPV, LIPV), which can be traced into the left atrium (LA).

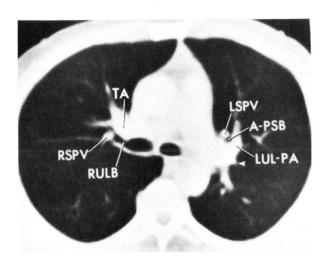

FIG. 10. Similar section to that shown in Fig. 9, showing minor variation in the anatomy of the upper portion of the left hilum. A-PSB, apical-posterior segmental bronchus; LSPV, left superior pulmonary vein; LUL-PA, left upper lobe pulmonary artery; RULB, right upper lobe bronchus; RSPV, right superior pulmonary vein; TA, truncus anterior. The *arrowhead* points to characteristic triangular configuration of a small branch of the pulmonary artery sectioned at its origin.

pulmonary artery as it courses over the left upper lobe bronchus (see also Fig. 6a). Posterior to the left upper lobe bronchus, the left pulmonary artery continues as the left interlobar pulmonary artery. The interlobar pulmonary artery usually appears triangular and irregular at this level; this is exactly analogous to the anatomy of the pulmonary artery on the right side. This normal variation is caused by a change in the course of the left pulmonary artery as it turns to descend toward the lower lung segments (Figs. 6a and b).

The left superior pulmonary vein invariably lies in front of the left upper lobe bronchus as it courses toward the left atrium (Fig. 11; compare with the injected anatomic specimens in Figs. 4b and c). This vein frequently has a horizontal course at this level; distinct branching usually can be identified peripherally within the pulmonary parenchyma.

Figure 12 is a section through the lower portion of the left upper lobe bronchus at the level of the left upper lobe spur, corresponding with level D in Fig. 1 (see also Fig. 5c). This spur divides the left upper lobe bronchus from the proximal portion of the left lower lobe bronchus. At this level, the left interlobar pulmonary artery has a nearly vertical course and always lies just lateral to the spur. The interface between the artery and the adjacent pulmonary parenchyma is generally smooth and rounded (Figs. 5c and 12). The lingular bronchus originates from the distal portion of the left upper lobe bronchus; adjacent and just lateral to the origin of the lingular bronchus, the pulmonary artery to the lingula fre-

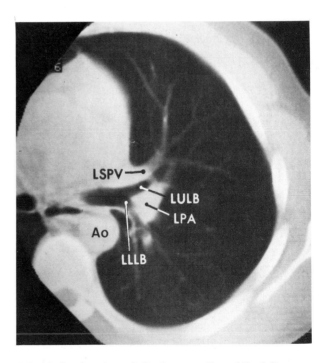

FIG. 11. Section through upper portion of the left upper lobe bronchus (LULB). LPA, left interlobar pulmonary artery; LSPV, left superior pulmonary vein. Note the smooth posterior border of the left upper lobe bronchus. Lung invaginates between the aorta (Ao) and the pulmonary artery to come into close proximity with the bronchus.

FIG. 12. Section through the lower portion of the left upper lobe bronchus (LULB). LLB, left lower lobe bronchus; LPA, left interlobar pulmonary artery; LSPV, left superior pulmonary vein; Ao, aorta.

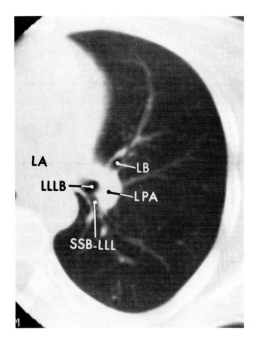

FIG. 13. Section through the lingular bronchus (LB). LLLB, left lower lobe bronchus; SSB, superior segmental bronchus; LPA, left interlobar pulmonary artery; LA, left atrium.

quently can be identified (Fig. 5c). Anteriorly, the inferior portion of the left superior pulmonary vein can be recognized; as shown at a higher level, this vein lies directly anterior to the left upper lobe bronchus.

Characteristically, pulmonary parenchyma can be seen between the pulmonary artery and the descending aorta at the level of the left upper lobe bronchus (Figs. 5c, 6a, 11, and 12). Webb et al. (8) have shown that this portion of lung frequently comes in close proximity to the posteromedial wall of the left upper and lower lobe bronchi at this level. Thickening and/or nodularity of this left "retro-bronchial stripe" is a sensitive sign for tumor infiltration and/or adenopathy in the left hilum, and should be searched for routinely.

Figure 13 is a section just below the left upper lobe bronchus. The left interlobar pulmonary artery has a smooth, rounded contour; the artery lies between the proximal portion of the left lower lobe bronchus (and, frequently at this level, the bronchus to the superior segment of the left lower lobe) and the proximal portion of the lingular bronchus. Not infrequently, small veins can be seen posteriorly, imparting a slightly nodular contour to the posterior portion of the left hilum at this level. This should not be confused with adenopathy.

Below this level, the anatomy of the inferior portion of the left hilum is essentially a mirror image of

that on the right side, corresponding to level E in Fig. 2 (see Figs. 7c and 8). Branches of the pulmonary artery to the left lower lobe lie lateral and posterior to the left lower lobe bronchus. The left inferior pulmonary vein is oriented horizontally and can routinely be traced into the lower portion of the left atrium (Fig. 8; compare with the injected anatomic specimen in Fig. 4d). The left inferior pulmonary vein courses alongside the lateral border of the descending aorta.

Cross-sectional anatomy of the major pulmonary vessels is simplified by the characteristic relationships of the vessels to the bronchial tree. Identification of smaller vessels is also possible, despite significant variation in their appearance, because smaller vessels can almost always be traced to larger vessels. When smaller vessels course horizontally, it is particularly simple to trace their origins to major segmental vessels (Fig. 10). This may be appreciated on almost every scan illustrated in this section. If a vessel courses obliquely, or in a cephalocaudal direction, visualization of the origin of these vessels may require examination of sequential images to verify that they are vascular.

This important principle is illustrated in Fig. 14. Figure 14a is a cone-down view of a slightly delayed image obtained from a selective left main pulmonary arterial injection in a patient with a solitary pulmonary atriovenous malformation (AVM). Note that the appearance of the enlarged draining vein in Fig. 14a corresponds with the appearance of this vein when tracked in sequential sections from the AVM to the left hilum (Figs. 14b–d). This same approach may be applied to any vascular structure emanating from or draining toward the pulmonary hila; furthermore, as shown in Fig. 14, such an analysis need not require the use of intravenous contrast material.

Of course, rapid intravenous injection of contrast medium is available as an ancillary means to study hilar vascular anatomy. Although this need not be routine, in select or equivocal cases, a bolus of contrast agent can quickly resolve any problem in interpretation (Figs. 15 and 18).

PULMONARY VASCULAR DISEASE

Differentiation between enlarged vessels and hilar adenopathy and/or hilar masses is frequently difficult with plain radiography. CT plays an important role in differentiating pulmonary vascular disease from other significant hilar pathology, largely because of the clarity of detail obtained with cross-sectional imaging.

O'Callaghan et al. (9) have shown that CT is an

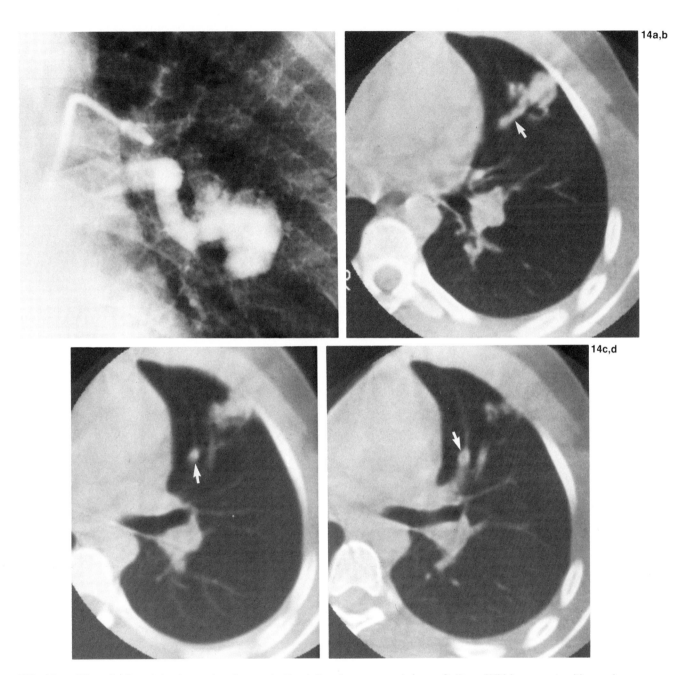

FIG. 14. a: PA projection; late-phase view from selective left pulmonary angiogram. Solitary AVM is present, with one large draining vein. **b:** Section through discrete mass in lingula. A large vascular structure can be seen in close proximity with this mass *(arrow)* Note that this conforms to the inferior horizontal configuration of the draining vein shown in (a). **c:** Section 1 cm above that shown in (b). The vascular structure seen in (b) has now changed course to become vertically oriented *(arrow)*. This corresponds with the vertical portion of the draining vein seen in (a). **d:** Section 15 mm above that shown in (c). This large vessel can be traced into the left superior pulmonary vein, confirming that this is a large draining vein *(arrow)*. This type of analysis can be applied to any structure in or near the hilum that is believed to be vascular in origin.

15a,b

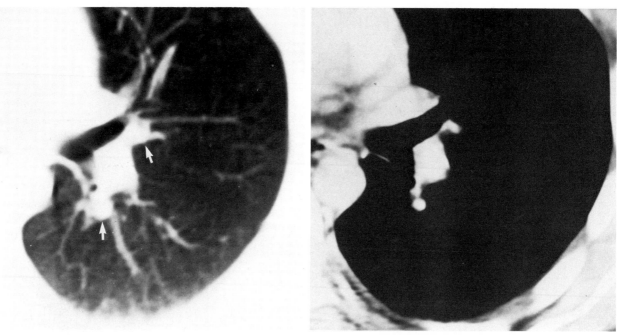

FIG. 15. a: Enlargement of a section through the left upper lobe spur. The *arrows* point to two densities, one anterior and one posterior to the left interlobar pulmonary artery, which are of questionable nature. **b:** Same section following a bolus of contrast medium, confirming the vascular nature of these densities.

accurate means for evaluating pulmonary artery size. This is important, since the size of the pulmonary arteries may be a useful indicator of pulmonary hypertension. O'Callaghan et al. measured the size of the intrapericardial portion of the right main pulmonary artery in 25 patients, and found a mean value of 13.3 mm for normal patients (with a standard deviation of 1.5 mm). The appearance of enlarged pulmonary arteries in a patient with pulmonary artery hypertension secondary to diffuse fibrotic lung disease is illustrated in Fig. 16. Interestingly, there may be enlargement of the main pulmonary artery without evidence of significant enlargement of the right and left pulmonary arteries, as illustrated in Fig. 17. While more typical of pulmonic valve stenosis, this patient had pulmonary hypertension with dilatation of the pulmonary outflow tract.

Occasionally, the configuration of the pulmonary outflow tract and the left pulmonary artery may appear to be abnormal in a normal patient. Mencini and Proto (10) have called attention to a variation in the configuration of the pulmonary outflow tract and the main left pulmonary artery in which these structures are higher than usual, lying adjacent and to the left of the aortic arch (Fig. 23, Chapter 3). This appearance may simulate a mediastinal mass. In cases in which the configuration of the pulmonary artery is unusual (particularly when associated with a paucity of mediastinal fat), the injection of a bolus of intravenous contrast medium may be indispensable (Fig. 18).

One potential use for CT is the evaluation of patients with suspected pulmonary thromboembolism. Overfors et al. (11) have shown experimentally that peripheral pulmonary emboli could be diagnosed in the descending pulmonary arteries in 4 of 5 living dogs. Godwin et al. (12) detected central pulmonary emboli in three patients; on the basis of this data it was concluded that CT scanning may supplement or even replace pulmonary arteriography in select cases.

Central pulmonary emboli appear as filling defects in the main pulmonary arteries on bolus contrast-enhanced scans. This appearance is illustrated in Fig. 19. Obstruction, of course, may also be secondary to tumor within the hilum or mediastinum (see Fig. 21).

Dynamic scanning of the pulmonary arteries has potential use in measuring pulmonary blood flow. A bolus of contrast agent is injected and sequential images at the same level through the main pulmonary arteries are obtained. The change of density within the pulmonary arteries can then be measured over time and the results displayed graphically. Further, if properly timed, circulation time between the appearance of contrast medium in the superior vena cava, the pulmonary arteries, and the aorta

16a

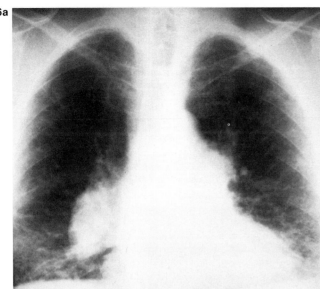

FIG. 16. Pulmonary artery dilatation: Sarcoidosis. **a:** PA chest radiograph demonstrates bilateral hilar prominence and diffuse, increased lung markings. **b:** Markedly enlarged main pulmonary artery (M), right pulmonary artery (RPA), and left pulmonary artery (LPA) are present. **c:** Very prominent right (RPA) and left (L) pulmonary arteries are seen. There is no hilar adenopathy. Pulmonary hypertension was secondary to chronic pulmonary fibrosis.

16b,c

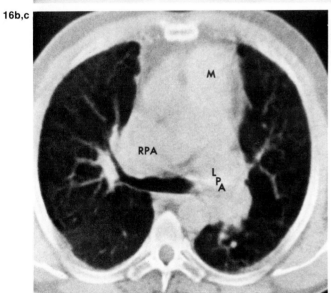
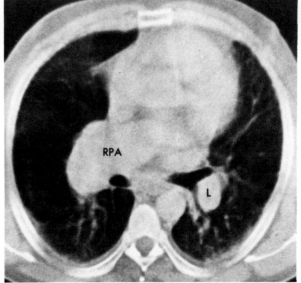

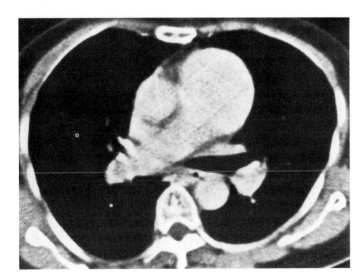

FIG. 17. Pulmonary hypertension dilatation of the main pulmonary artery. The main pulmonary artery is markedly dilated; notice the normal caliber of the right main pulmonary and the left interlobar pulmonary artery.

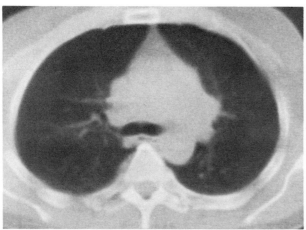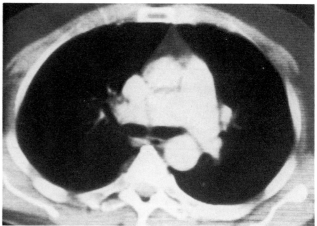

FIG. 18. Normal variant: Pulmonary arteries. **a:** Unenhanced scan shows unusual configuration of the left hilum and apparent effacement of normal mediastinal tissue planes. **b.** Post-contrast scan shows prominent pulmonary arteries and no significant pathology.

may also be measured (13). Theoretically, such a display may allow detection and quantification of intracardiac shunting. The manner in which this data may be generated and displayed is shown in Fig. 20.

In our experience, with current commercially available scanning capabilities, insufficient data are usually accumulated within allowable time to generate truly accurate flow measurements, particularly in the pulmonary arteries. The overall value of CT in analyzing pulmonary blood flow dynamics must await future developments in technology (see Chapter 1).

Tumorous involvement of the pulmonary arteries may also be detected with CT (14) (Fig. 21). Tumor encasement of hilar vessels and mediastinal invasion are best visualized following a bolus of intravenous contrast medium. Interestingly, as shown in this case, the ipsilateral pulmonary parenchymal markings may appear slightly more prominent when tumor encases and obstructs a major pulmonary artery (Fig. 21). This probably reflects a combination of venous engorgement and lymphatic obstruction. While tumor obstruction of hilar vessels is most often secondary to bronchogenic carcinoma, other lesions, both benign and malignant, have been re-

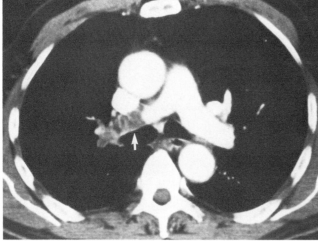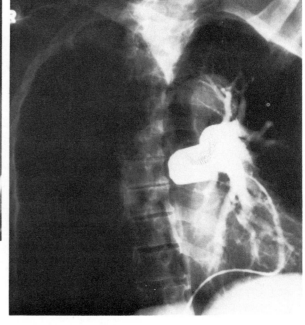

FIG. 19. Pulmonary embolus: Right main pulmonary artery. **a.** A large, filling defect is apparent in this contrast-enhanced section through the right main pulmonary artery (*arrow*). There is no evidence of tumor surrounding the artery. **b:** Oblique projection; main pulmonary arteriogram. Obstruction of the right main pulmonary artery is confirmed. The angiographic appearance suggested tumor occlusion: none was found at surgery.

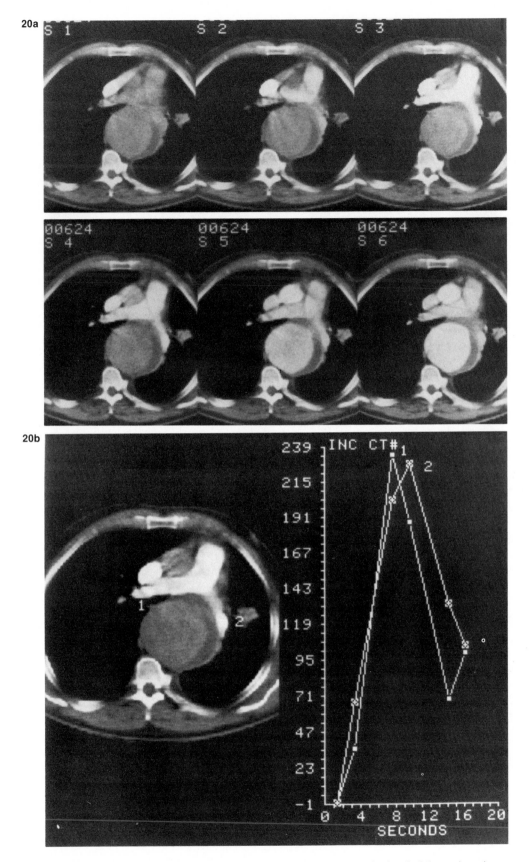

FIG. 20. Dynamic scanning of the pulmonary arteries. **a:** Six sequential images at the level of the main pulmonary arteries in a patient with a large aneurysm of the descending thoracic aorta. Preoperatively, the question of impingement of the left pulmonary artery was raised. This study shows sequential dense opacification first of the superior vena cava, then the pulmonary arteries, and finally the ascending and descending aorta. **b:** Graphical display of pulmonary arterial blood flow from study illustrated in (a). Cursors are present overlying the main right and left pulmonary arteries. To the right, changes in contrast density over time are plotted. While of great potential value, at present this methodology is insufficiently precise for accurate determination of pulmonary blood flow, largely because insufficient datum points can be acquired in available time sequences.

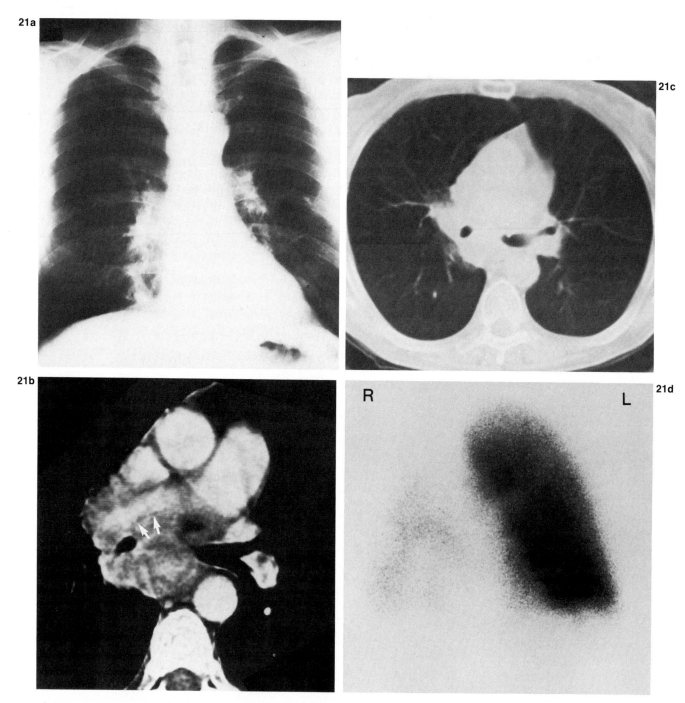

FIG. 21. Tumor compression: right main pulmonary artery. **a:** PA radiograph shows enlargement of the right hilum and infiltrate in the medial portion of the right lower lobe. **b:** Section through the main right pulmonary artery following contrast enhancement. There is extensive tumor involving the right hilum and extending into the mediastinum. The right main pulmonary artery is encased by tumor *(arrows),* (compare with Fig. 19). **c:** Section at the same level as (b), imaged with wide windows. There are prominent parenchymal markings in the right lung, probably secondary to a combination of venous and lymphatic obstruction. **d:** Anterior view from a lung scan shows almost no initial flow into the right lung.

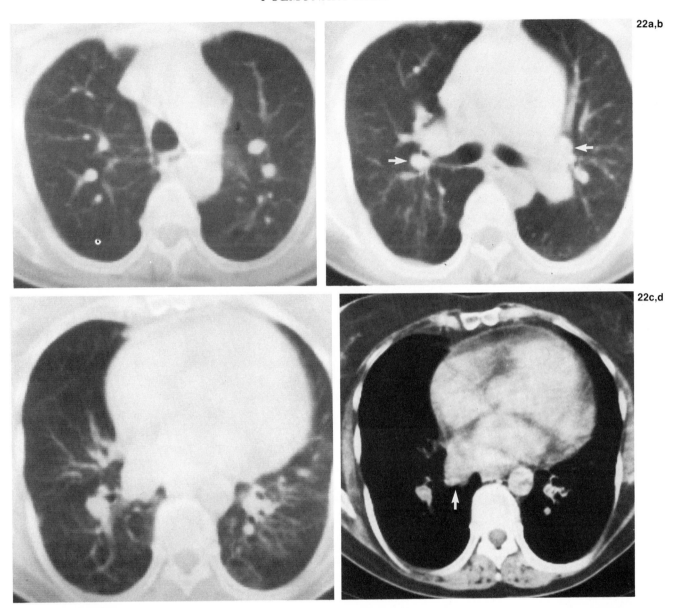

22a,b

22c,d

FIG. 22. Mitral stenosis: Pulmonary venous distension. **a:** Section through the upper lobes shows markedly dilated upper lobe pulmonary veins. Notice the branching patterns, confirming these as vessels. **b:** Section through the right upper lobe bronchus. The right and left superior pulmonary veins are dilated *(arrows)*. The upper lobe veins seen in (a) could be traced into these veins on sequential scans (not shown). **c,d:** Section through the right inferior pulmonary vein, imaged with wide and narrow windows. This vein is aneurysmally dilated just proximal to the left atrium *(arrow)*.

ported to cause pulmonary arterial obstruction. Accurate diagnosis requires histologic evaluation (15,16).

Pulmonary venous distension, such as may occur in congestive heart failure or valvular heart disease, may also be defined with CT. Detailed knowledge of normal cross-sectional anatomy is critical for accurate interpretation. As illustrated in Fig. 22 (an example of pulmonary venous engorgement in a patient with relatively mild mitral valve stenosis), enlarged pulmonary veins can be identified as branching structures in the pulmonary parenchyma

(Fig. 22a). On serial sections, these can be traced into the main pulmonary hilar veins (Fig 22b). These central veins are easy to identify, since they occupy characteristic positions in the pulmonary hila. As has been shown by Borkoweski et al. (17) CT is a sensitive, noninvasive method for establishing the diagnosis of a pulmonary varix, obviating the need for angiography. This is of particular interest in those cases in which a pulmonary varix may masquerade as a pulmonary nodule or even an AVM (Fig. 22).

Anomalies of the pulmonary arteries, while rare,

23a,b

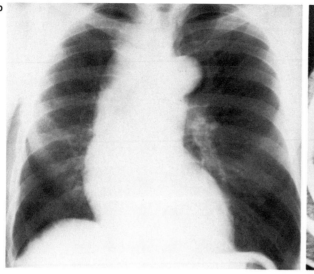

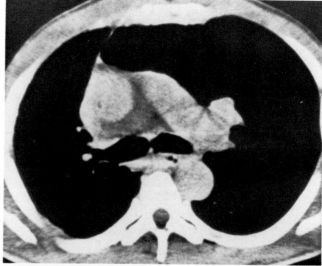

23c

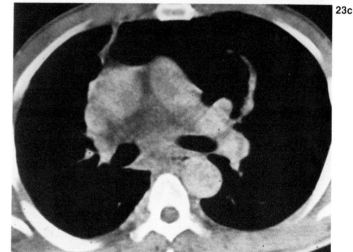

FIG. 23. Congenital absence of the right pulmonary artery. **a:** PA radiograph shows decreased volume in the right lung and a small right hilum. **b:** CT scan at the level of the right upper lobe bronchus. Fat occupies the precarinal, retroaortic space, normally filled by the truncus anterior. **c:** Section through the bronchus intermedius. Fat fills the space anterior to this bronchus, normally filled by the main right pulmonary artery.

are also easily diagnosed with CT. The radiologic features of absence of a pulmonary artery are frequently characteristic and include a small hemithorax, ipsilateral displacement of the mediastinum, absence of the corresponding pulmonary artery, and reticular densities in the lung, usually attributed to bronchial collaterals (18). If confusion or doubt persists about the diagnosis, CT is especially efficacious in establishing the diagnosis (Fig. 23).

Another rare pulmonary arterial anomaly is the pulmonary artery sling, or anomalous left pulmonary artery. The appearance on CT of this condition has been described by Stone et al. (19). In these cases, the left pulmonary artery arises from the right pulmonary artery and enters the left hilum by passing between the trachea and esophagus. Generally these cases are found in neonates and young infants and are associated with tracheobronchial or cardiovascular anomalies; rarely they are found as mediastinal masses later in life (Fig. 24).

HILAR MASSES/ADENOPATHY

The same criteria applicable in the interpretation of routine tomography (both antero-posterior (AP) and 55° oblique hilar tomography) apply as well in CT (20,21). The criteria are as follows: generalized hilar enlargement; focal hilar enlargement (focal hilar mass); compression, displacement, and/or infiltration of the bronchial tree; and nodularity in the contour of the hilum, usually indicating hilar lymph node enlargement. In any given case, the presence of multiple findings will undoubtedly increase confidence and diagnostic precision.

As outlined in the section in this chapter on general principles and methodology, initial imaging should be performed without intravenous contrast medium administration. Close scrutiny of the criteria outlined above indicates that most abnormalities may be detected either as a consequence of distortion of the general configuration of the hilum (i.e., a

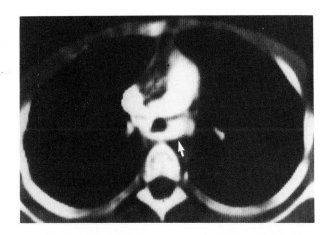

FIG. 24. Anomalous left pulmonary artery. Contrast-enhanced scan outlining the anomalous course of the left pulmonary artery swinging behind the trachea to reach the left hilum *(arrow)*. (From Ref. 40.)

change in the nature of the lung–hilum interface) or of alterations in the bronchial tree. In both cases, the emphasis is on visualization of structures and/or interfaces that are best seen with wide windows. Use of intravenous contrast media should be reserved for those cases in which additional information concerning the hilum or mediastinum is necessary and could not be appreciated on the initial precontrast scans.

In this section, each of these criteria will be illustrated by detailed analysis of representative case material. In this manner, clues to the recognition of pathology can be most efficaciously defined and emphasized.

Generalized Hilar Enlargement

Large hilar masses cause characteristic alterations in the anatomy of the hila, easily perceived

25a

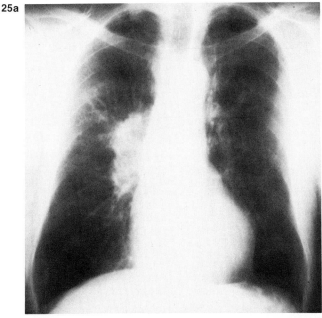

FIG. 25. Bronchogenic carcinoma: Right hilum. **a:** PA radiograph showing enlarged right hilum. **b:** Section at the level of the carina. The apical segmental bronchus is engulfed by tumor. Mediastinal adenopathy is apparent even on this nonenhanced image *(arrow)*. **c:** Section through the right upper lobe bronchus. Irregular tumor mass infiltrates the right hilum, causing nodularity in the contour of the hilum. Tumor is infiltrating the mediastinum *(arrow)*, apparent even on this nonenhanced scan.

25b,c

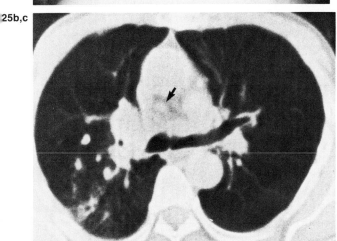
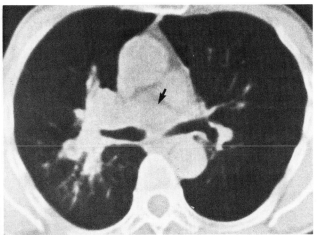

26a,b

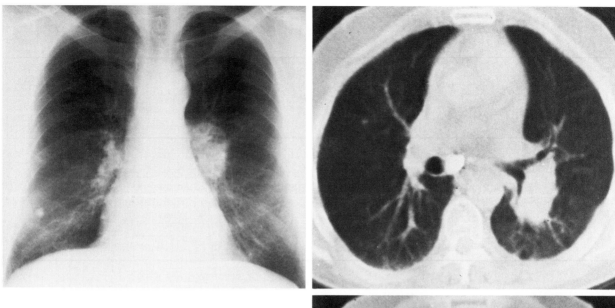

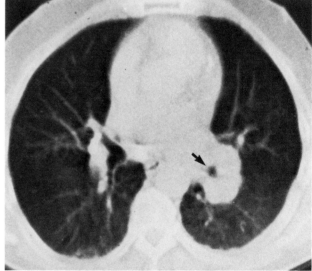

26c

FIG. 26. Small cell carcinoma: Left hilum. **a:** PA radiograph shows enlarged left hilum. **b:** Section through the left upper lobe spur. The left hilum is enlarged; there is splaying of the left upper and lower lobe bronchi. **c:** Section through the proximal portion of the left lower lobe bronchus, which is engulfed by tumor *(arrow).*

with CT. Invariably, such masses cause alterations in the configuration of the lung–hilum interface, as well as of the bronchial tree. It is worthwhile to illustrate such cases as a prelude to the recognition of subtler CT abnormalities.

Figure 25a is a PA radiograph of a patient with an enlarged right hilum. Figures 25b and c are sections through the carina and the right upper lobe bronchus, respectively. In Fig. 25b, the apical-segmental bronchus of the right upper lobe is encircled by tumor mass. The normally visualized pulmonary artery and vein that surround this bronchus are effaced. The back wall of the right main stem bronchus is thickened and irregular, indicating tumor infiltration. Additionally, enlarged mediastinal nodes can be visualized. In Fig. 25c, a mass surrounds the distal portion of the right upper lobe

bronchus, obscuring visualization of the right superior pulmonary vein and the right upper lobe pulmonary artery. There is distinct nodularity in the contour of the right hilum at this level. The posterior wall of the right upper lobe bronchus is thickened, akin to the changes seen along the posterior wall of the right main bronchus shown in Fig. 25b. There is clear extension of tumor into the middle mediastinum; this is most marked centrally behind the superior vena cava and the ascending aorta.

Figure 26a is a PA radiograph of a patient with an enlarged left hilum. Figure 26b is a section at the level of the left upper spur. The hilum is enlarged (compare with the overall size and configuration of the hilum on the right side). The bronchi are splayed by "tumor mass" in the left hilum, with widening of the normally smaller angle found between the left

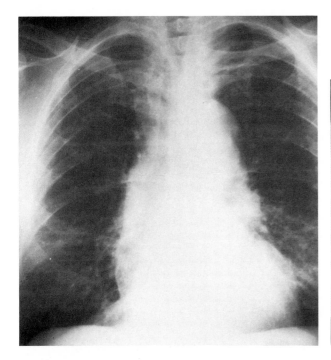

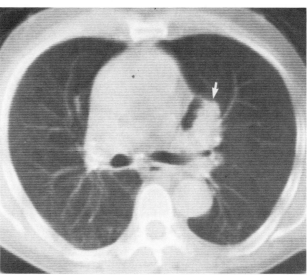

27a,b

FIG. 27. Small cell carcinoma: Left hilum. **a:** PA radiograph shows increased density in the left hilum. The bulge below the aortic knob proved to be enlarged ductus nodes. **b:** Section at the level of the left upper lobe bronchus. Nodular tumor can be identified anterior to the left superior pulmonary vein *(arrow)*. (Same case as shown in Fig. 10, Chapter 1.)

upper and lower lobe bronchi (compare with Fig. 12). Figure 26c is a section 2 cm below that shown in Fig. 26b. The left lower lobe bronchus can be identified and is entirely surrounded by soft-tissue density. Normally, at this level, the left lower lobe pulmonary arteries are discrete vessels that can be identified posterior and lateral to the lower lobe bronchus (compare with Fig. 7c).

Differentiation between mass *per se* and massively enlarged, tumor-filled hilar lymph nodes may be problematic, although the significance of this differentiation is of little consequence in most cases. The appearance of the left hilum shown in Fig. 27 would be characteristic of either situation; in this case, enlargement of the left hilum was secondary to massive, tumor-filled lymph nodes in a patient with a peripheral small cell carcinoma.

Focal Hilar Enlargement

Solitary hilar masses have the same general characteristics as have more diffuse hilar disease (Figs 25 and 26). The only significant difference is that abnormalities may be restricted to only one level or section (Fig. 28). As a general rule, any solitary density within the hilum not clearly vascular in origin should be suspect. Any doubt may be dispelled by use of intravenous contrast medium.

Bronchial Alterations

Perhaps the most sensitive indicator to the presence of tumor within the pulmonary hila is alterations in the course, configuration, or caliber of the bronchi (Fig. 28). Accurate interpretation of bronchial abnormalities requires meticulous scanning technique, as discussed in Chapter 4.

Broncial alterations may be exceedingly subtle, and may represent the only clear abnormality in an otherwise normal-appearing hilum (see Fig. 30). Especially significant are abrupt changes in the overall caliber of the bronchial tree. This may be indicative of diffuse, circumferential, submucosal tumor infiltration. Figures 29a, b, and c are sequential 10-mm thick sections through the right upper lobe bronchus, and the upper and lower portions of the bronchus intermedius, respectively. There is slight nodularity in the contour of the right hilum, especially anterior to the right upper lobe bronchus. The most significant finding, however, is the abrupt change in caliber of the bronchus intermedius, as compared with the right upper lobe bronchus or the bronchi on the left side. In this case, the entire length of the bronchus intermedius was found on bronchoscopy to be thickened by infiltrating squamous cell carcinoma.

Bronchial pathology may, of course, lead to changes within the pulmonary parenchyma, which

28a,b

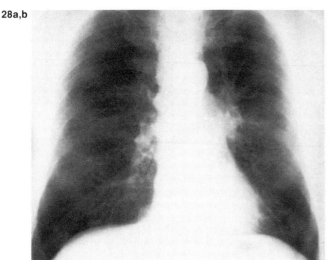

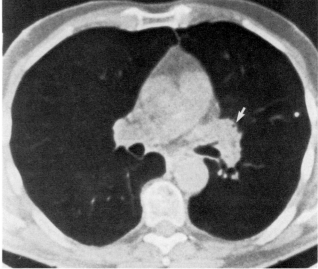

28c

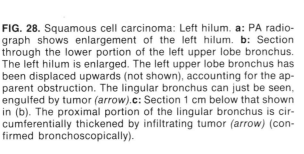

FIG. 28. Squamous cell carcinoma: Left hilum. **a:** PA radiograph shows enlargement of the left hilum. **b:** Section through the lower portion of the left upper lobe bronchus. The left hilum is enlarged. The left upper lobe bronchus has been displaced upwards (not shown), accounting for the apparent obstruction. The lingular bronchus can just be seen, engulfed by tumor *(arrow).***c:** Section 1 cm below that shown in (b). The proximal portion of the lingular bronchus is circumferentially thickened by infiltrating tumor *(arrow)* (confirmed bronchoscopically).

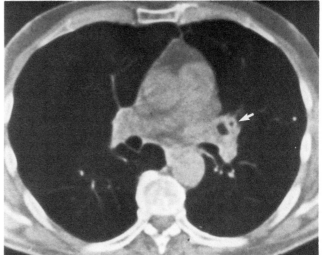

is easily identified with CT. This is illustrated in Fig. 30.

Hilar Adenopathy

While CT is efficacious in defining the presence and extent of tumor involvement in the pulmonary hila and mediastinum, of greater clinical concern is the value of CT in identifying the presence of hilar adenopathy. Differentiation between pulmonary vascular "prominence" and adenopathy probably accounts, more than any other indication, for the necessity of further study of the hila beyond routine radiographs.

The hallmark of hilar adenopathy on CT is the finding of nodularity in the contour of the hilum. The characteristic appearance of hilar adenopathy is illustrated in Fig. 31 (a patient with sarcoidosis). Figures 31 a–d are sequential 10-mm thick sections

through the hila; at each level, both on the right and left side, the interface between the pulmonary parenchyma and the hilum is distorted. For example, in Fig. 31a, a discrete, rounded density is present just behind the posterior wall of the right upper lobe bronchus. In the same figure, on the left side, there is subtle obliteration of the left retrobronchial stripe. In Fig. 31b, the contour of both the right and left hilum is distinctly nodular; there is, in addition, effacement of the azygo-esophageal recess by subcarinal adenopathy. The same appearance can be noted in Fig. 31c. Also note that there is slight medial displacement and subtle attenuation of the middle lobe bronchus. In Fig. 31d, the proximal portions of both lower lobe bronchi are surrounded by nodular, soft-tissue densities (compare with Fig. 26c). In general, recognition of adenopathy, as shown in Fig. 32, presents no special difficulties, provided that characteristic sections are obtained.

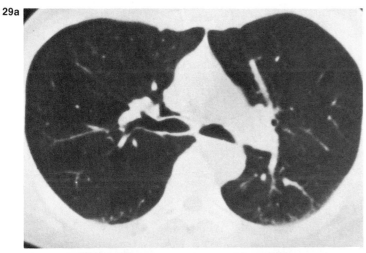

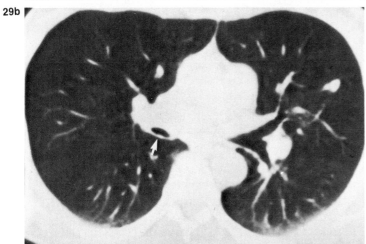

FIG. 29. Infiltrating squamous cell carcinoma. **a–c:** Sequential images through the right upper lobe bronchus, and the upper and lower portions of the bronchus intermedius. There is an abrupt change in caliber of the bronchus intermedius *(arrow)*. Compare with caliber of the right upper lobe bronchus. At bronchoscopy, the bronchus intermedius was circumferentially infiltrated with tumor.

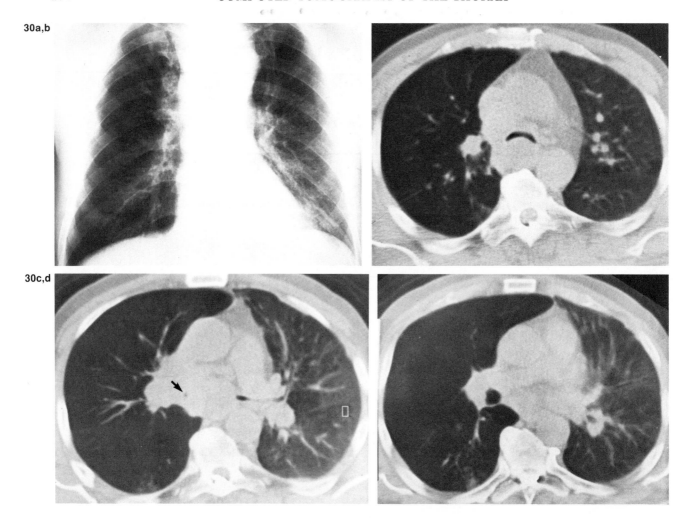

FIG. 30. Small cell carcinoma: Right hilum and mediastinum. **a:** PA radiograph shows widened mediastinum, and decreased vascularity of the right lung, initially thought to be possibly secondary to tumor infiltration of the right pulmonary artery. **b,c,d:** Sequential images through the carina, bronchus intermedius, and origin of the middle lobe bronchus. Extensive tumor mass fills the mediastinum, narrowing and displacing the carina (b). The bronchus intermedius is encased with tumor, narrowed to a pinpoint (c; *arrow*). The hilum at the level of the middle lobe bronchus is grossly normal. At all levels, there is marked hyperinflation of the right lung with decreased vascularity. In this case, this was caused by tumor involving the bronchus intermedius that acted as a ball valve mechanism.

Adenopathy need not be apparent on plain radiographs to be visualized with CT (Fig. 32). In our experience, CT is most efficacious in detecting unsuspected posterior hilar adenopathy. First, the posterior hilar–lung interface seen in cross section is especially characteristic. Alterations in this portion of the hila, such as, for example, effacement of the posterior wall of the right upper lobe bronchus, the bronchus intermedius, or obliteration of the azygo-esophageal recess or the left retrobronchial strip, may be exceedingly subtle yet still distinctive when seen in cross section (8) (Fig. 32b). Second, posterior hilar adenopathy does not distort the lateral margin of the hila, and hence is usually undefinable on a PA radiograph. Posterior hilar

adenopathy usually has to be quite pronounced to be visualized on a lateral radiograph.

Adenopathy restricted to the anterior portions of the hila is more difficult to define than are posterior nodes. This is because the pulmonary–hilar interface anteriorly is somewhat less characteristic than these same interfaces posteriorly. For this reason, suspected adenopathy, if anterior, may require the use of i.v. contrast media somewhat more frequently.

Adenopathy may be present and definable without evidence of either bronchial distortion or nodularity in hilar contour. This fact is illustrated in Fig. 33 (a patient with calcified granulomatous hilar lymph nodes). While some of these nodes cause an

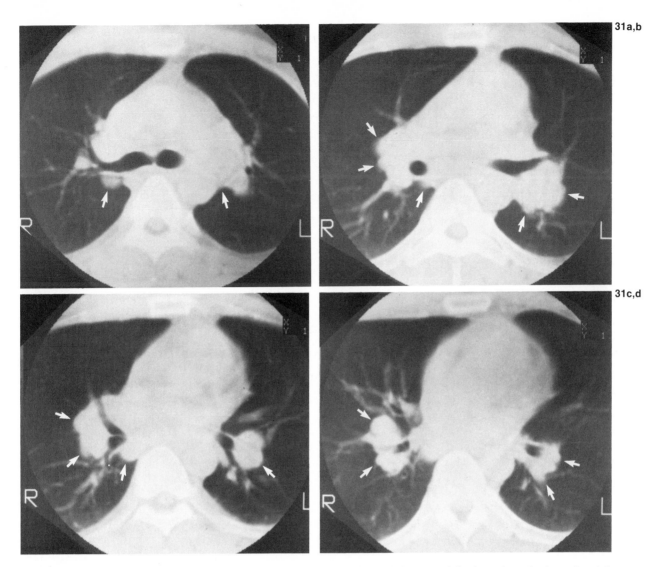

FIG. 31. Hilar adenopathy: Sarcoidosis. **a–d:** Sequential images through the right upper lobe bronchus, the bronchus intermedius, the middle lobe bronchus, and the lower lobe bronchi, respectively. At each level, bilaterally enlarged lymph nodes can be identified, without the use of intravenous contrast medium. The key to identification of adenopathy is the change in the normal contour of the lung–hilum interface (arrows). Such alterations are easiest to identify when sections are obtained through the hilum–bronchi at the characteristic levels shown above.

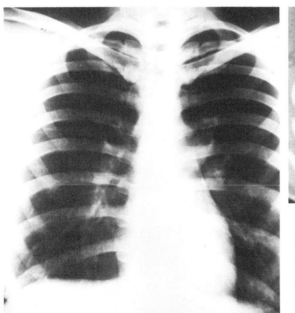

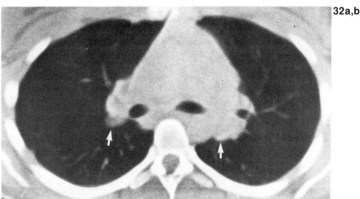

FIG. 32: Hilar adenopathy: Sarcoidosis. **a:** Normal PA radiograph. **b:** Nonenhanced section through the bronchus intermedius. Bilateral hilar adenopathy is present, deforming the contour of the right hilum posteriorly (right arrow), filling the azygoesophageal recess, and obliterating the left retrobronchial stripe (left arrow).

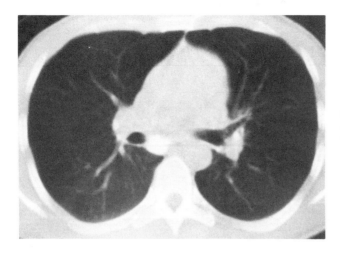

FIG. 33. Calcified hilar nodes. Except for the large subcarinal nodes, none of these nodes would be identified if it were not for calcification.

alteration in the hilar configuration, especially the large calcified subcarinal node, it is equally apparent that many of the smaller nodes would not be definable were it not for the presence of calcification.

Identification of subtle, small hilar nodes requires the use of i.v. contrast media; nodes as small as 3 mm may be defined with bolus scanning (Fig. 34). The value of this, however, must be weighed carefully in light of the clinical problem to be investigated. CT is essentially an anatomic imaging modality, and cannot differentiate inflammatory, reactive adenopathy from other causes of enlarged nodes, specifically tumor. In our experience, many patients, especially in the older age groups, have small hilar nodes. The significance of these in a large proportion of patients is debatable.

Even when nodes are known to be tumorous,

such as, for example, in patients with lymphoma, the significance of adenopathy may pose problems, especially in the assessment of follow-up studies after therapy. Lewis et al. (26) have reported four cases in which CT disclosed residual retroperitoneal "adenopathy" in patients with known lymphoma following therapy, in whom biopsy revealed fibrous tissue with no evidence of viable neoplasia. The same problem exists in patients with known metastatic disease. Libshitz et al. (27) have reported their experience with so-called "sterilized metastases," in which follow-up biopsies in patients with known tumors revealed only necrosis and/or fibrosis in persistent masses. It is to be anticipated that similar problems will be encountered in evaluating tumorous nodes in the hila. This is significant as the presence of hilar adenopathy does affect staging according to the TNM classification (22–

34a,b

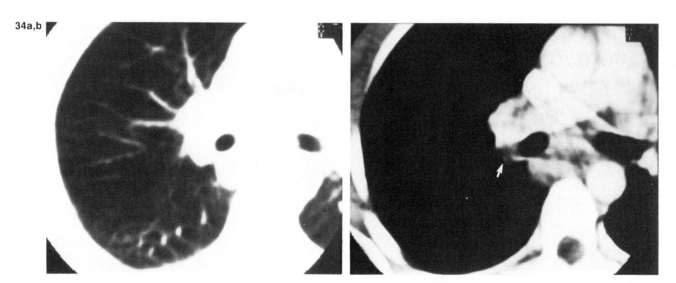

FIG. 34. Subtle hilar adenopathy disclosed by contrast enhancement. **a:** Enlargement of a section through the right hilum. Subcarinal adenopathy is apparent. The remainder of the right hilum is grossly normal. **b:** Following a bolus of contrast agent, a discrete 3 mm node lateral to the bronchus intermedius is present *(arrow)*.

25). Positive hilar nodes do not exclude surgery, although their presence rules out a segmental resection and necessitates pneumonectomy.

It is therefore clear that detection of hilar lymphadenopathy *per se* may be of limited value unless it is carefully correlated with the clinical indications for the study. For convenience, we define "significant" in a "routine" setting as adenopathy sufficiently large to only deform or distort the contour of the lung–hilar interface. In general, this corresponds to lymph nodes that are 1–1.5 cm in size. This is in keeping with most reports of established criteria for significant mediastinal adenopathy (28–32), considering that the range in size of normal hilar nodes is usually considered slightly greater than that for mediastinal nodes. It cannot be overemphasized, however, that this definition is intentionally "practicable," and subject to the limitations outlined above. That is, the significance of adenopathy can only be interpreted with reference to the clinical history, and, perhaps more important, absolute verification of the significance of any sized lymph node requires histologic correlation.

An example in which detailed evaluation of the hilus with a bolus study is of value is illustrated in Fig. 35. In this case, the patient presented with symptoms of weight loss, anorexia, and malaise; the findings suggested occult malignancy, Routine radiographs were initially interpreted to be normal. Because of a long history of cigarette smoking, a chest CT was obtained. Figure 35a is a section through the bronchus intermedius. While some fullness in the right hilum may be suspected, this image is nondiagnostic. Figure 35b is a section at the same level as that shown in Fig. 35a, following a bolus of contrast agent. A discrete mass can be identified in the right hilum, deforming the right main pulmonary artery. At biopsy, these proved to be nodes infiltrated with small cell carcinoma.

In addition to the value of CT in detecting adenopathy, CT occasionally can be used to differentiate "ordinary" from "vascular" lymph nodes. In select cases, this may suggest a specific diagnosis, as for example, A.I.L.D. (see Fig. 36).

The distribution of intravenous contrast medium within tumors is a reflection of several parameters, including blood flow, total quantity and concentration of contrast medium, distribution between the vascular and extravascular spaces, and renal function. These matters are considered in detail in Chapter 1. Marked enhancement of lymph nodes following intravenous contrast medium administration has been noted in a variety of tumors (33,34). In addition to the case of angioimmunoblastic lymphadenopathy illustrated in Fig. 36, vascular lymph nodes have been noted in cases of small cell carcinoma of the lung, vascular metastases from renal cell and papillary thyroid carcinoma, viral infections, vaccinations, and drug reactions (33,34) (see Fig. 10 in Chapter 1).

CONCLUSIONS

As has been emphasized throughout this chapter, cross-sectional imaging of the pulmonary hila is a sensitive method for detection of hilar abnormalities. CT can be used reliably to differentiate

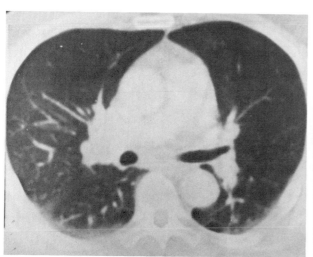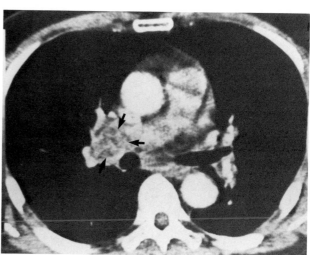

35a,b

FIG. 35. Occult carcinoma: Right hilum. **a:** Section through the right hilum, imaged with wide windows. There is some fullness in the right hilum. This image is nondiagnostic. **b:** Following a bolus of contrast agent, a discrete mass is present in the right hilum *(arrows)*.

36a,b

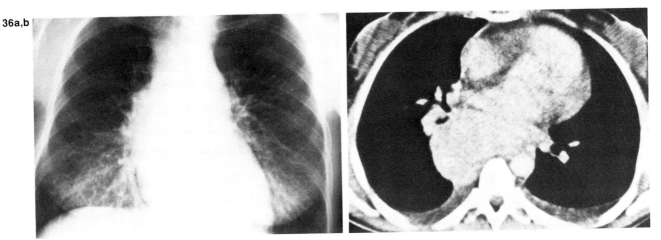

FIG. 36. Angioimmunoblastic lymphadenopathy. **a:** PA radiograph shows enlarged hila and a subcarinal mass. **b:** Post-contrast scan at level of the middle lobe bronchus. Massive adenopathy is present, showing significant contrast enhancement (compare, visually, the density of these nodes with the superior vena cava).

pulmonary vascular disease from hilar masses and adenopathy. The major limitation of CT is lack of histologic specificity. This is more than compensated for by the exquisite anatomic depiction of the extent of disease that may be uniformly obtained.

Invariably, any discussion of CT of the pulmonary hila provokes questions about the efficacy of CT as compared to routine tomography (both AP and 55° oblique). Initial comparisons were critical of CT; these studies are generally invalid, however,

37a,b

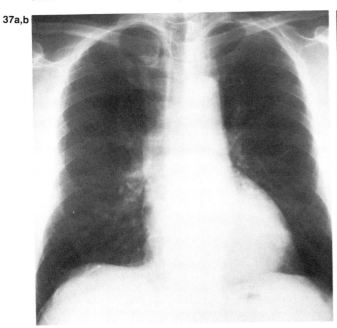

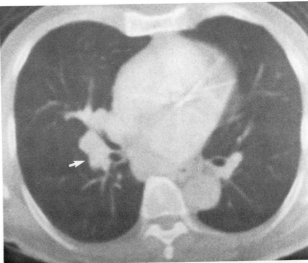

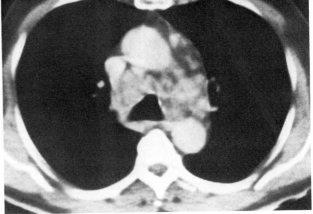

37c

FIG. 37. Lymphoma. **a:** PA radiograph shows enlarged right hilum. There is questionable mediastinal fullness on the left side. **b:** Section through the middle lobe bronchus. Characteristic nodularity can be identified *(arrow)*. Left hilum is normal. **c:** Section through the aortico-pulmonary window shows massive mediastinal adenopathy.

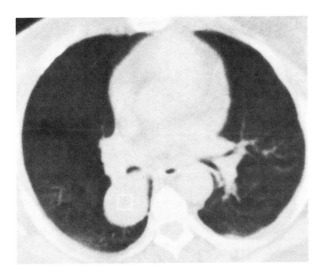

FIG. 38. Bronchogenic cyst. A discrete mass deforms the posterior wall of the bronchus intermedius. Density measurements within this lesion revealed numbers in the range of water. There was no evidence of increased density following contrast enhancement.

since many of them were performed with older units (frequently with 18-sec scan times), and more important, were conducted prior to detailed anatomic evaluation of normal cross-sectional hilar anatomy (25,30,35,36). Few prospective studies with large series of patients comparing CT with routine tomography have been conducted. Osborne et al. (37) found near-equivalence in the utility of both modalities in a large series of patients preoperatively staged for resection of bronchogenic carcinomas. It should be noted, however, that this study was confined to 42 patients with fairly advanced, stage-T2 lesions.

There are several advantages inherent in CT imaging. The first of these is the clarity of anatomic detail that can be obtained with cross-sectional imaging. The ability to visualize the hilum without intervening or superimposed structures allows precise visualization and evaluation of structures that previously were difficult to see. As has been discussed, this is especially important in assessing posterior hilar abnormalities.

Another, and perhaps more important, advantage inherent in CT scanning is that every image provides detailed information about every anatomic structure in the thorax with equivalent clarity. This frequently provides important information that otherwise could be overlooked. An example of this attribute of CT is illustrated in Fig. 37.

Finally, CT can be used to analyze tissue by means of differential density measurements. Occa-

sionally, tissue-specific characteristics allow definitive diagnosis. This is illustrated in Fig. 38 (an example of a bronchogenic cyst). Care must be taken in analyzing these lesions, since, unlike the case shown in Fig. 38, many bronchogenic cysts do not measure within the range of water. This is probably secondary to the presence of debris from exfoliated lining cells and mucoid material within the lung. However, as shown by Mendelson et al. (38) even those bronchogenic cysts with high-density measurements show no evidence of enhancement following a bolus of contrast agent. This is distinct from most solid pulmonary hilar lesions, which, even if relatively avascular, will show some increase in density following contrast enhancement.

The major use of contrast media, of course, is to differentiate between otherwise inseparable structures lying adjacent to one another. In the hilum, use of contrast medium allows definition of lymph nodes as small as 3 mm in size (Fig. 34). The problem with CT, as compared with other diagnostic modalities, is precisely its advantage of enhanced delineation of anatomy. The significance of hilar adenopathy, for example, will probably require redefinition in light of increased diagnostic accuracy.

The final role of CT in the work-up of patients with hilar disease still awaits definitive investigation. In this regard, CT will ultimately have to be compared not only with conventional radiologic technique, but with newer modalities, including nuclear magnetic resonance (39).

REFERENCES

1. Naidich DP, Khouri NF, Scott WW, Wang KP, and Siegelman SS. Computed tomography of the pulmonary hila: 1. Normal anatomy *J Comput Assist Tomogr* 5:459–467, 1981
2. Naidich DP, Khouri NF, Stitik FP, McCauley DI, Siegelman SS. Computed tomography of the pulmonary hila: 2. Abnormal anatomy. *J Comput Assist Tomogr* 5:468–475, 1981
3. Webb WR, Glazer G, Gamsu G. Computed tomography of the normal pulmonary hilum. *J Comput Assist Tomogr* 5:476–484, 1981
4. Webb WR, Gamsu G, Glazer G. Computed tomography of the abnormal pulmonary hilum. *J Comput Assist Tomogr* 5:485–490,1981
5. Glazer G, Francis IR, Gebarski K, Samuels BI, Sorensen KW. Dynamic incremental computed tomography in evaluation of the pulmonary hila. *J Comput Assist Tomgr* 7:59–64, 1983
6. Naidich DP, Terry PB, Stitik FP, Siegelman SS. Computed tomography of the bronchi: 1. Normal anatomy. *J Comput Assist Tomgr* 4:746–753, 1980
7. Yamashita H. *Roentgenologic Anatomy of the Lung*. Tokyo, Igaku-Shoin, 1978
8. Webb WR, Gamsu G. Computed tomography of the left retrobronchial stripe. *J Comput Assist Tomogr* 7:65–69, 1983
9. O'Callaghan JP, Heitzman ER, Somogyi JW, Spirt BA. CT evaluation of pulmonary artery size. *J Comput Assist Tomogr* 6:101–104, 1982

10. Mencini RA, Proto AV. The high left and main pulmonary arteries: A CT pitfall. *J Comput Assist Tomogr* 6:452–459, 1982

11. Ovenfors C-O, Godwin JD, Brito BS. Diagnosis of peripheral pulmonary emboli by computed tomography in the living dog. Work in progress *Radiology* 141:519–523, 1981

12. Godwin JD, Webb WR, Gamsu G, Ovenfors C-O. Computed tomography of pulmonary embolism. *AJR* 135:691–695, 1980

13. Godwin JD, Webb RW. Dynamic computed tomography in the evaluation of vascular lung lesions. *Radiology* 138:629–635, 1981

14. Lewis E, Bernardino MD, Valdivieso M, Farha P, Barnes PA, Thomas JL. Computed tomography and routine chest radiography in oat cell carcinoma of the lung. *J Comput Assist Tomogr* 6:739–745, 1982

15. Shields JJ, Cho KJ, Geisinger KR. Pulmonary artery constriction by mediastinal lymphoma simulating pulmonary embolus. *AJR* 135:147–150, 1980

16. Westcott JL, DeGraff AC. Sarcoidosis, hilar adenopathy, and pulmonary artery narrowing. *Radiology* 108:585–586, 1973

17. Borokowski GP, O'Donovan PB, Troup BR. Pulmonary varix: CT findings. *J. Comput Assist Tomogr* 5:827–829, 1981

18. Kleinman PK. Pleural telangiectasia and absence of a pulmonary artery. *Radiology* 132:281–284, 1979

19. Stone DN, Bein ME, Garris JB. Anomalous left pulmonary artery: Two new adult cases. *AJR* 135:1259–1263, 1980

20. Favez G, Willa C, Heinzer F. Posterior oblique tomography at an angle of 55 degrees in chest roentgenology. *Am J Roentgenol Radium Ther Nucl Med* 120:907–915, 1974

21. McLeod RA, Brown LR, Miller WE, DeRenee RA. Evaluation of the pulmonary hila by tomography. *Radiol Clin North Am* 14:51–84, 1976

22. Carr DT, Mountain CF. The staging of lung cancer. *Semin Oncol* 1:229–234, 1974

23. Carr DT. The staging of lung cancer. Editorial. *Am Rev Resp Dis* 117:819–823, 1978

24. TNM classification of malignant tumors. Joint publication of International Union Against Cancer and American Joint Committee on Cancer Staging and End Results Reporting, Geneva, 1972

25. Hughes RL, Mintza RA, Shields TW, Jensik RJ, Cugell DW. Management of the hilar mass. Clinical Conference in Pulmonary Disease. *Chest* 79:85–91, 1981

26. Lewis E, Bernardino ME, Salvador PG, Cabanillas FF, Barnes PA, Thoms JL. Post-therapy CT–detected mass in lymphoma patients: Is it viable tissue? *J Comput Assist Tomogr* 6:792–795, 1982

27. Libshitz HI, Jing BS, Wallace S, Logothetis CJ. Sterilized metastases: A diagnostic and therapeutic dilemma. *AJR* 140:15–19, 1983

28. Ekholm S, Albrechtsson U, Kugelberg J, Tyler U. Computed tomography in preoperative staging of bronchogenic carcinoma. *J Comput Assist Tomogr* 4:763–765, 1980

29. Underwood GH, Hooper RG, Axelbaum SP, Goodwin DW. Computed tomographic scanning of the thorax in the staging of bronchogenic carcinoma. *N Engl J Med* 300:777–778, 1979

30. Mintzer RA, Malave SR, Neuman HL, et al. Computed vs, conventional tomography in evaluation of primary and secondary pulmonary neoplasms. *Radiology* 132:653–659, 1979

31. Rea HH, Shevland JE, House AJS. Accuracy of computed tomographic scanning in assessment of the mediastinum in bronchial carcinoma. *J Thorac Cardiovasc Surg* 81:825–829, 1981

32. Baron RL, Levitt RG, Sagel SS, et al. Computed tomography in the pre-operative evaluation of bronchogenic carcinoma. *Radiology* 145:727–732, 1982

33. Khouri NF, Eggelston JE, Siegelman SS. Angioimmunoblastic lympadenopathy: A cause for mediastinal nodal enlargement. *Am J Roentgenol* 130:1186–1188, 1978

34. Shapeero LG, Blank N, Young SW. Contrast enhancement in mediastinal and cervical lymph nodes. *J Comput Assist Tomogr* 7:242–244, 1983

35. McCloud TC, Wittenberg J, Ferrucci JT. Computed tomography of the thorax and standard radiographic evaluation of the chest: A comparative study. *J Comput Assist Tomogr* 3:170–180, 1979

36. Hirleman J, Yiu-Chiv V, Chiv L, Shapiro R. The resectability of primary lung carcinoma: A diagnostic staging review. *CT* 4:146–163, 1980

37. Osborne DR, Korobkin M, Ravin CE, Putman CE, Wolfe WG, Sealy WC, Young WG, Breiman R, Heaston D, Ram P, Halber M. Comparison of plain radiography, conventional tomography, and computed tomography in detecting intrathoracic lymph node metastases from lung carcinoma. *Radiology* 143:157–161, 1982

38. Mendelson DS, Rose JS, Efremidis SC, Kirschner PA, Cohen BA. Bronchogenic cysts with high CT numbers. *AJR* 140:463–465, 1983

39. Webb WR, Gamsu G, Birnberg FA, Goodman P, Hedgcock M, Moon K, Hinchcliffe, WA. Nuclear magnetic resonance imaging of the thorax. *Radiology* 149:December, 1983

40. Moncado R, Demos TC, Churchill R, Reynes C. Case report. Chronic stridor in a child: CT diagnosis of pulmonary vascular sling. *J Comput Assist Tomogr* 7:713–715, 1983

Chapter 7

Pulmonary Nodule

The solitary pulmonary nodule, a circumscribed mass lesion of the lung detected by chest roentgenography, is a common diagnostic problem. Since a nodule may represent the first detectable manifestation of bronchogenic carcinoma, its discovery is a source of major concern for patient and physician alike, especially in view of the epidemic proportions reached by lung cancer over the last four decades. In 1983, approximately 135,000 new cases of bronchogenic carcinoma will be discovered, a four- to fivefold increase in incidence compared with 1940 (1).

A significant percentage of lung cancers is first discovered as solitary pulmonary nodules on a chest radiograph. In a review of 1,267 lung cancers by Theros (2), 507, or 40% of the cases were initially manifested as peripheral lung masses. In an asymptomatic individual, a bronchogenic tumor is even more likely to be located in the mid- or outer lung regions. Such was the case in 71.7% of the patients with lung cancer, detected by radiographic screening, in the series of Stitik and Tockman (3).

A lung nodule is also the most common manifestation of pulmonary granulomas and benign neoplasms, and thus represents a challenge to the radiologist from two standpoints. The first is reliable *detection*, so that early therapy can be initiated for malignant lesions, and the other is *assessment* of the nature of the lesion, so that unnecessary procedures can be avoided for benign conditions. With CT, the radiologist contributes to both of these functions, since the method depicts nodules better than conventional techniques and also provides quantitative data on X-ray attenuation values,

which can help determine the etiology of a pulmonary nodule. These two distinct roles of CT will be discussed in this chapter.

THE IMAGING ROLE OF CT

The plain chest roentgenogram remains the initial procedure of choice in the thorax. CT is not likely to become a routine screening procedure because of the associated financial and radiation costs; however, it can assist the radiologist to overcome the inherent limitations of conventional radiography in selected groups of patients.

Limitations of Conventional Radiography

There is a direct correlation between the size of a lesion and its detectability on chest radiographs. Lesions 5 mm or smaller are rarely seen unless they are densely calcified. Successful visualization of a lesion is more likely if its surroundings are not complex, its margins are sharp, and its density is high. Overlying structures, such as bones or blood vessels, can obscure nodules in front of or behind them (Fig. 1). High kVp chest radiographs, now commonly used, enhance the ability to see nodules by decreasing the prominence of the ribs. Despite this improvement, areas such as the lung apices, the costophrenic recesses, the perihilar regions, and the subpleural zones remain difficult to investigate. Conventional tomography improves the detectability of nodules in these areas by "blurring" overlying structures, thus "simplifying" the nodule environment. In the subpleural zones, conventional

1a,b

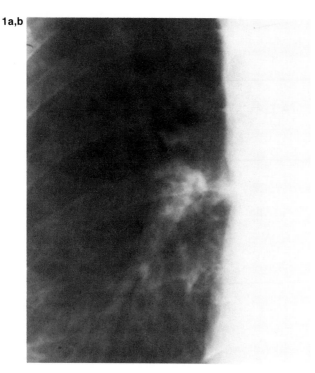

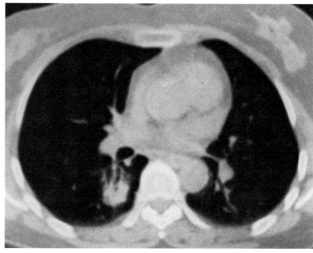

FIG. 1. Limitations of conventional radiography: overlapping structures (63-year-old female with positive sputum cytology for cancer and negative chest X-ray films). **a:** Cone-down view of the right hilum. Retrospectively, a questionable prominence of the hilum was noted. **b:** CT scan at the level of the right hilum. A large mass is appreciated. The mass overlaps the hilum in the posteroanterior (PA) axis and the spine on the lateral axis which explains why it was not detected on plain films.

tomography remains limited because of the proximity of the ribs.

Lastly, observer errors are still a major problem with conventional techniques. The "gray-on-gray" format of plain films and our inability to manipulate image contrast leads to frequent diagnostic misses. Muhm et al. (4) indicated that 90% of the peripheral cancers detected by systematic screening were present, in retrospect, for months or even years on previous films. Reading of chest radiographs by a single radiologist is associated with a "miss rate" of 30–40%. Double reading improves this figure, but only to about 20% (3).

Imaging Advantages of CT

Computed tomography reduces the error associated with conventional techniques. The cross-sectional plane of CT imaging eliminates structural overlap. Nodules in the subpleural regions or areas of complex anatomy are easily depicted. Contrast resolution is approximately 10 times greater with CT than with conventional techniques, and nodules are well-differentiated from the surrounding lung. Furthermore, the CT image can be manipulated on the display monitor. With proper electronic windows, nodules appear white on a black background, which greatly reduces errors of detection.

In the lungs, unlike other organs, the partial volume effect is sometimes advantageous. As discussed in Chapter 1, there is such a great difference in the intrinsic CT numbers of normal lung and soft tissue that even tiny nodules can be seen with sections of 10 mm or more (Figs. 3 and 4, Chapter 1). The thickest section available should be used when searching for pulmonary nodules. Thick slices allow recognition of blood vessels, by demonstrating their tubular and branching nature (see Fig. 3, Chapter 1). Small nodules that are close to vessels running perpendicularly to the scan plane are sometimes difficult to identify with CT. Examination of adjacent scans can generally solve this problem. If there is still doubt, changing the patient from a supine to a prone position will demonstrate a change in the diameter of vessels, thereby excluding a nodule. Another possible differentiating point is that, sometimes, the pulsation of vessels may create star-like artifacts around them, revealing their vascular nature (5).

The most significant disadvantage of CT is the risk of missing a pulmonary nodule because of unequal respiratory cycles or undetected patient displacement during the examination (6). Extreme care should be exercised to ensure the patient's understanding of and compliance with breathing instructions. Careful analysis of the CT images in a sequential manner is mandatory to identify discrepancies in anatomical levels. In practice, the problem of positional mis-registration does not seem very important. In a series of 52 children, who are less likely to fully cooperate, Cohen et al. (7) missed only two lesions previously demonstrated by conventional techniques. Muhm et al. (8) observed false-negative CT examinations in 4 of 91 patients with nodules. However, all four occurred early in their experience. Thus, a reasonable amount of experience and caution would seem sufficient to reduce this source of error. Control of respiratory excursion by simple feedback monitoring devices may become a practical way to solve this problem (9). When searching for pulmonary nodules, we examine patients at suspended resting lung volume, which is the most reproducible phase of the respiratory cycle.

Clinical Applications

The advantages of CT over conventional techniques apply to two clinical subgroups: patients in whom a nodule is questionably present on conventional radiographs, and patients with extrathoracic malignancies in whom undetected metastases may be present.

Questionable Nodule on Conventional Studies

An often understated advantage of CT is its ability to exclude a suspected pulmonary nodule when plain film techniques are equivocal.

Pathological data explain the better performance of CT. In a study of serial sections of resected lungs containing metastatic nodules, Scholten and Kreel (10) found 67% of the lesions in a pleural or subpleural location and 25% in the outer third of the lungs, regions which are difficult to investigate with conventional radiography. In another pathologic study by Crow et al. (11), 59% of the metastases measured 5 mm or less, sizes rarely detected with standard radiography.

In a clinical series of 91 patients with extrathoracic malignancies, Muhm et al. (8) confirmed the higher sensitivity and usefulness of CT. In 35% of the cases, they found more nodules with CT than with whole-lung tomography. In 14%, bilateral nodules were demonstrated when conventional tomography had shown only unilateral disease, and, in 5.5%, nodules were detected when none were seen with conventional techniques. Eighty-three percent of the additional nodules detected with CT were found to represent metastatic disease at surgery. These investigators concluded that CT should replace whole-lung tomography in patients with occult metastases.

Schaner et al. (12), in a prospective radiological–pathological study, confirmed that CT defined more nodules than did conventional tomography, especially in the 3–6 mm range, but 60 % of these nodules proved to be granulomas and pleural-based lymph nodes at resection. In addition, nearly one-third of the nodules discovered by CT could not be found by the surgeon. Schaner et al. stated that "until CT can be made more specific, its ability to visualize small additional nodules may not justify its substitution for conventional linear tomography."

Indeed, small lesions pose a real dilemma. They are difficult to biopsy percutaneously. Their physical consistency, which determines whether they will be palpable at surgery, cannot be predicted radiologically. Furthermore, the prevalence of granulomas in a given population will influence the likelihood of such nodules being metastatic. In areas where pulmonary granulomatous infection is endemic, the radiologist should exercise caution in reporting small lesions as metastatic.

Despite these limitations, CT remains, in our opinion, the modality of choice for detecting occult metastases, and it should not be discarded in favor of the less sensitive whole-lung tomography for the following reasons: (a) CT detects not only small nodules, but also large ones that can be overlooked on conventional studies (Figs. 1 and 5). (b) The radiation exposure is lower with whole-lung CT than with whole-lung tomography. (c) Because it is more sensitive, CT is ideal for baseline studies to monitor patients with a high probability of lung metastases. (d) Quantitative analysis of nodular density, as discussed later in this chapter, reduces the specificity problem. (e) If nodules of questionable significance are found, a follow-up CT study to determine growth will provide an answer in most cases.

Not all patients with extrathoracic malignancies should undergo thoracic CT. Additional considerations intervene in the selection of patients who would benefit from CT. The findings on the chest radiograph can guide such a decision process as follows.

Extrathoracic Malignancies and Suspected Occult Metastases

Soon after the introduction of total body scanners, the superior sensitivity of CT in the detection of pulmonary nodules was documented (14–18), and

2a,b

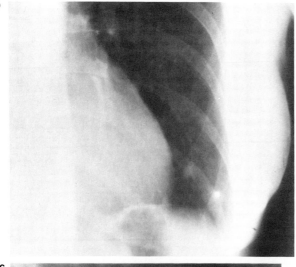
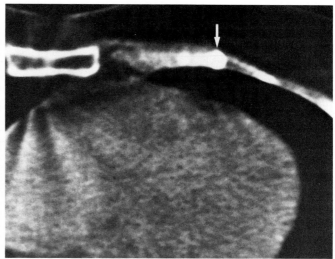

2c

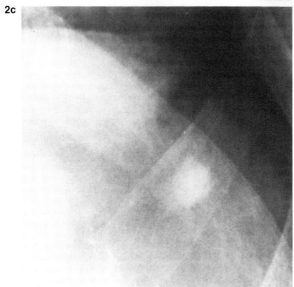

FIG. 2. Limitations of conventional radiography: chest wall lesions (58-year-old female with history of right mastectomy for carcinoma and an apparently new left lower lobe nodule). **a:** Chest radiography with nipple marker. A definite nodule density is present in the lower left lung field. **b:** CT scan. No lung nodule is seen, but in the projected area of the radiographic abnormality, a focal density in the overlying rib is noted *(arrow)*. A diagnosis of bone island was suggested. **c:** Fluorographic spot view. The diagnosis of bone island is confirmed.

the demonstration of occult pulmonary metastases in patients with known extrathoracic malignancies became a primary indication for thoracic CT.

CT should be used when the discovery of an occult lesion may have an impact on clinical management, such as when surgical resection of the primary neoplasm is not performed, when chemotherapy or radiotherapy are added to the therapeutic regimen, and when any lung metastasis found is surgically resected.

The propensity of tumors to metastasize to the lungs should also be taken into account. Gilbert and Kagan (19) have provided us with the estimated incidences of lung metastases for various primary neoplasms at presentation and at autopsy. Choriocarcinoma, renal cell carcinoma, and bone and soft tissue sarcomas are the types most likely to metastasize to the lung. CT is more likely to be of benefit in patients with such tumors (Table 1).

Patients with extrathoracic malignancies and a normal chest roentgenogram.

Pleural, skeletal, and chest wall abnormalities can simulate intraparenchymal nodules. CT easily clarifies the nature of such lesions (Figs. 2–4). Confluence of shadows may lead to the appearance of a lung nodule on plain films. CT can help define the true nature of the abnormality by showing, for instance, focal areas of linear fibrosis, vascular structures, or intralobar pleural plaques (13). Conversely, in areas in which interpretation of standard radiographs is difficult, such as the lung bases and apices, the paraspinal areas, or near the hila, CT may confirm the nodular nature of a questionable abnormality (Figs. 1 and 5). A potential pitfall with CT is the possibility of mistaking pleural nodules in the minor fissure for intraparenchymal nodules, as illustrated in Fig. 6.

3a,b

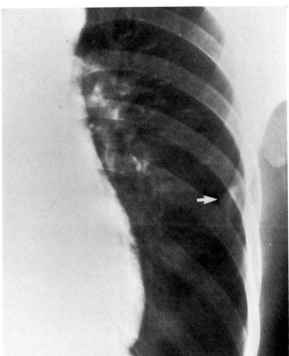 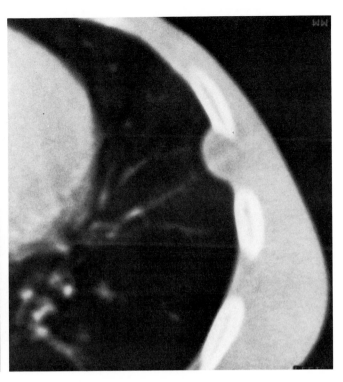

FIG. 3. Limitations of conventional radiography: extrapleural lesions. **a:** Radiographs showing a semicircular density on the lateral aspect of left chest *(arrow)*. **b:** CT demonstrates a pleural mass with smooth margins and obtuse angles. The CT numbers were low and a lipoma was diagnosed. No confirmation was obtained. By clearly showing the extrapulmonary locations of radiographic abnormalities, CT obviates the need for more invasive testing.

Patients with extrathoracic malignancies and a solitary nodule newly discovered on a chest radiograph.

CT is usually indicated in these patients for two major reasons. First, a new, solitary nodule, found a year or more after the discovery of an extra-thoracic primary tumor, is more likely to represent a primary lung neoplasm than a metastasis. In a series of 800 such patients studied by Cahan et al. (20) 63% proved to have a new, primary lung tumor and fewer than 25% had a solitary metastasis. In only 1.5% did the nodule prove to be benign. Thus, if no other lesion is found with CT, the solitary nodule should be considered to be a primary lung cancer until proven otherwise. If other lesions are seen, the nodule is more likely to be a metastasis.

Second, the patient with a solitary nodule on chest X-ray films is much more likely to harbor other lesions than is the patient without chest X-ray film abnormalities. For instance, Neifeld et al. (21) discovered additional metastases at thoracotomy in 21% of patients with extrathoracic malignancies in whom a solitary nodule was found on whole-lung tomography.

Patients with extrathoracic malignancies and multiple nodules on chest radiography.

CT is of limited usefulness in this situation unless the nodules are unilateral and clinical management would be affected by the presence of nodules in the other lung; CT can then help by excluding bilateral disease.

ASSESSMENT OF THE ETIOLOGY OF PULMONARY NODULES

Traditional Approach

One of the most challenging tasks facing the ra-diologist is distinguishing benign from malignant lung nodules. Over the years, many criteria have been developed.

The *size* of a lesion is a rough guide, with lung cancers as a group exhibiting a diameter much larger than the diameter of the group of benign le-sions. Masses larger than 3.5 cm are generally ma-lignant (22). Although smaller nodules are more likely to be benign, small size cannot be used as a

4a,b

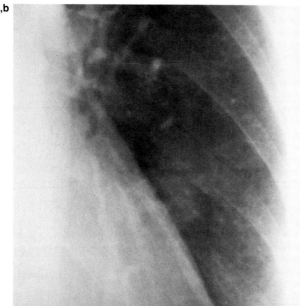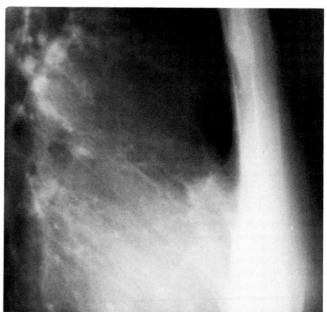

4c

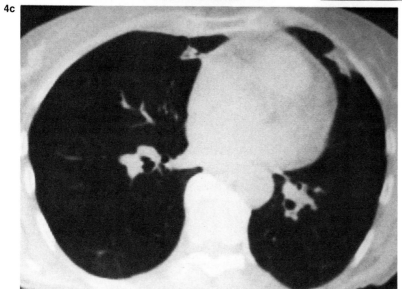

FIG. 4. Limitations of conventional radiography: pleural plaque and fibrosis. **a,b:** PA and lateral radiographs, coned down views. An irregular, spiculated, round density is seen on both views that gives the impression of a mass. **c:** CT definitely demonstrates that the mass is, in fact, an irregular, flat, pleural plaque, which does not warrant suspicion of carcinoma and should be followed conservatively. It is because the plaque is obliquely oriented relative to the PA as well as the lateral axis that it appears mass-like on PA and lateral plain films.

5a,b

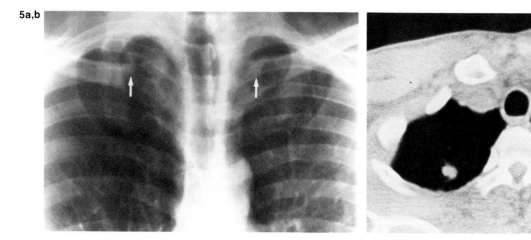

FIG. 5. CT in questionable abnormalities (42-year-old asymptomatic male smoker). **a:** Close-up view of apices reveals a small density on the right side and a similar one on the left *(arrows)*. **b:** CT reveals that the right density represents a true intrapulmonary lesion, which subsequently was proved to be an adenocarcinoma, and that the left lesion represents a tortuous subclavian artery.

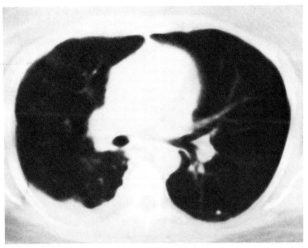
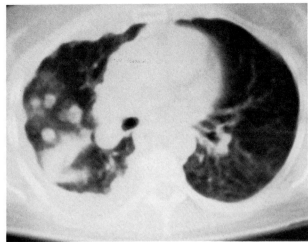

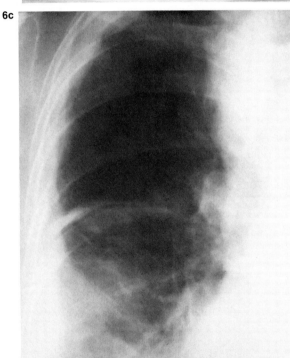

FIG. 6. A CT pitfall. The minor fissure is a potential pitfall with CT of pulmonary nodules because the CT section is parallel to the plane of the minor fissure. Pleural nodules within the fissure may be mistaken for intraparenchymal lesions (53-year-old female with malignant pleural effusion). **a:** CT scan of 10-mm-thick section. Small nodules are scattered in the right lung field. A pleural effusion is present and the pleura appears slightly lobulated medially and posteriorly. Note the absence of vascular structures (normally visible with thick sections) in the areas of the nodules. Lack of vessels is a clue to the location of the minor fissure on CT scans. The nodules were mistakenly interpreted as intraparenchymal in this case. **b:** Follow-up CT scan taken 4 months after that in (a). The nodules have grown and lobulation of the pleura is apparent. Again, note the paucity of vessels in the area of the nodules. **c:** AP chest radiograph. Large pleural nodules are apparent along the lateral wall and minor fissure. At autopsy, no intraparenchymal lesion was found.

criterion because a significant number of smaller lesions will be malignant and prognosis of lung cancer is related to size. Steele et al. (22) point out a 53% 4-year survival rate in patients with cancers less than 2 cm in size. Buell (12) predicts an 80% survival rate at 5 years for lesions measuring 1 cm or less. Detecting cancers when they are still small, therefore, is critical, and small size should not be considered evidence of benignancy. Today, awareness of better prognosis with smaller lesions is leading to the more frequent discovery of lung cancers measuring 0.5–2 cm, a distinctly unusual event in surgical series published in the 1950s (24).

Morphological characteristics, such as lobulation, notches, irregular contours, and lines extend-

ing from the nodule to the pleura, suggest malignancy, but they are not specific enough (25). It is not unusual to find benign lesions with the same characteristics.

A malignant nodule is considered unlikely below the *age* of 40, but, as pointed out by Rigler, the epidemiology of lung cancer is changing and it can no longer be safely assumed that a nodule in an individual under the age of 35 is invariably benign (25).

The *growth rate* of a nodule is a reliable indicator of its nature. Nathan et al. (26) measured the doubling times of 177 malignant and 41 benign nodules. The longest doubling time for malignancy was 6–7 months. Lesions with doubling times of 18 months

TABLE 1. *Incidence of pulmonary metastases from extrathoracic primaries (at presentation and autopsy)[a]*

Primary lesion	Presentation %	Autopsy %
Choriocarcinoma (female)	60	70–100
Kidney	5–30	50–75
Rhabdomyosarcoma	21	25
Wilm's tumor	20	60
Ewing's sarcoma	18	77
Osteosarcoma	15	75
Testicular (germinal)	12	70–80
Melanoma	5	66–80
Thyroid	5–10	65
Breast	5	60
Hodgkin's lymphoma	5	50–70
Colon/rectum	5	25–40
Head and neck	5	13–40
Bladder	5–10	25–30
Prostate	5	13–53
Non-Hodgkin's lymphoma	1–10	30–40

[a] Modified from ref. 19.

or over were invariably benign. Weiss and colleagues (27) found doubling times ranging between 1.8 and 10 months for malignancies. Active inflammatory lesions are prone to appreciable changes in size that occur in less than 1 month. Such rapid evolution is unlikely in malignancies, except for metastases from very aggressive primary lesions such as choriocarcinomas or sarcomas. Absence of growth for over 18 months to 2 years, documented by comparing previous and current chest radiographs, is the most definite indication of benignancy. In contrast to patients with extrathoracic malignancies and questionable metastases, monitoring growth rate with sequential examinations is undesirable for patients with solitary nodules which represent potential primary lung cancers. Good (28) opposed such a policy of watchful waiting because it amounts to a trade-off between prognosis, which is more favorable the smaller the lesion, and diagnostic accuracy, which would be increased when growth is demonstrated (but at the potential cost of jeopardizing prognosis).

The radiographic detection of *calcification* in pulmonary nodules indicates a very high probability of benign disease. Several series published in the 1950s reported large numbers of surgically resected calcified solitary masses that proved to be uniformly benign (28,29). Specimen radiographs of lung nodules reveal four different patterns of calcification: (a) laminated and concentric, (b) dense central nidus, (c) "popcorn" type, and (d) punctate (30). The first three types are characteristic of be-

nign lesions. The fourth type can be seen in unusual cases of malignancy. Theros (2) found only seven radiographically calcified cancers in a series of 1,267 cases. Only 2 of the 7 appeared intrinsically calcified; the remainder seemed to have engulfed nearby granulomatous calcifications.

Using all of the traditional criteria, the radiologist can, to a certain extent, reduce the number of patients with benign disease who undergo invasive procedures. In mass screening of the general population, only 3–6% of the nodules found turn out to be malignant (31,32). In surgical series, however, the percentage of malignant lesions is higher, Higgins et al. (33), in a 10-year study at the Veterans Administration, found that 36% of resected nodules were malignant. In individuals over 50 years of age, the percentage rose to 55%. Reviewing large surgical series, Siegelman et al. (24) found that benign lesions made up 60% of the resected solitary pulmonary nodules. Thus, it is evident that a significant percentage of benign lesions cannot be distinguished from malignant ones by using conventional techniques alone, which leads to a high percentage of unnecessary, invasive procedures. Because the presence of calcification in a nodule is a reliable indicator of benignancy, conventional tomography has been extensively relied on to detect calcified nodules, but, in the series of Stitik and Tockman (3), linear tomography showed unsuspected calcification in less than 4% of the cases. In a series of 294 masses considered noncalcified by standard chest roentgenography, tomography revealed unsuspected calcium deposits in five, or less than 2% (34). A more sensitive technique to assess the calcification of pulmonary nodules seems to be needed. CT, with its much better density resolution, can be utilized for this purpose.

Quantitative CT Analysis of Pulmonary Nodules

The basic assumptions underlying the use of CT to distinguish benign from malignant nodules are that (a) granulomas contain more calcium more often than do malignant tumors and (b) a large number of calcified granulomas cannot be identified as such by conventional techniques. Dystrophic calcification—the type found in granulomas—is a common end-result of many types of tissue injury. Suppurative liquefaction, coagulation, and enzymatic necrosis can all lead to the deposition of calcium salts, mostly calcium carbonates and calcium phosphates (35). Calcium and phosphorus, which are elements with high atomic numbers, increase attenuation coefficients and lead to higher CT numbers for calcified nodules.

Sagel et al. (9) first reported this phenomenon in an asymptomatic patient with two nodules apparently not calcified on conventional tomography. One of the nodules, a granuloma, had CT numbers much higher than the other nodule, a carcinoma. Similar observations were made in subsequent series by Jost et al. (17), Muhm et al. (16), and McLoud et al. (18).

Raptopoulos et al. (36), in the first systematic analysis of CT density in 31 solitary lung nodules, found five high-density nodules in which no calcification was apparent on conventional tomography. All nodules seen to contain calcification with standard techniques had calcification demonstrated by CT also, and no malignant lesion had high CT numbers.

These early studies confirmed the potential of CT in the evaluation of the pulmonary nodule, but were hampered by the absence of thin sections on the scanners used. With thick sections, partial volume averaging of surrounding air prevents the determination of the "true" CT numbers of a nodule. The thinner the sections, the more pixels will be representative of the nodules (37). CT density measurements are also dependent on the shape and orientation of the nodule, which determine the location of the pixels free of partial volume effect as well as calcification patterns (Fig. 7). Given the variations of size, shape, and orientation of lung nodules, one cannot predict which pixels will be free of partial volume effect. Thus, reliable measurements of nodule density require thin sections and a method of selecting the pixels which truly represent the nodule.

Siegelman and colleagues (38) addressed this problem and established the fundamentals of a technique to measure the density of lung nodules.

After locating the nodule with thick sections, a series of thin-section scans are obtained at suspended respiration, with slice thicknesses varying between 2 and 5 mm and not exceeding half the diameter of each nodule. To achieve more reproducible respiratory cycles, respiration is suspended at resting lung volume. The breathing instructions are "breathe in, breathe out, relax, hold your breath." For each nodule, several sections are obtained. The CT numbers representing the nodule are then printed on paper for subsequent analysis. By comparing the printouts of malignant and benign lesions in a series of 91 nodules, Siegelman et al. found that the average of the 32 highest contiguous pixels was the criterion which best dis-

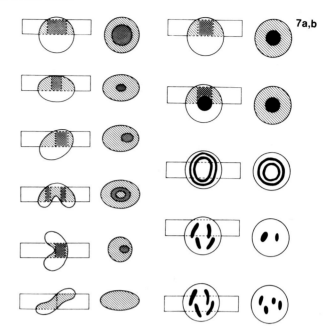

FIG. 7. Influence of shape, orientation, and calcification patterns. **a:** Homogeneously calcified nodules of different shapes are represented on the left, with the location and thickness of the CT slice used. Cross-hatched areas represent regions with no partial volume averaging. Hatched areas represent regions of the nodule where partial volume averaging with air is taking place. On the right are the resultant CT images of the theoretical nodules. Two observations can be made: first, even though the density of the nodules is homogeneous, the nodules rarely appear homogeneous with CT; and second, the location, size, and distribution of the pixels without partial volume effect will vary for the same nodule according to the orientation and position of the nodule relative to the CT slice. **b:** Round nodules with different patterns of calcification are represented on the left. The corresponding CT images are represented on the right. A dense, central nidus, as seen in the two top right models, does not systematically indicate central calcification; it may also be seen in homogeneously calcified nodules (top left). Concentric rings of calcium should also appear concentric on CT. A "popcorn" pattern, as illustrated in the lower two models on the left, may lead to a "stippled" appearance on CT, depending on the location of the slice relative to the nodule. When interpreting high-density pixels, the radiologist should be aware that the appearance and position of calcium deposits on CT does not always correlate with the plain film or tomographic patterns.

criminated between benign and malignant nodules. They defined this average as the "representative CT number" of each nodule (Fig. 8).

When the representative CT number was above 164 Hounsfield units (HU), the nodules were uniformly benign. All 58 malignant nodules had representative CT numbers lower than 147 HU, and 20 of the 33 benign lesions had representative CT numbers higher than 164 HU. Twelve additional nodules apparently calcified on chest radiographs or linear tomographs had representative CT numbers higher than 600 HU.

In three of the malignant lesions, plain film inter-

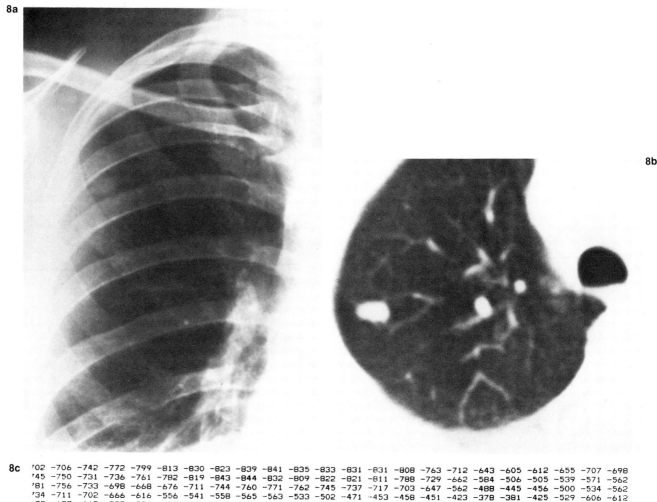

8a

8b

8c

'02	-706	-742	-772	-799	-813	-830	-823	-839	-841	-835	-833	-831	-831	-808	-763	-712	-643	-605	-612	-655	-707	-698
'45	-750	-731	-736	-761	-782	-819	-843	-844	-832	-809	-822	-821	-811	-788	-729	-662	-584	-506	-505	-539	-571	-562
'81	-756	-733	-698	-668	-676	-711	-744	-760	-771	-762	-745	-737	-717	-703	-647	-562	-488	-445	-456	-500	-534	-562
'34	-711	-702	-666	-616	-556	-541	-558	-565	-563	-533	-502	-471	-453	-458	-451	-423	-378	-381	-425	-529	-606	-612
,98	-697	-669	-598	-501	-435	-377	-331	-291	-264	-228	-213	-210	-214	-217	-214	-190	-192	-273	-403	-556	-650	-696
,21	-589	-525	-450	-371	-290	-186	-94	-35	-9	-2	-29	-23	-12	3	9	-5	-23	-136	-328	-526	-673	-750
,14	-421	-356	-295	-219	-110	-12	60	107	128	112	121	134	142	126	122	111	64	-48	-240	-460	-643	-738
,09	-298	-219	-138	-40	49	113	162	194	209	208	221	235	237	225	215	202	157	54	-112	-337	-570	-719
,65	-211	-87	22	101	139	166	179	193	237	269	257	242	260	290	313	305	255	150	-15	-254	-507	-700
,23	-136	15	105	139	151	135	144	164	182	198	214	247	276	298	305	294	273	189	29	-202	-468	-668
,28	-109	32	95	102	116	135	166	166	174	183	210	238	252	293	312	287	276	222	79	-147	-397	-621
,62	-193	-55	54	114	157	166	159	165	196	199	196	225	282	317	333	325	280	213	97	-102	-347	-555
,41	-276	-131	-17	61	110	155	184	201	238	230	238	283	344	364	354	346	319	263	151	-31	-279	-504
,26	-411	-272	-143	-39	39	96	148	174	193	204	251	294	335	342	343	330	314	264	161	-31	-281	-524
,95	-505	-397	-284	-165	-64	8	49	84	109	166	183	214	259	279	272	258	240	214	117	-75	-319	-564
'06	-623	-526	-414	-327	-242	-170	-101	-35	25	68	95	119	156	163	160	161	150	106	-11	-173	-415	-631
,29	-775	-699	-602	-537	-477	-403	-295	-204	-120	-59	-28	-29	-10	26	61	95	64	-24	-150	-318	-521	-685
,85	-844	-796	-770	-749	-705	-654	-564	-439	-321	-225	-195	-191	-184	-164	-122	-109	-155	-199	-298	-452	-593	-669
,94	-892	-896	-886	-876	-872	-829	-747	-629	-522	-426	-360	-356	-384	-395	-380	-360	-375	-441	-526	-596	-667	-702
,88	-903	-896	-888	-892	-893	-860	-790	-692	-620	-553	-507	-527	-575	-593	-571	-557	-568	-607	-673	-729	-749	-736
,92	-884	-877	-857	-863	-872	-864	-823	-774	-706	-663	-656	-681	-701	-718	-701	-685	-689	-714	-759	-795	-796	-755

FIG. 8. Numerical method of CT analysis of lung nodules. **a:** Chest X-ray film. A nodule was seen in the right upper lobe. No definite calcification was appreciated on plain films or tomography. **b:** CT scan of a 4-mm-thick section. Several sections of the nodule are obtained at suspended respiration. The section in which the highest CT numbers are observed is selected for analysis. **c:** A printout of the CT numbers representing the nodules is obtained. The highest numbers are identified within the section and the average of the 32 highest contiguous numbers is calculated; when above 164 HU, the nodule can be considered benign, as in this case.

pretation suggested the presence of calcification, but the CT numbers were below the range of calcified lesions. The investigators concluded that CT was more objective and sensitive than conventional techniques in assessing the density of solitary pulmonary nodules (38).

Attempting to confirm these results, other inves-

tigators met with varying degrees of success. Freundlich and Horsley (39) were able to use the method on a different type of scanner after defining criteria different from those of Siegelman et al. (39). Sagel (40), using a threshold CT number of 140 HU, was able to diagnose benign disease in 15% of all the cases in which conventional tomography did not suggest calcification, as compared to 22% (20 of 91 cases) for Siegelman et al.

Godwin et al. (41) measured the density of 36 nodules. All 14 malignant lesions had low CT numbers, but although 6 of the 22 benign nodules had CT numbers higher than 165 HU, only 1 of those 6 did not appear calcified using conventional techniques. Justifiably, these latter investigators questioned the usefulness of CT in the assessment of the solitary nodule.

At the time of the above-mentioned studies, partial volume effect, daily scanner variations, and the method used to compute the "representative" density of the nodule were the only elements thought to be of importance in quantitative CT measurements. The divergent results obtained by separate groups of investigators using different types of scanners led to the suspicion that other machine-related or patient-related factors were at play. Indeed, the knowledge that CT numbers are defined relative to physically constant substances such as water or air leads to the widely held belief that CT numbers are independent of scanner or patient variations. How-

ever, very early on, physicists realized that CT numbers could be influenced by a multitude of parameters (42). A systematic study of these factors, as they apply to the pulmonary nodule, explains the discrepancies noted in clinical series.

Factors Influencing Density Measurements of Pulmonary Nodules

In the chain of events leading from the interaction of the X-ray beam with the patient to the measurements of X-ray attenuation by the detectors and the computation of CT numbers, several sources of variance can be introduced. To understand the influence of these factors, we performed a series of simple experiments that clarify the effects of such variables on the CT numbers of lung nodules (43). Each experiment was designed to answer a basic question.

Experiment 1.

Are CT numbers for the same object independent of the CT numbers of the surrounding medium? If

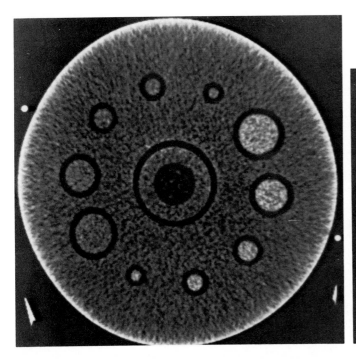
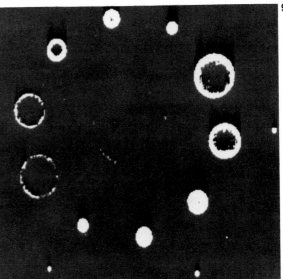

9a,b

FIG. 9. Dependence of CT numbers on surrounding medium. **a:** Syringes of different sizes and with calcium chloride solutions of different concentrations were placed within a tissue-equivalent material measuring approximately 40 HU. The appearance of the syringes is homogeneous; the CT numbers are equal, regardless of size; and the CT numbers for the higher concentration were approximately 80 HU, and for the lower concentration, 45 HU. **b:** Same syringes as in (a), scanned in air. The syringes no longer appear to be homogeneous. A rim of high numbers is seen at the edges of the syringes. Furthermore, the CT numbers of the syringes were higher than in the tissue-equivalent phantom and the smaller syringes had much higher numbers than did the larger ones. For instance, the high-density solution measured 150 HU in the large syringe and 250 HU in the small syringe. The CT numbers of the substance surrounding given objects have an influence on the CT numbers of those objects. Therefore, a CT value that may be valid in the abdomen may not be valid in the thorax. One can easily verify this fact by measuring the density of the aorta in the abdomen and the density of pulmonary arteries within the lung fields. On most scanners, their CT numbers will be different, even though the composition of the pulmonary artery and the aorta are identical.

identical syringes of different sizes containing the same substance are scanned in an abdomen phantom and in air, the CT numbers will be equal for all syringes regardless of size in the body phantom, but unequal and different in air (Fig. 9).

Experiment 2.

Are CT numbers influenced by surrounding structures? If the same syringes are now scanned within a chest phantom, the CT numbers will again be different than those measured in air or in the abdomen phantom. Furthermore, the size of the phantom will also affect CT numbers (Fig. 10).

Experiment 3.

Are CT numbers affected by machine software? On most scanners, different computer programs for image reconstruction are available. These programs are more properly called reconstruction algorithms. Some are designed to yield images with high *spatial*

resolution and some to yield images with high *contrast* resolution. If the images of Experiment 2 are processed with a high spatial resolution algorithm, the syringes will generally have high CT numbers, especially at their periphery, and the smaller syringes will appear more dense than the larger ones (Fig. 11).

With a high contrast resolution algorithm, the syringes will appear homogeneous, but their CT numbers will be low and the smaller syringes will be of lower density than the larger ones. If the same experiment is done with the syringes placed within the abdomen phantom, no difference between the CT numbers of the various syringes is noted.

Experiment 4.

Are CT numbers independent of position within the gantry? On some scanners, if a syringe is placed in various positions within the field of view, CT number values may vary as a function of position (Fig. 12).

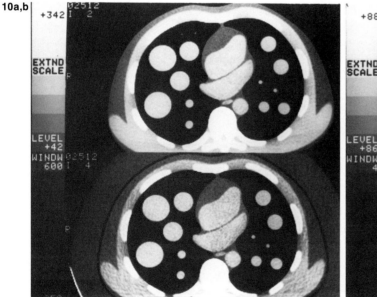
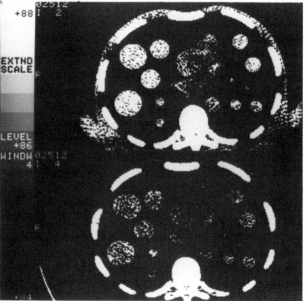

FIG. 10. Influence of surrounding structures on CT numbers. **a:** Specially designed phantom (see also Fig. 16) scanned with same technical factors but with the addition of a ring of fat-equivalent material in the lower image. The test objects are of identical composition. Note the lesser density of the "muscles" in the phantom scanned with the additional ring. The test nodules are also less dense. **b:** Same image as in (a), but at a narrower window width. The differences in CT number are more apparent, with CT densities being higher in the upper image (most probably because of a lesser beam-hardening effect). Likewise, syringes scanned in air have higher CT numbers than do syringes scanned in a chest phantom. Because of beam hardening and the different corrections included in each type of scanner, CT numbers of lung nodules will be variably affected by the patient's size and the type of scanner used, as well as by changes in the spectral energy of the X-ray tube.

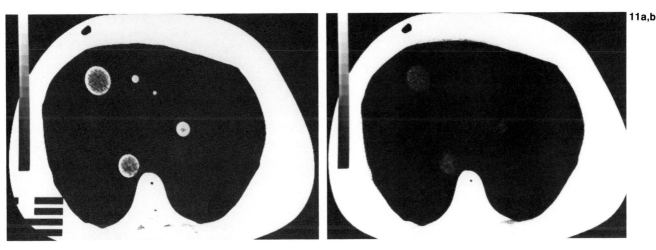

11a,b

FIG. 11. Influence of reconstruction software on CT numbers. The same set of raw data was processed with two different types of algorithms. **a:** Processing with a high spatial resolution algorithm. These algorithms are also called "sharp" because they enhance edges of structures. Spheres were scanned within a chest phantom. One can see a rim of high numbers at the edges of the spheres. The smallest sphere demonstrates numbers higher than the largest one. **b:** Image processed with high contrast resolution algorithm. These programs are sometimes called "smooth," and improve the detection of small differences in contrast. The smaller spheres have now completely disappeared from the image because their CT numbers have been mathematically averaged with the CT numbers of the surrounding air-containing pixels by the smoothing process. The CT numbers of the larger spheres have decreased markedly. The effects of the different reconstruction software programs are dependent on the density gradient between the nodules and the surrounding tissue. In the lungs, this density gradient is very large, and marked differences will be appreciated with different types of software. In the abdomen, the differences are minimal, and no significant changes in CT numbers will be observed (see also Fig. 14).

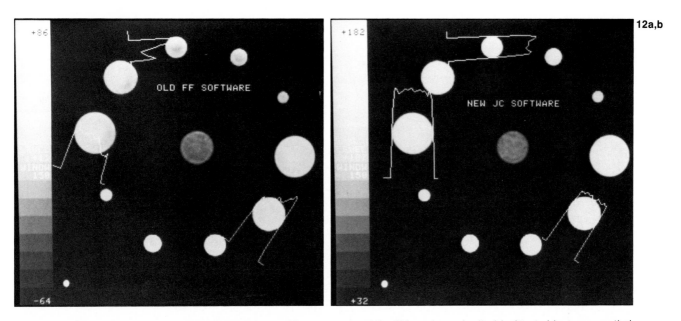

12a,b

FIG. 12. Influence of position within the field of view. **a:** Measurements of the CT numbers of cylindrical test objects across their diameter have been plotted. The plots indicate abnormally low CT numbers on the side of the test nodules nearer the center of the field of view, even though the test objects are homogeneous in composition. Depending on the position of the test object in the field of view, more or fewer variations will be seen. The least amount of variation is seen at the center of the field of view. The data were processed with a reconstruction program designated "FF software" by the manufacturer (General Electric Medical Systems). The test objects were scanned on a GE 8800. **b:** Same image as in (a), but reprocessed with a newer reconstruction program designated "JC." Made aware of the problem of positional variations, the manufacturer was able to correct this artifact by improving the performance of the reconstruction algorithms. These improvements have greatly enhanced the ability to perform quantitative studies on this type of scanner. (Partially reprinted from ref. 43 and courtesy of General Electric Medical Systems.)

Experiment 5.

Can substances of different density always be compared on the same scanner using identical measurement factors? If two identical syringes filled with substances of different densities are tested successively on the same scanner—with all other factors being equal—the absolute CT numbers of the syringes will be seen to vary over time or with different technical parameters, but the *relative* change in CT number between the two syringes will remain unchanged and we will always be able to tell which one is more dense.

These experiments reveal quite surprising results. The CT numbers of the same objects are seen to vary even though partial volume effect was eliminated by using cylindrical objects like syringes. With the thin slices (1–2 mm) now available on most scanners, volume averaging is not a significant problem except for the smallest nodules (3–5 mm). However, the true slice thickness may be different from the selected one and should always be directly verified when performing quantitative analysis to avoid errors secondary to poor collimation (Fig. 13). The experimental results here described call for a revision of the usual concepts we, as radiologists, associate with measuring CT numbers.

Interpretation of experiments.

Experiments 1, 2, and 3 identify two major facts. First, the type of reconstruction algorithm will affect CT numbers variably; second, the medium and structures surrounding a nodule influence its CT numbers.

Influence of Reconstruction Algorithm

The algorithm is a set of computer instructions used to reconstruct an image from the multiple measurements of the body sections obtained at various angles. On current scanners, each projection is transformed into a series of sinusoidal curves, which can fairly represent the original projection when added together. The process of adding and subtracting such curves is extremely easy and fast with computers. The application of such algorithms to CT reconstructions has greatly reduced image processing time. With these methods, an interesting phenomenon is seen at edges where abrupt changes in density occur: there is an overestimation of the change on the high-density side of the edge and an underestimation on the lower-density side. This "overshoot–undershoot" artifact is proportional to the amount of density change at such edges. Therefore, for a lung nodule for which density differential between surrounding air and nodule is very large, the CT numbers at the edge of the nodule (the high-density side) will be overestimated by an amount proportional to the density gradient between lung and nodule. The CT numbers of the lung immediately surrounding the nodule will be underestimated (Fig. 14). This property of CT scanner algorithms

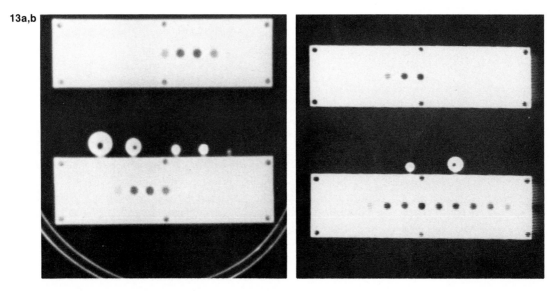

13a,b

FIG. 13. Importance of slice thickness verification. **a:** Example of properly collimated slice thickness. The thickness selected was 4 mm. Four holes are seen in the upper and lower parts of the slice thickness measuring device, indicating proper calibration. **b:** Example of poorly collimated slice thickness. For the selected thickness of 4 mm, three holes are seen in the upper part of the phantom and nine holes in the lower part, indicating inaccurate and unequal slice thickness across the field of view, probably due to poor alignment of the collimators and the X-ray tube.

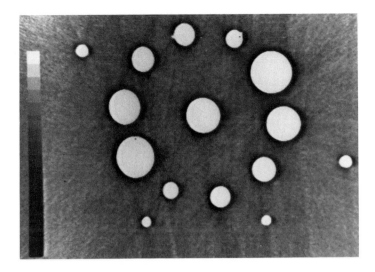

FIG. 14. The overshoot–undershoot artifact. [This figure should be viewed in conjunction with Fig. 8b.] With high spatial resolution algorithms and the current methods of image reconstruction for CT scanners, an increase in CT numbers is seen on the high-density side of edges where abrupt changes in density occur. Such an edge exists between nodules and surrounding lung. These changes are also proportional to the density gradient between nodule and surrounding tissue. This is why a rim of high numbers is seen at the edges of a nodule, as illustrated in Figs. 8b and 10a, representing the overshoot aspect of the artifact. To further support this view, the windows were manipulated on the same image as 8b to demonstrate the undershoot aspect of the artifact that is illustrated here. A dark rim of CT numbers lower than the value of the surrounding air (seen here as a gray background because of the window selection) can be identified.

has the advantage of enhancing edges, which is beneficial to *spatial* resolution. CT designers take advantage of this property by exaggerating it to further improve spatial resolution. In CT jargon, this is sometimes called "sharpening." In the lungs, the density of nodules will be overestimated with such "sharp" algorithms. Also, if an infiltrate develops around a nodule—thereby changing the lung–nodule gradient—different readings may be obtained for the same nodule. It should be noted that, in the series of Siegelman et al. (38), nodules with infiltrates were excluded from consideration. In the abdomen phantom, where the gradient between syringes and the surrounding soft tissue density is small, overshoot is minimal and the syringes appear homogeneous, as demonstrated in Figs. 9 and 15. Also, smaller nodules will appear more dense because their edges are closer together, which leads to a compounding of overshoot effects.

The random variations in CT numbers due to noise are also enhanced with sharp algorithms. Since noise decreases our ability to see structures that differ from the surroundings by only a few CT numbers, high spatial resolution algorithms are undesirable in such situations (detecting liver metastases or brain infarcts, for instance). Fortunately, noise in CT is peculiar in that it usually varies from point to point in opposite directions, i.e., if there is a positive variation at one pixel, the neighboring pixel is very likely to show a negative variation. By averaging the values of an even number of neighboring pixels, attributing this average to one of those pixels, and repeating the process for the entire image, noise can be reduced and low contrast resolution improved, as demonstrated by Joseph et al. (44). This manipulation of CT data is called "smoothing." Obviously, when this is done in a

body part in which no marked changes in density are present, CT numbers will not be much affected. On the other hand, for a lung nodule, a marked decrease in CT numbers will be observed because neighboring lung and nodule pixels will be averaged together, amounting to an effect similar to the well-known partial volume effect. The smaller the nodule, the more likely are its pixels to be averaged with the surrounding low-density lung pixels, leading to spuriously low CT numbers (Figs. 11 and 15).

There is no ideal algorithm for CT image reconstruction. Most scanners offer a choice of programs from which the radiologist can choose. None of these algorithms has been designed to properly measure the density of lung nodules. Furthermore, the degrees of smoothing and sharpening applied by each manufacturer are different, and threshold CT numbers for lung nodules will not apply from one type of scanner to another.

Influence of Surrounding Structures

As we have just discussed, certain variations in CT numbers noted between the measurements made in different media are, in part, related to the effect of the reconstruction algorithm. In Experiment 2, however, the addition of a chest phantom around the syringes also changed the CT numbers, even though the same algorithm was used. "Beam hardening," the shift toward a higher energy spectrum of the polychromatic X-ray beam as it traverses the body, accounts for this observation. As the X-ray beam becomes more penetrating near the center of the body it will be less attenuated, and the CT number of the structures near the center should decrease. With larger bodies, this effect is more

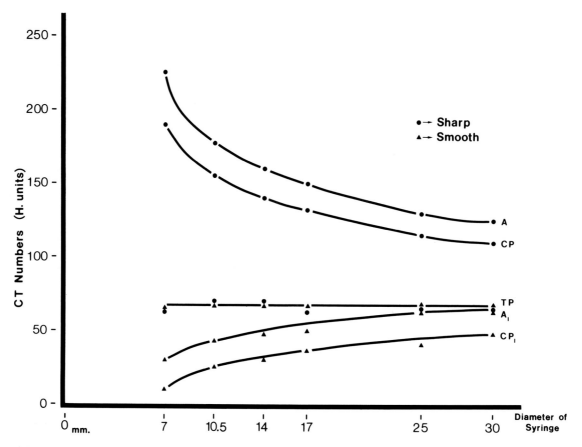

FIG. 15. Combined effects of surrounding medium, surrounding structures, and reconstruction algorithms. Plastic syringes varying in size from 7 to 30 mm in outer diameter were filled with a solution of $CaCl_2(H_2O)_2$ of 40 mg/ml of water and scanned in air, chest phantom, and tissue phantom. The raw data were processed separately with "sharp" and "smooth" algorithms. Within the tissue phantom, the CT numbers are equal and independent of size for both algorithms. CT numbers are approximately 20 HU lower in the chest phantom than in air. This is seen with both types of algorithms and is due to beam hardening. Relative to the values in the tissue phantom, CT numbers are higher with a sharp algorithm and lower with a smooth algorithm. This illustrates the effect of the surrounding medium on the performance of the reconstruction algorithm. A, air "sharp"; A_1 air "smooth"; CP, chest phantom "sharp"; CP_1 chest phantom "smooth"; TP, tissue phantom, both algorithms.

pronounced. With some scanners, increased beam hardening may lead to a decrease in CT numbers, whereas in others, an increase in CT numbers can be seen. Rao and Alfidi (45), who termed this effect the "environmental density artifact," observed a rise in CT numbers, whereas, with our scanner, we observed a decrease (43). These contradictory observations are due to beam-hardening corrections included in the reconstruction programs by the manufacturers. CT designers introduce certain assumptions of shape and density in their programs to correct for beam-hardening effects. This explains why for all scanners there are separate programs for head and body examinations. For the body programs, the shape and density assumptions are based on the abdomen and not the thorax. Depending on the difference between the body part examined and those assumptions, CT numbers will be more or less accurate, and will vary either positively or nega-

tively from their expected value. In any individual patient or scanner, it is difficult to predict whether the CT numbers of a particular object will be accurate. In our experience, CT numbers are more accurate in the abdomen than in the chest.

Positional Changes

Experiment 4 indicates another possible source of error that is difficult to ascribe to a particular cause. The lack of positional uniformity may be due to a combination of factors, such as the geometry of the scanner, the stability of the detectors, the homogeneity of the X-ray beam, and scattered radiation. If the clinical importance of CT number accuracy is given proper consideration, manufacturers can drastically improve the quantitative abilities of their programs, as demonstrated in Fig. 12.

In summary, many variables other than slice

thickness and daily electronic drifts affect the measurement of CT numbers. The specifics of the reconstruction algorithm, the size of the nodule, the structures surrounding it, and the design and stability of the scanner all prevent a meaningful comparison of data among scanners, as well as among patients. Levi et al. (46) reached similar conclusions and stated that "direct extrapolation of quantitative data between scanners, even of the same manufacturer and model, is not possible." They stressed the unreliability of CT numbers as absolute values. Sagel (40) suggested that each radiology department develop its own CT number for distinguishing calcified from noncalcified pulmonary nodules. This would be difficult and would require adequate reconstruction programs and a scanner with exceptional stability over time, ensured by stringent quality controls. These capabilities are available only in major centers.

Other Options

Analysis of pulmonary nodule density at two different kVp values, or dual-energy scanning, would, theoretically, be a better alternative to direct measurements of CT numbers. Cann et al. (47) have demonstrated the ability of dual-energy CT to quantify calcium content in phantom studies of pulmonary nodules. At lower kVp values, the CT numbers of nodules containing calcium should increase relative to the CT number obtained with higher kVp values, whereas, in noncalcified nodules, the CT number should not change. This method would have the advantage of using only relative measurements and would therefore be more reliable. However, the value of dual-energy CT in clinical testing is still unknown. Because of respiratory displacement of lung nodules, dual-energy CT methods would have to ensure that the same portion of the nodule is sampled. Dual-energy CT would also require extensive modifications of current scanners.

Another approach would be to standardize scanner designs and reconstruction programs for thoracic CT, but manufacturing standardization is unlikely to occur and would not solve the problem of time-related and patient-related variations.

Since relative measurements of the CT density of one object against another are always possible on any scanner (Experiment 5), we hypothesized that a practical way to overcome intra- and inter-scanner variations would be to use an external standard. Density assessment of nodules in patients would be done relative to such an external standard and would therefore become possible on any scanner at any given time. This external standard would have to take into account the body shape and density assumptions included in the reconstructed algorithms, as well as the nodule size and position dependence of numbers, and would simulate the patient's anatomy within acceptable limits to allow a meaningful comparison of CT numbers. A reproducible standard of density to distinguish benign from indeterminate nodules would also have to be defined. We developed such a reference phantom system to test the validity of the concept of quantitative CT analysis of lung nodules relative to an external physical standard.

Reference Phantom for Quantitative CT Analysis of Lung Nodules

Most current devices to calibrate CT scanners have well-defined geometric shapes and test patterns, with substances of known densities for assessing the physical performance of CT scanners. However, they do not take into account the numerous variables affecting the measurement of CT numbers in patients. Given the complexity of quantitative CT analysis, as discussed in this chapter, more appropriate phantoms would seem desirable. Fullerton and White (48) proposed the use of anthropomorphic test objects in CT to detect machine specific artifacts. White et al. (49) suggested the use of epoxy resin–based tissue substitutes to duplicate the shape and density of body parts for dosimetric purposes.

Based on these concepts, we designed and built a chest phantom[1] made of plastics specially formulated to simulate the CT density of the bones, muscle, and fat within two representative sections of the thorax, with dimensions and densities derived from average measurements of a series of patients (Fig. 16). Various attachments allow sufficient reproduction of the patient's anatomy at the level of the nodule to simulate the influence of surrounding structures. Lung tissue was not reproduced, since its effect on CT measurements is negligible. Within the phantom, rods of various sizes can be placed in positions similar to those of the nodules in the patient's chest. Plastic rods were selected to serve as "reference nodules" because they are not affected by partial volume averaging, due to their cylindrical shape.

The composition of the reference nodules was ad-

---

[1] Manufactured by Computerized Imaging Reference Systems, Inc., Virginia Beach, Virginia (patent pending).

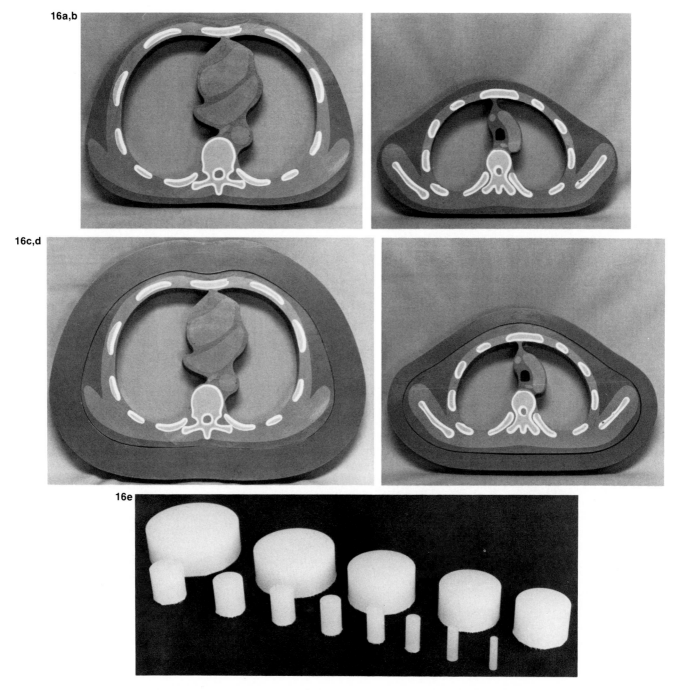

FIG. 16. Prototype model of reference phantom. **a:** Lower section of the phantom. **b:** Upper thorax section of the phantom. The average anatomy of a series of patients was reproduced using plastic materials of shapes and densities close to the shape and density of normal anatomical structures. These two sections were found to be adequate in simulating most clinical situations within the accuracy of current scanners. **c,d:** To correct for beam-hardening, rings of fat-equivalent plastic were made to fit around the phantom sections to equate the chest wall thickness of patients with the wall thickness of the phantom. An example of the medium ring is seen in (d) and a large ring is seen in (c). **e:** "Reference nodules" made of plastic rods of special composition (courtesy of Computerized Imaging Reference Systems, Inc., Virgina Beach, Virginia).

justed until a CT density of 164 HU on the scanner used by Siegelman and colleagues (38) was measured for the 1-cm (in diameter) reference nodule. On that scanner, more than 100 patients with nodules classified as benign by CT have been followed for more than 2 years, without any errors.

The Phantom Technique

The essentials of the technique are similar to those described by Siegelman et al. (38), except that all patients are scanned with the thinnest section available on the scanner, i.e., 1–2 mm. Several sections of the nodule in suspended respiration are obtained first. Immediately thereafter, the phantom parts are mounted on a scanning support in a configuration that is as similar as possible to the patient's anatomy at the level of the nodule. A plastic reference nodule of a size equal to the average diameter of the patient's nodule is then placed within the phantom in the same position as the actual nodule in the patient's chest (Fig. 17). The phantom with reference nodule in place is then scanned immediately after completion of the patient's study and with the same technical factors as those used for the patient.

The images of the patient's nodule and the images of the phantom reference nodule are then compared on the display monitor. Numerical printouts are not necessary with this method.

By using a very narrow window width, it is easy to determine whether the patient's nodule is more or less dense than the reference nodule (Fig. 18).

We have reported preliminary results with the phantom method from a series of 35 patients with 41 apparently noncalcified nodules, and found that all 24 malignant lesions had CT numbers lower than those of the reference nodule within the phantom, and that 11 of the 17 benign lesions had CT numbers higher than those of the reference nodule (50). More than 250 patients have now been examined at different centers with different scanners, and preliminary results support the view that CT assessment of lung nodule density relative to an external standard is a practical and generally applicable method that can reliably detect calcified nodules.

The role of CT in the assessment of pulmonary nodules is still evolving. Further investigations will

17a,b

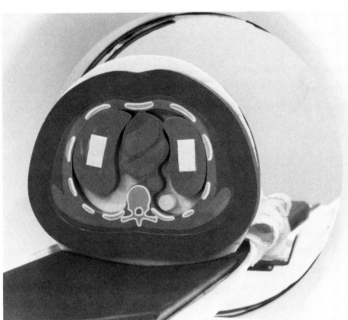 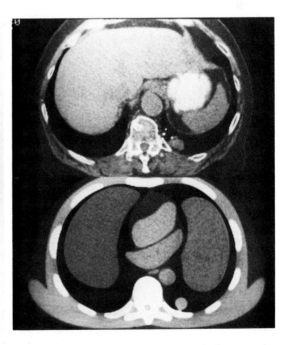

FIG. 17. Examples of patient simulation. **a:** The phantom can be mounted on a vertical board covered with Velcro. In the example illustrated, the lower thorax section is used with a large fat ring, which would correspond to an obese patient. Attachments can be added within the lung fields to simulate the effect of the diaphragms when the lung nodule is situated low in the thorax. A reference nodule made of a plastic rod of special composition can also be placed in any position within the lung fields of the phantom, using Velcro backing. The phantom and the nodule can be shifted in position to reproduce the same position as that of the patient and the nodule being examined. **b:** A clinical example somewhat similar to (a) is illustrated. In the top image, the CT scan of the patient is displayed. A mass is seen in the left costophrenic angle. In the bottom image, the lower thorax section of the phantom was used with diaphragm simulators in place and a nodule in a position similar to that of the patient's nodule. No additional fat rings were necessary in this case, the chest wall thickness of the patient and the wall thickness of the phantom being adequately matched. Even though the simulation is not anatomically perfect, it allows comparison within the accuracy of current CT scanners (5–10 HU).

18a,b

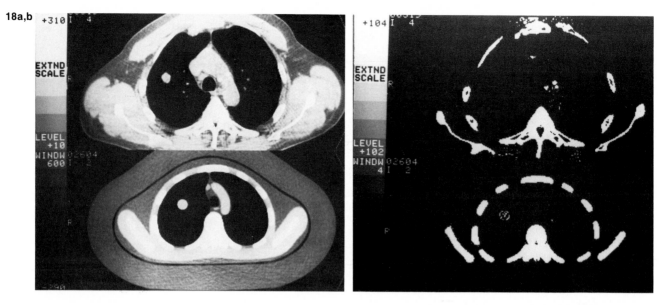

FIG. 18. Phantom method for CT analysis of lung nodules (53-year-old male with right upper lobe adenocarcinoma). **a:** The patient's scan is displayed in the upper image. The scan of the reference phantom with ''reference nodule'' in position is shown in the lower image. A fat-equivalent ring of appropriate thickness was added to the upper thorax section of the phantom to simulate the chest wall thickness of the patient. The same technical factors were used to scan patient and phantom. The phantom was scanned immediately after completion of the patient's study to avoid time-related drifts. To interpret the images no computer printouts are needed. **b:** Method of interpretation. The same image as in (a) is displayed, but the window width is reduced to a minimum, 4 HU in this case. The window level is then progressively moved up until either the patient's nodule or the phantom's nodule disappears from view. In the case illustrated, the patient's nodule is no longer visible at 102 HU, whereas the phantom's nodule is still visible. This indicates that the patient's nodule is not sufficiently dense to be considered benign and should be investigated further. If simultaneous double display is not available on the scanner, the phantom can be viewed first, and the window level moved up until the reference nodule disappears; then the patient's images are displayed using that particular window level and the narrowest window width.

19a,b

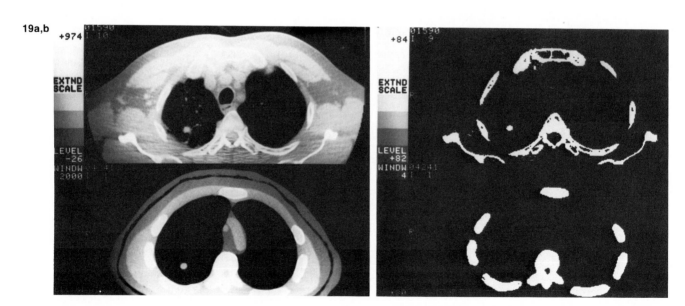

FIG. 19. Definite diagnosis of benign disease (63-year-old patient with right upper lobe nodule found on routine examination). **a:** Patient's scan is the upper image. The nodule is clearly identified and its irregular margins noted. A phantom simulation is the lower image. (The phantom illustrated here is an older prototype.) **b:** In an intrepretation at a window width of 4 HU and a window level of 82 HU, the phantom reference nodule has completely disappeared, but the patient's nodule is still entirely visible. In such cases, we are most confident of the diagnosis of benign disease. Note that the level at which the reference nodule disappeared is 82 HU, whereas in the case illustrated in Fig. 18, the reference nodule is still visible at 102 HU, illustrating the variation in threshold CT numbers.

be required to definitively address all the issues related to this technique. For instance, the definition of "significant calcification" is a most important consideration. Some carcinomas contain small foci of intrinsic calcification or exhibit calcium deposits within prior granulomas engulfed by the growing neoplasm. CT, being more sensitive in detecting calcification, may also be more likely to visualize calcium deposits in cancers where none would have been seen with conventional techniques. How does one distinguish benign calcified masses from cancers with calcification? All current criteria have been empirically derived from clinical experience, and more basic work, such as histopathologic determination of calcium content in lung neoplasms, would have to be done.

We are most confident of the diagnosis of benign disease when the entire lesion exhibits attenuation

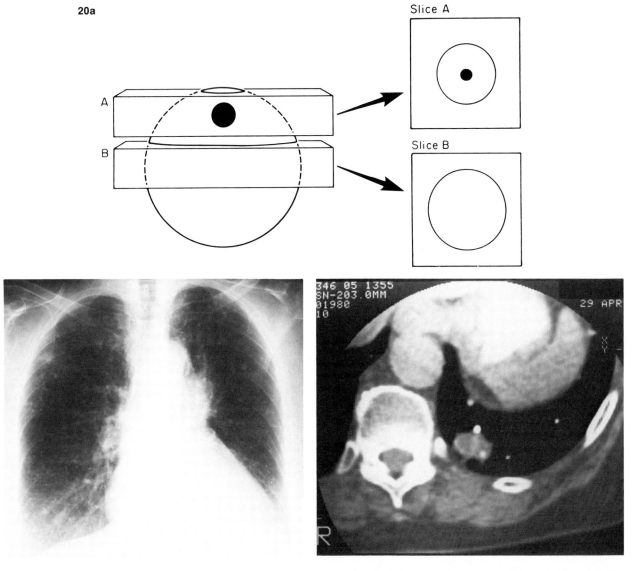

FIG. 20. Eccentric calcifications and need for visualization of high-density pixels on several sections. **a:** Theoretical model. If a nodule with an eccentric calcification is scanned with slice A, a zone of high density will be seen in the center of the nodule, giving the impression of a central nidus that is very suggestive of a benign lesion. However, if contiguous sections, such as slice B, do not show any evidence of calcification, a pattern of "central nidus" calcification cannot be assumed. Analysis of several sections is mandatory. **b:** Chest X-ray film of a patient with history of chicken pox pneumonia in childhood. Numerous, small, calcified granulomata are seen. **c:** CT scan of an incidentally discovered left lower lobe mass. (This is the same patient as the patient illustrated in Fig. 17b, but the sections are different.) Note that several eccentric foci of calcifications are seen on separate sections, but are not contiguous. This case is presented to demonstrate the need for careful analysis of contiguous sections. In this case, an adenocarcinoma has grown to involve several surrounding calcified granulomata. The foci of calcification are eccentric and represent only a small portion of the lesion. Benign disease is more likely when areas of high CT numbers are contiguous on several sections.

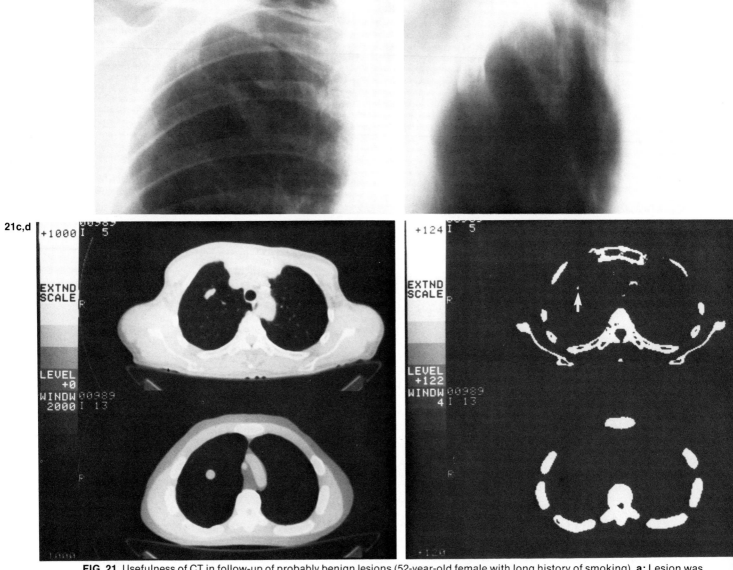

FIG. 21. Usefulness of CT in follow-up of probably benign lesions (52-year-old female with long history of smoking). **a:** Lesion was discovered on a routine chest X-ray film in the right upper lobe. **b:** A tomogram was performed, which showed no evidence of significant calcification. **c,d:** A density analysis was performed relative to a reference phantom. At a level of 122 HU, a cluster of high-density pixels was noted in the patient's nodule *(arrow)*. We made a diagnosis of probable benign disease and recommended close follow-up or needle biopsy. Close follow-up was selected.

values in excess of the reference standard (Fig. 19). Lesions larger than 1 cm in diameter should contain a dense zone which measures at least 3.5 mm in diameter and exceeds the density of the reference standard. For lesions 1 cm or smaller in diameter, partial volume effects become significant. In the initial study of Siegelman et al. (38), the numbers of voxels chosen for calculating the representative CT number varied with the size of the nodule. Since a 304.8 mm field of reconstruction was used in conjunction with a 512 × 512 matrix, each voxel had

dimensions of .6 × .6 mm. For evaluating lesions of 10, 9, 8, 7, 6, and 5 mm in diameter, 32, 24, 20, 16, 12 and 8 contiguous voxels were used. Using the computer printout and the designated number of voxels, a reference CT number was calculated for each lesion. Since the representative CT number is an average, many cases had some voxels with CT numbers below the critical level of 164 HU. In the vast majority of cases, however, two-thirds of the chosen voxels had values exceeding 164 HU. Hence, in evaluating small lesions against a reference stan-

FIG. 21 (*cont.*). **e:** A follow-up chest X-ray film 2 months after the initial examination showed apparent growth of the lesion. The patient was then admitted with the working diagnosis of carcinoma. **f,g:** A repeat study of the nodule with CT was elected. The patient's scan is the upper image and the phantom scan is the lower image. In (f), interpretation at narrow window width demonstrated more pixels of high density relative to the reference nodule in the patient's lesion than on the previous examination shown in (c). Because more than half of the lesion was calcified centrally, we made the diagnosis of calcifying granuloma in evolution. Surgery was nonetheless performed and the diagnosis was confirmed. This case illustrates two points: First, the appearance of increase in size on the chest X-ray film was probably due to slight changes in orientation and an intrinsic increase in density due to increasing calcification. If the tomogram obtained on the first examination in (b) is compared to the follow-up chest X-ray film in (e), no large difference in size is noted. Because CT can avoid errors of projection, it is more reliable in assessing growth. Second, because we used an external standard such as the phantom we felt very confident that, indeed, more calcium had deposited in the lesion and that technical variations were not responsible for the finding of a larger number of high-density pixels.

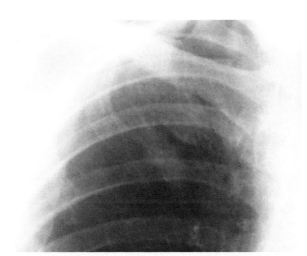

21e

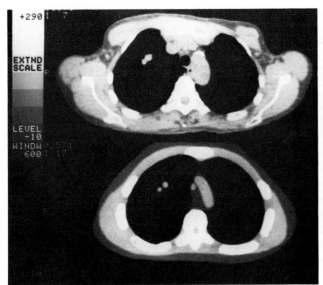 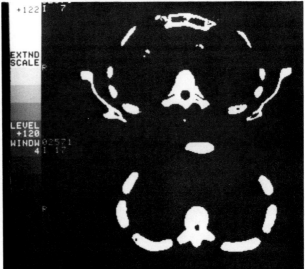

21f,g

dard, the equivalent of 21, 16, 12, 10, 7, and 5 (.6 × .6 mm) voxels should exceed the attenuation values of the standard.

If the dense voxels are centrally located, the diagnosis of benign disease is firmer. Central location of the dense voxels is not, however, a necessary condition, because the shape, orientation, and reconstruction software may affect the location of the denser pixels even in uniformly calcified lesions as demonstrated in Fig. 7.

High attenuation values should be seen on several different sections to avoid confusion with an eccentric granuloma adjacent to a malignant lesion (Fig. 20).

The appearance of the margins of lesions is also an important factor in cases which do not fit all the criteria for definitely benign lesions. Occasional borderline cases will be encountered in which the lesion is small, smooth and with clusters of CT numbers slightly lower than the reference nodule or threshold number, therefore not quite satisfying the criteria for benignancy. In such cases, we discuss the situation with the patient and the referring physician, indicating that a slight but definite risk of malignancy exists and advising either needle biopsy or more careful observation with repeat chest X-ray films at 2 and 4 months and repeat CT scan at 6 months. We believe that repeat CT studies are more reliable than chest roentgenograms in determining the presence or absence of growth in questionable cases, as illustrated in Fig. 21.

There is a remote possibility that a scar carcinoma developing in association with a prior granuloma may completely encircle it, thus creating the appearance of central calcification. We have seen such a case, but the lesion had fuzzy, irregular margins and was not considered to be definitely benign. An eccentric small cluster of high attenuation values in a predominantly low-density lesion with irregular margins is suggestive of scar carcinoma.

There have been cases of central carcinoid tumors that presented as mass lesions with definite foci of calcification. In each instance, however, a carcinoid tumor was correctly diagnosed because the mass was immediately contiguous to a secondary bronchus (51). We have not seen calcified carcinoid tumors in the lung periphery. In rare instances, intrinsically calcified carcinomas can be observed, but they are usually very large and the amount of calcification represents a small portion of the total lesion (Fig. 22). More commonly, a carcinoma is found adjacent to a calcified granuloma (Fig. 20).

In patients with bone sarcomas, metastatic nodules may be calcified, and CT is not helpful in assessing the nature of lesions in such patients. Calcified metastases can also be seen with synovial sarcoma (52).

Obviously, when no high-density pixels are found in a lesion, the diagnosis is indeterminate, and further investigations are necessary. This is especially true in patients with small, benign-appearing lesions on conventional studies in whom an indeterminate CT examination helps prompt timely invasive procedures (Fig. 23).

As experience with the technique increases, more precise criteria will be defined. Likewise, limitations will become more apparent. For example, X-ray attenuation measurements of cavitated lesions can be misleading, with spuriously high CT numbers often being observed (Fig. 24). We do not attempt to make a definite assessment of cavitated lesions. Cavitation places a nodule in the indeterminate category.

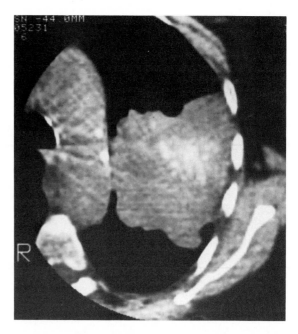

FIG. 22. Intrinsically calcified carcinoma (patient with large adenocarcinoma with centrally located cluster of calcifications). Truly calcified carcinomas can be seen with CT, and more such cases are likely to be detected. The process of dystrophic calcification is not specific to benign lesions; it can be seen in necrotic tumors. This was the case in the patient illustrated here. However, despite the presence of relatively large amounts of calcium, this lesion cannot be considered to be benign if we apply our criteria.

Motion artifacts are another technical limitation, and are very difficult to control when the nodule is located near the left heart border because of transmitted cardiac pulsations. Motion artifacts can also interfere with density measurements in other parts of the lung and create falsely high attenuation values (Fig. 25). One cannot reach a valid conclusion about the nature of a nodule if persistent motion artifacts are present.

CONCLUSIONS

Computed tomography is a valuable technique for assessing the density of pulmonary nodules. Complex technical factors prevent us from defining a single CT value applicable to all scanners. Measurements relative to an external standard are more reliable, are simpler to apply, and permit a generalization of the method.

When reliable CT measurements can be obtained, CT should replace conventional tomography, not only because it may be the only technique indicating calcification in a significant percentage of cases but also for the following reasons: (a) Lesions that are thought to be calcified on conventional studies

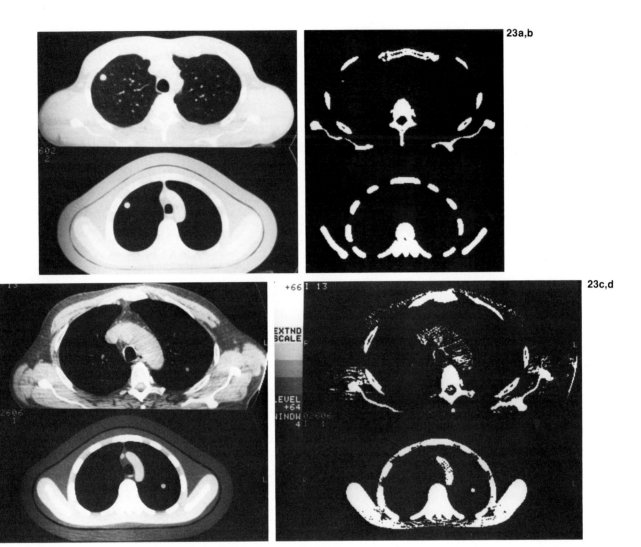

FIG. 23. Advantage of CT in small lesions. Two apparently similar lesions are illustrated. **a,b:** A 58-year-old male with newly discovered, small right upper lobe nodule, measuring approximately 1 cm in diameter. In (a), patient and phantom are scanned at usual window widths. In (b), a comparison is made. At 122 HU, a cluster of high-density pixels is still visible in the patient's nodule, whereas no reference nodule pixels are seen, indicating a very high probability of benign disease. The patient was conservatively followed for more than 12 months without change. **c,d:** 62-year-old male with an even smaller lesion newly discovered in the left upper lobe. In (c), patient and phantom images are displayed simultaneously. Visual density analysis relative to the phantom in (d) shows complete disappearance of the patient's nodule at a level of 64 HU, which indicates total absence of significant calcification. The diagnosis is indeterminate in this case. More invasive tests were recommended. Because of the size of the lesion, needle biopsy could not be performed. At surgery, a small cell carcinoma was found.

24a,b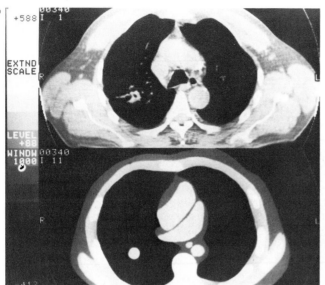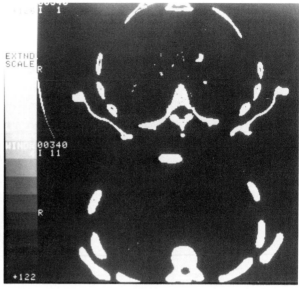

FIG. 24. Misleading effect of cavitation. During investigation for a right upper lobe mass, a CT study was performed, which revealed cavitation within the mass. Evaluation of the density of the mass with reference to a lung nodule phantom was performed. **a:** The cavitated lesion is seen in the right upper lobe (top image). An early prototype phantom is displayed in the lower image. **b:** Patient–phantom comparison. At a level of 124 HU, two clusters of high-density pixels are seen in the lesion. At surgery, this lesion proved to be a squamous cell carcinoma. Histopathologic examination revealed no evidence of calcium. For as yet unclear reasons, cavitated lesions seem to generate falsely high CT values. Density assessment of such lesions should not be attempted. The finding of cavitation in a lung nodule, even in the presence of high-density pixels, cannot be interpreted as benign disease.

can sometimes be shown to be noncalcified by CT, which helps justify the prompt use of more invasive procedures, to the benefit of the patient. (b) With the proper technique, nodules that are calcified on conventional studies are invariably found to be calcified with CT, and the risk of misinterpreting a lesion that is calcified on conventional studies as indeterminate with CT appears minimal. Thus, CT does not need to be performed in addition to conventional tomography. (c) Some lesions that seem to be intrapulmonary on conventional studies can be shown to be extrapulmonary, or to represent areas of focal fibrosis with CT, thereby preventing more invasive procedures. (d) CT provides additional useful information in planning for needle biopsy of indeterminate lesions when necessary.

The better depiction of pulmonary nodules due to the cross-sectional plane of imaging, the higher contrast resolution of CT, and the ability to manipulate the display format help overcome the limitations of conventional techniques. From the imaging standpoint, CT is useful in excluding or confirming the presence of pulmonary nodules questioned on plain films.

Because it is more sensitive than conventional techniques in detecting occult metastases, CT plays an important role in patients with extrathoracic malignancies, which have a high propensity to metastasize to the lungs. With a moderate amount of experience, reliable examinations of the thorax can be achieved, which provide a greater degree of diagnostic confidence when looking for additional lesions in patients having extrathoracic malignancies with solitary or multiple unilateral nodules.

After an initial period of some confusion due to unappreciated technological problems, it now appears that quantitative CT analysis of lung nodules can be a valuable tool in the investigation of patients with solitary pulmonary nodules. The problem of technical variations within the same scanner, among scanners, and among patients can be solved by the use of an external standard, such as an anthropomorphic phantom with "reference nodules," relative to which the density of pulmonary nodules can be reliably and easily assessed. Further experience in larger series of patients is still needed to refine the particulars of the technique and the interpretation of quantitative CT studies of pulmonary

25a

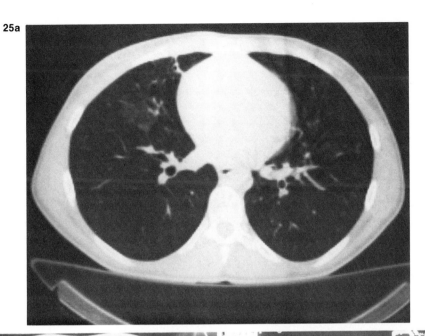

5b,c

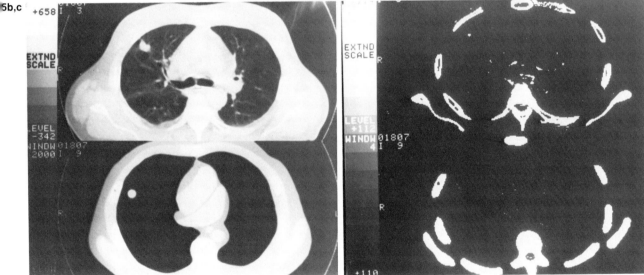

FIG. 25. The motion artifact problem. **a:** Because of the more prominent pulsations of the left side of the heart, significant motion artifacts can be created, especially when high exposure factors are used (over 250 MaS). Three linear bands of lucency are seen adjacent to the left heart border in this case, for which the exposure was 600 MaS. **b:** Motion artifacts can also be a problem in other areas of the lungs and, when present, can sometimes create falsely high CT numbers. The upper image is the patient's scan. The vessels appear blurred and the outline of the lesion is also fuzzy. These findings suggest that significant motion occurred during the scan. **c:** Density assessment at a level of 112 HU. A large cluster of high-density pixels is seen in the patient's lesion (top), strongly suggesting benign disease. Follow-up chest radiography showed an increase in the lesion size, which was confirmed by CT. Adenocarcinoma was diagnosed by needle biopsy. Pathologic examination after surgical removal showed no evidence of calcium in the lesion. If motion artifacts are present on a CT section, density assessment should not be attempted with that particular section.

nodules. A generalization of the CT method may, it is hoped, reduce the number of unnecessary procedures in patients with calcified nodules not characterized as calcified by traditional techniques.

REFERENCES

1. American Cancer Society. Cancer statistics 1983. *CA* 33: 16–17, 1983
2. Theros EG. Caldwell lecture: Varying manifestations of peripheral pulmonary neoplasms. A radiologic-pathologic correlative study. *AJR* 128:893–914, 1977
3. Stitik FP, Tockman MS. Radiographic screening in the early detection of lung cancer. *Radiol Clin North Am* 16:347–366, 1978
4. Muhm JR, Miller WE, Fontana RS, Sanderson DR, Woolner LB, Uhlenhopp MA. The radiologic appearance of lung cancer detected by four monthly screening chest X-rays in the Mayo lung project. Presented at the Radiological Society of North America Meeting, Chicago, November 1982
5. Kuhns LR, Borlaza G. The "twinkling star" sign. An aid in differentiating pulmonary vessels from pulmonary nodules on computed tomograms. *Radiology* 135:763–764, 1980
6. Krudy AG, Doppman JL, Herdt JR. Failure to detect a 1.5 centimeter lung nodule by chest computed tomography. *J Comput Assist Tomogr* 6:1178–1180, 1982
7. Cohen, M, Grosfeld J, Baehner R, Weetman R. Lung CT for detection of metastases: Solid tissue neoplasms in children. *AJR* 139:895–898, 1982
8. Muhm JR, Brown LR, Crowe JK, Sheedy PF, Hattery RR, Stephens DH. Comparison of whole lung tomography and computed tomography for detecting pulmonary nodules. *AJR* 131:981–984, 1978
9. Robinson PJ, Jones KR. Improved control of respiration during computed tomography by feedback monitoring. *J Comput Assist Tomogr* 6:802–806, 1982
10. Scholten ET, Kreel L. Distribution of lung metastases in the axial plane: A radiological-pathological study. *Radiol Clin (Basel)* 46:248–265, 1977
11. Crow, J, Salvin G, Kreel L. Pulmonary metastasis: A pathologic and radiologic study. *Cancer* 47:2595–2602, 1981
12. Schaner EG, Chang AE, Doppman JL, Conkle DM, Flye MW, Rosenberg SA. Comparison of computed and conventional whole lung tomography in detecting pulmonary nodules: A prospective radiologic-pathologic study. *AJR* 131:51–54, 1978
13. Webb WR, Cooper C, Gamsu G. Interlobar pleural plaque mimicking a lung nodule in a patient with asbestos exposure. *J Comput Assist Tomogr* 7:135–136, 1983
14. Sagel SS, Stanley RJ, Evans RG. Early clinical experience with motionless whole-body computed tomography. *Radiology* 119:321–330, 1976
15. Stanley RJ, Sagel SS, Levitt RG. Computed tomography of the body: Early trends in application and accuracy of the method. *AJR* 127:53–67, 1976
16. Muhm JR, Brown LR, Crowe JK. Detection of pulmonary nodules by computed tomography. *AJR* 128:267–270, 1977
17. Jost RG, Sagel SS, Stanley RJ, Levitt RG. Computed tomography of the thorax. *Radiology* 126:125–136, 1978
18. McLoud TC, Wittenberg J, Ferrucci JT. Computed tomography of the thorax and standard radiographic evaluation of the chest: A comparative study. *J Comput Assist Tomogr* 3:170–180, 1979
19. Gilbert HA, Kagan AR. Metastases: Incidence, detection and evaluation without histologic confirmation. In: *Fundamental Aspects of Metastasis*, ed. by L Weiss. Amsterdam, North-Holland Publishing Co, 1976
20. Cahan WG, Shah JP, Castro ELB. Benign solitary lung lesions in patients with cancer. *Ann Surg* 187:241–249, 1978
21. Neifeld JP, Michaelis LC, Doppman JL. Suspected pulmonary mestastases—Correlation of chest X-ray, whole lung tomograms and operative findings. *Cancer* 39:383–387, 1977
22. Steele JD, Kleitsch WP, Dunn JE, Buell P. Survival in males with bronchogenic carcinomas resected as asymptomatic solitary pulmonary nodules. *Ann Thorac Surg* 2:368–373, 1966
23. Buell PE. The importance of tumor size in prognosis for resected bronchogenic carcinoma. *J Surg Oncol* 3:539–551, 1971
24. Siegelman SS, Stitik FP, Summer WR. Management of the patient with a localized pulmonary lesion. In: *Pulmonary System. Practical Approaches to Pulmonary Diagnosis*, ed. by SS Siegelman, FP Stitik, WR Summer. New York, Grune and Stratton, 1979
25. Rigler LG. An overview of cancer of the lung. *Semin Roentgenol* 12:161–164, 1977
26. Nathan MH, Collins VP, Adams RA. Differentiation of benign and malignant pulmonary nodules by growth rate. *Radiology* 79:221–227, 1962
27. Weiss W. Boucot KE, Cooper DA. Survival of men with peripheral lung cancer in relation to histologic characteristics and growth rate. *Am Rev Respir Dis* 98:75–92, 1968
28. Good CA. The solitary pulmonary nodule: A problem of management. *Radiol Clin North Am* 1:429–437, 1963
29. Good CA, Hood RT, McDonald JR. Significance of a solitary mass in the lung. *Am J Roentgenol Radium Ther Nucl Med* 70:543–554, 1953
30. O'Keefe ME Jr, Good CA, McDonald JR. Calcification in solitary nodules in the lung. *Am J Roentgenol Radium Ther Nucl Med* 77:1023–1033, 1957
31. Holin SM, Dwork RE, Glaser S, Rikli AE, Stocklen JB. Solitary pulmonary nodules found in a community-wide chest roentgenographic survey: A five year follow-up study. *Am Rev Tuberculosis* 79:427–439, 1959
32. McClure CD, Boucot KE, Gilliam AG, Milmore BK, Lloyd JW. The solitary pulmonary nodule and primary lung malignancy. *Arch Environ Health* 3:127–139, 1961
33. Higgins GA, Shields TW, Keehn RJ. The solitary pulmonary nodule. Ten year follow-up. Veterans Administration–Armed Forces cooperative study. *Arch Surg* 110:570–575, 1975
34. Good CA, Wilson TW. The solitary circumscribed pulmonary nodule. *JAMA* 166:210–214, 1958
35. Robbins SL. *Pathology*, 3rd ed. Philadelphia, W.B. Saunders, 1968, pp 403–407
36. Raptopoulos V, Schellinger D, Katz S. Computed tomography of solitary pulmonary nodules: Experience with scanning times longer than breathholding. *J Comput Assist Tomogr* 2:55–60, 1978
37. Godwin JD, Fram EK, Cann CE, Gamsu GG. CT densitometry of pulmonary nodules: A phantom study. *J Comput Assist Tomogr* 6:254–258, 1982
38. Siegelman SS, Zerhouni EA, Leo FP, Khouri NF, Stitik FP. CT of the solitary pulmonary nodule. *AJR* 135:1–13, 1980
39. Freundlich IM, Horsley WW. Evaluation of pulmonary masses by CT number: A modification of the Siegelman method. Presented at the 67th Radiological Society of North America Meeting, Chicago, November 1981
40. Sagel SS. Lung, pleura, pericardium and chest wall. In: *Computed Body Tomography*, ed. by JKT Lee, SS Sagel, RJ Stanley, New York, Raven Press, 1983, pp 99–101
41. Godwin DJ, Speckman JM, Putman CE, Korobkin M, Breiman RS. CT densitometry: Distinguishing benign from malignant pulmonary nodules. *Radiology* 144:349–351, 1982
42. McCullough EC. Factors affecting the use of quantitative information from a CT scanner. *Radiology* 124:99–107, 1977
43. Zerhouni EA, Spivey JF, Morgan RH, Leo FP, Stitik FP, Siegelman SS. Factors influencing quantitative CT measurements of solitary pulmonary nodules. *J Comput Assist Tomogr* 6:1075–1087, 1982
44. Joseph PM, Hillal SR, Schultz MS, Kelcz F. Clinical and experimental investigation of a smoothed CT reconstruction algorithm. *Radiology* 134:508–516, 1980

45. Rao SP, Alfidi RJ. The environmental density artifact: A beam hardening effect in computed tomography. *Radiology* 141:223–227, 1981
46. Levi C, Gray JE, McCullough EC, Hattery RR. The unreliability of CT numbers as absolute values. *AJR* 139: 443–447, 1982
47. Cann CE, Gamsu G, Birnberg FA, Webb RW. Quantification of calcium in solitary pulmonary nodules using single and dual energy CT. *Radiology* 145:493–496, 1982
48. Fullerton GD, White DR. Anthropomorphic test objects for CT scanners. *Radiology* 133:217–227, 1979
49. White DR, Martin RJ, Darlison R. Epoxy resin based tissue substitutes. *Br J Radiol* 50:814–821, 1977
50. Zerhouni EA, Boukadoum M, Siddiky MA, et al. A standard phantom for quantitative analysis of pulmonary nodules by computed tomography. *Radiology* (in press)
51. Naidich DP, McCauley DI, Siegelman SS. Computed tomography of bronchial adenomas. *J Comput Assist Tomogr* 6:725–732, 1982
52. Zollikofer C, Castaneda-Zuniga W, Stenlund R, Sibley R. Lung metastases from synovial sacroma simulating granulomas. *AJR* 135:161–163, 1980

Chapter 8

Pulmonary Parenchyma

Chest radiography traditionally has been an excellent method for delineating pulmonary pathology, largely because of the naturally high contrast provided by aeration within the lungs. As a consequence CT has played a far less critical role in evaluating the pulmonary parenchyma, as compared with its use for the mediastinum, for example, in which there is intrinsically far less contrast.

Despite considerable controversy, it is generally accepted that the key to the radiologic interpretation of pulmonary parenchymal disease is pattern recognition. Proponents of this approach claim that it represents the only rational means of radiologic diagnosis, given the great number of disease entities that are manifested by diffuse pulmonary abnormalities. Critics point out that pattern recognition may be misleading because so many diseases represent admixtures of patterns, and equally important, because radiologic–pathologic correlation is poor in many cases.

Given the diversity of pulmonary parenchymal disease, some systematic approach to differential diagnosis is warranted, and it seems reasonable to use pattern recognition as a point of departure, provided, as pointed out by Heitzman (1), that this method is properly applied in a "conservative manner."

Computed tomography can have a potentially im-portant role in the characterization of patterns of parenchymal disease. This is because there are limitations in both the detection and characterization of lung disease with routine radiographs. Although chest radiography provides far superior spatial resolution, as compared with CT, subtle focal parenchymal abnormalities are more reliably detected with CT because of the greatly enhanced contrast resolution it affords, as well as the important advantage of unobstructed, cross-sectional visualization of the lung.

As discussed in Chapter 7, the increased efficiency of CT, as compared to chest radiography, has already been established for the detection of pulmonary nodules. In our experience, CT also plays an important role in the evaluation of widespread lung disease, the interpretation of which is frequently problematic with routine radiographs. Two-dimensional representation of three-dimensional pathology is the most serious drawback encountered with interpreting chest X-ray films. This problem is obviated with CT.

Pulmonary parenchymal disease has conventionally been divided into two large groups: those diseases that radiographically appear to involve the terminal air-spaces (i.e., alveolar disease), and those diseases that primarily involve the tissues that surround the air-spaces (i.e., interstitial disease). This division is generally accepted, although controversy continues as to what are the anatomic and pathologic correlates of these patterns.

In this chapter, the value of CT in refining this traditional approach to pulmonary parenchymal disease will be discussed. A great deal of this material is necessarily speculative, considering that the application of CT to the interpretation of diffuse lung disease is so recent. Additionally, the value of CT in assessing patterns of destructive lung disease, that is, cystic and cavitary lung disease, will be discussed.

GENERAL PRINCIPLES AND METHODOLOGY

Detailed knowledge of technique is probably most important in evaluating, of all areas in the thorax, the pulmonary parenchyma. This is a reflection of the great variability of pathology that may be encountered, as well as the wide range of tissue-density alterations that are frequently present. While the principles of chest CT have been reviewed in Chapter 1, some of the most important concepts necessary to accurate interpretation will be reviewed here.

Slice Spacing

The manner in which the lung is evaluated with CT depends on the nature of the pathology to be examined. Routine chest radiographs are always used as a guide. If occult disease is to be ruled out, such as, for example, metastases, contiguous sections from the lung apices to the diaphragm are necessary. Localized pulmonary pathology generally requires less detailed examination, although additional sections through the mediastinum, the airways, or varying portions of the pleura may be necessary, depending in any given case on the suspected nature of pathology.

Slice Thickness

Generally, disease within the lung is best evaluated with 10-mm-thick sections (see Chapter 1). The detection of a lesion with CT depends on the density gradient between the lesion and its surrounding normal tissue. The larger this difference, the less pathologic tissue needs to be included in the slice to create a significant difference in CT number between the lesion and normal tissue. In the low-density environment of the lung, a large slice thickness is advantageous because most pathologic processes are of a much higher density than normal lung. If only a small portion of such an abnormality is included in the slice, averaging of densities will be sufficient to render the abnormality visible.

Thick sections also provide a greater sense of orientation in the lung. In particular, obliquely coursing structures, such as blood vessels, are better defined with thick sections, making their differentiation from pathology easier (see Figs. 3 and 4, Chapter 1).

Despite these advantages, there exists an important role for thinly collimated sections on the order of 1.5 mm. As discussed in Chapter 7, thin sections are mandatory for the determination of the density of pulmonary nodules. Additionally, thin sections may be used to evaluate diffuse pulmonary pathology. This has been most applicable to analysis of interstitial disease processes, for which fine detail of lung parenchyma may provide precise characterization of the nature of the underlying disease process. The technique and indications for this approach to interstitial lung disease will be discussed in detail in the appropriate sections of this chapter.

Information Display

There are no predetermined "best" windows and levels to image the lung. Precise settings are often a matter of subjective preference. However, as a general guide, the window width should be set at twice the CT number range of the particular area of interest. In the lungs, the average range of densities extends from approximately −800 Hounsfield units (HU) to 60 HU, and therefore a window width of 1,800–2,000 HU will be appropriate. As reported throughout the literature, window widths of 1,000 HU are generally considered to be "appropriate" lung settings. As illustrated in this chapter, a wide range of settings is employed, depending on the particular nature of the pathology to be illustrated. Narrowing the window width enhances visual resolution. This may be particularly helpful when assessing both focal increases and decreases in parenchymal densities (Figs. 1 and 2). Conversely, wide window widths are often more informative when the disease process occupies a large area and involves a wide range of tissue-density alterations (see Fig. 3). In these cases, the panoramic view afforded by a wide window width improves visual comprehension. Furthermore, wide windows have a "smoothing" effect on the image, also rendering evaluation somewhat simpler.

Attempts have been made to image both the lung parenchyma and the soft-tissue structures of the mediastinum and chest wall simultaneously (2,3). This is accomplished by use of reverse images. Low-density organs, such as the lungs, are exposed

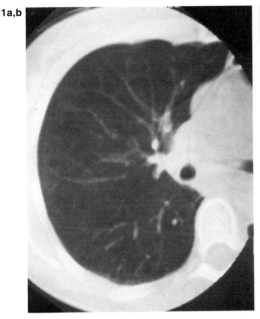
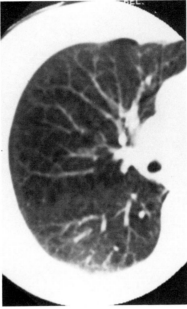

FIG. 1. Centriacinar emphysema: variations in visibility with alterations of window width. **a,b:** Enlargements of a section through the right midlung field in a patient with extensive centriacinar emphysema, imaged with window widths of 2,000 HU (a) and 1,000 HU (b). While the abnormalities can be defined with 2,000-HU windows, the abnormalities are easier to decipher visually with narrower windows.

in the negative mode; high-density structures as are found in the mediastinum, are exposed in the positive mode. While in theory such an approach would be advantageous, in practice, the quality of the images obtained with double-exposure techniques is seriously degraded because of edge enhancement at the points of interface between the positive and negative modes. At present, it is usually simpler and more valuable to examine each section with at least two, and optimally three, settings individually monitored and recorded as hard copy.

Lung-Density Measurements

Considerable interest has been focused on the use of CT to obtain quantitative information concerning

the density of lung tissue (4–6). Assessment of lung density on a plain radiograph is subjective and requires relatively gross derangements to be reliable. Alternative methods, such as fluorodensitometry, radiographic densitometry, and Compton backscatter measurements, have been investigated, but none can differentiate the relative contributions made by lung, pleura, or chest wall. Furthermore, it is impossible to obtain values with any of these techniques that allow comparison to be made among patients.

Computed tomography represents the first imaging modality that facilitates evaluation of quantitative variations in actual lung density in both normal and pathologic states. This is of great potential value, especially in diseases causing a generalized al-

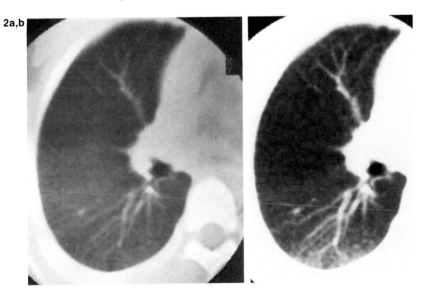

FIG. 2. Miliary sarcoid: variations in visibility with alterations of window width. **a,b:** Enlargements of a section through the right midlung field in a patient with biopsy-proven miliary sarcoid, imaged with window widths of 2,000 HU (a) and 1,000 HU (b). Visualization of individual nodules is easier with narrower windows, although the abnormalities can be defined with a wide window.

3a,b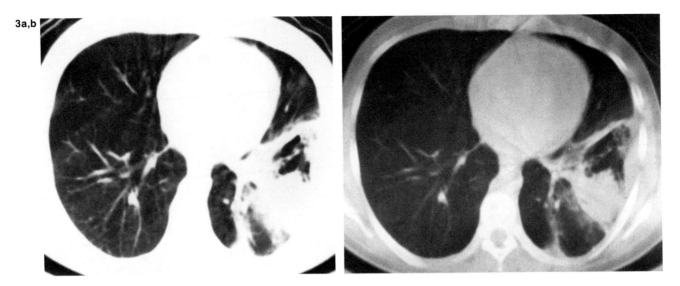

FIG. 3. Anaerobic lung abscess: variations in visibility with alterations of window width. **a,b:** Section through the left midlung field imaged with window widths of 1,000 HU (a) and 2,000 HU (b). A large, necrotic lung abscess can be defined on the left side. Detailed evaluation of the morphology of the abscess, as well as adjacent pleural disease, is easier with wider windows. Compared with Figs. 1 and 2, wider windows are usually better-suited to evaluate pathology when the range of abnormal densities is great. Additionally, wider windows have a "smoothing" effect on the image, also rendering evaluation visually easier.

teration in lung density, such as diffuse interstitial fibrosis, interstitial pulmonary edema, or diffuse emphysema.

Lung is composed of a variety of tissue densities, including air-spaces, the interstitium, and blood vessels, and is therefore inherently nonhomogenous. As a consequence, two CT methods for determining lung density have been investigated: a sector method, in which regions of interest are selected at various sites within the pulmonary parenchyma, and a whole-lung field method, in which the entire volume of lung contained within a given section is analyzed (4–6). These methods are illustrated in Fig. 4.

On the basis of their study of 69 random subjects, Rosenblum et al. (5) described a normal range of mean density values for patients examined during quiet respiration and during inspiratory breath holding, using both sector and whole-lung methods. They found that mean lung density is a function of the phase of respiration; the overall density of lung is significantly less when patients are examined during inspiratory breath holding, compared with scans obtained during quiet respiration. Additionally, there is a significant anteroposterior lung-density gradient that can be reversed when patients are scanned in the prone position. Similar findings have been reported by Robinson and Kreel (4), who showed that the magnitude of the anteroposterior density gradient decreases with increasing lung volumes, but that even with deep inspiration the gradient is not abolished.

Further refinements in the technique of CT lung densitometry have been advocated in an attempt to improve quantitative analysis. Hedlund et al. (7) have suggested automating density calculations by computer methods that isolate the lung area of a CT scan. Most promising is the use of a computer method that searches all contiguous pixels of lung that fall within the CT number range of air and water and that further excludes all densities within the parenchyma that cause strong density gradients. This method has potential use in the estimation of the density of lung parenchyma exclusive of pulmonary blood vessels, and has the inherent advantage of excluding operator subjectivity from lung-density calculations (see Fig. 4).

Another refinement in the measurement of lung density has been suggested by Wegener and Oeser (6), who advocate the use of frequency distribution analysis of attenuation values within a region of interest rather than mean attenuation values as an index of lung density. Theoretically, examining frequency distributions of CT numbers may disclose abnormalities where mean attenuation values are normal. This approach would obviously be most applicable when larger volumes are analyzed.

Despite the initial enthusiasm generated by use of quantitative lung measurements, in fact, such an approach has proven to be of little practical benefit to date. There are numerous technical difficulties involved.

Problems may be encountered in obtaining reproducible lung volumes, which is a critical factor

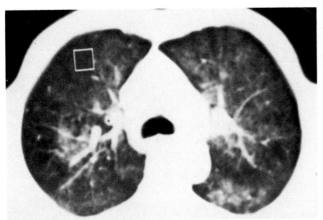
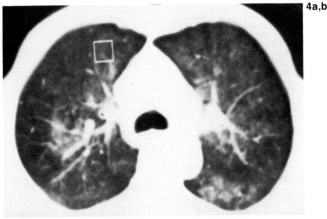

4a,b

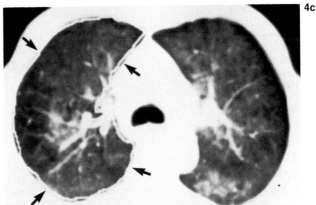

4c

FIG. 4. CT lung densitometry. **a,b:** Sector method. Section through the carina in a patient with diffuse interstitial pneumonia. The only difference between these two images is the position of the cursor in the right upper lung field. Note that very small differences in positioning may be associated with large changes in mean tissue density. The mean density in the region of interest (ROI) in (a) measured −761.04 HU (SD 19.62); the mean density in the ROI in (b) measured −690.87 HU (SD 36.19), for a difference of 70 HU. It is apparent that one limitation of the sector method as illustrated is dependence on the operator for the positioning of the ROI. **c:** Whole-lung field method. This is the same section as in (a) and (b). The perimeter of the right lung has been manually outlined *(arrows)*. The mean density averaged for the entire right lung measured −681.19 HU (SD 109). This method is less prone to operator bias than the sector method. However, regional changes in lung density cannot be analyzed. Ideally, some combination of both the sector and whole-lung field methods should be employed.

in quantitative analysis. As shown by Robinson and Kreel (4), there is a significant inverse correlation between lung volume and the mean attenuation values of lung. This is important, since there is considerable variation in lung expansion relative to midtidal volume not only during breath holding in neutral respiration but even during breath holding in deep inspiration.

Most significant is the problem encountered with the use and reliability of absolute CT numbers. As shown by Levi et al. (8), absolute density measurements vary widely when the same phantom is scanned on different machines. Significant fluctuations in absolute CT numbers occur with variations in kilovoltage, orientation and positioning of patients within the scanner, and the size of lesions and/or structures examined, as well as the nature of surrounding tissue (for example, the density of lung immediately adjacent to a rib) and the type of reconstruction algorithm employed.

Finally, quantitative analysis in our experience has proven no more sensitive in the detection of diffuse pulmonary abnormalities than simple visual inspection of individual scans. CT has the advantage over other imaging modalities of a greater sensitivity and a wider dynamic range, enabling accurate identification of even subtle abnormalities. We have yet to encounter a case of diffuse and/or focal parenchymal disease that was detected by quantitative evaluation when the scan abnormalities could not be detected visually.

More important, reliance on quantitative evaluation overlooks the critical role of pattern recognition. As will be illustrated throughout this chapter, cross-sectional imaging provides a unique method for assessing the pattern of distribution and configuration of pulmonary parenchymal disease. This is a time-honored approach, which, further, provides new insights into the recognition of pulmonary disease by allowing close correlation with conventional radiographic patterns of parenchymal abnormalities.

The role of quantitative analysis has yet to be determined clinically. It is to be anticipated that, eventually, visual and quantitative assessment of parenchymal disease will prove to be complementary. In this regard, there is considerable promise for the use of CT in determining regional pulmonary ventilation using xenon. As shown by Gur et al. (9,10), changes in regional lung ventilation may be mapped experimentally by observing temporal changes following enhancement of the pulmonary parenchyma caused by inhalation of subanesthetic concentrations of nonradioactive xenon. To date, the clinical utility of this method has not been determined. It should be noted that similar information concerning variations in regional lung ventilation may be obtained without the use of an inhalational contrast agent (see Fig. 5).

Normal Lung: Variations of the Respiratory Cycle and Patient Positioning

Accurate interpretation of the pulmonary parenchyma presupposes knowledge of the normal appearance of the lung on CT scans. Examples of normal lung at various levels of the thorax are illustrated in Fig. 6. As discussed previously, the appearance of the lung will vary depending on the width of the slice, the scan speed, and particular window widths and levels. Additionally, the appearance of the lung is dramatically altered by the phase of respiration. Thoracic scanning is usually performed at full lung capacity or end-inspiratory volume. This has the effect of reducing crowding of the pulmonary vessels and potentially improving resolution of fine pathologic abnormalities within the lung. However, the reproducibility of end-inspiratory scans may be less reliable than breath holding at resting lung volumes, especially if the anticipated length of the study is great. A simple strain-gauge device has been employed to improve control of respiration during CT by feedback monitoring; this has yet to be proven to be of definitive clinical value (11).

End-expiratory scans at resting lung volume should be utilized whenever anatomic reproducibility is important, such as when sequential thin sections through a pulmonary nodule are obtained. At resting lung volume, there is considerable crowding of pulmonary vessels in the dependent portion of the lung. This should not be confused with pathology (see Fig. 7).

As with variations in the respiratory cycle, variations in patient positioning also may be critical in analyzing the lungs. Generally, scans are obtained with the patient in the supine position. This may lead to an accentuation of vascular markings in the dependent portions of the lung, rendering evaluation of pathology difficult (Fig. 7). By scanning patients in the prone position, the normal distribution of pulmonary vascularity is altered; this has been shown to be effective in improving detection of pulmonary nodules in the posterior lung bases (12,13). Prone and/or decubitus scans also may be valuable as guides to the interpretation of generalized parenchymal abnormalities. Differentiation between fine diffuse parenchymal fibrosis and interstitial pulmonary edema, for example, may be possible with alterations of patient position (Fig. 8).

As has been briefly discussed in this section, scanning the pulmonary parenchyma involves detailed knowledge of the various techniques available to maximize obtainable, useful information. Thoracic CT should be thought of as interactive; on-line viewing of scans should improve diagnostic accuracy. While generally true, this is especially

5a,b

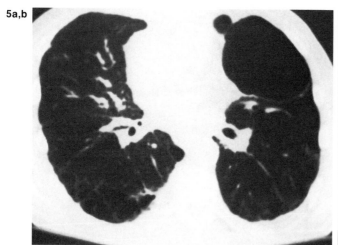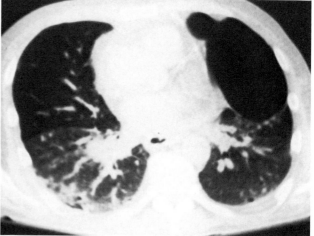

FIG. 5. CT evaluation of regional lung ventilation. **a,b:** Sections through the lower lobes in full inspiration (a) and expiration (b). A large bulla is present anteriorly on the left. Note that, with expiration, the overall density of both lower lobes increases as the overall volume of these lobes decreases, a change easily perceived visually. In comparison, the volume of the middle lobe has increased slightly, without a corresponding increase in tissue density. In this case, tumor partially obstructed the middle lobe bronchus and acted as a ball valve.

6a,b

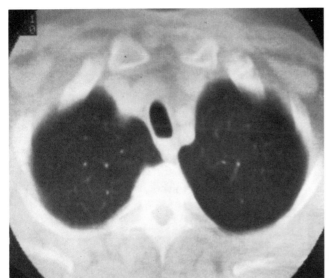

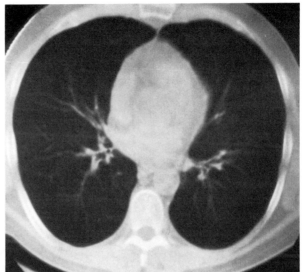

6c

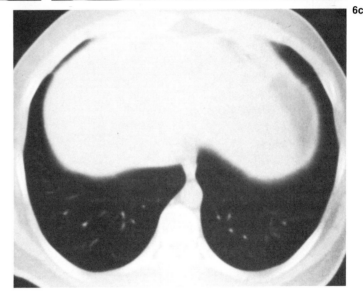

FIG. 6. Normal pulmonary parenchyma. **a–c:** Sections through the upper lobes (a), midportions of the lung (b), and lower lobes (c) in three different, normal cases. Each section is 10 mm thick. Pulmonary vascular markings can be defined in each section. The overall configuration of pulmonary vessels varies from predominantly vertical in the upper and lower lung fields to horizontal in the midlung fields. In each case, a distinct branching pattern characteristic of pulmonary vasculature can be identified. No other discrete structures can be identified within the parenchyma except for the proximal airways, seen only in (b). Notice that the overall density of the lungs, apart from the vessels, is still greater than air, as seen within the trachea. This density is due to subliminal pulmonary tissue, and is exceedingly uniform throughout the lung fields.

important in evaluating the pulmonary parenchyma.

AIR-SPACE (ALVEOLAR) DISEASE

The characteristic patterns of air-space disease as seen with plain radiographs have been defined. These include lobar and/or segmental distribution; poor margination and/or coalescence of disease; air-bronchograms and/or air-alveolograms; and a "bat's-wing" or "butterfly" distribution. While these patterns are easily recognizable in most cases, the underlying anatomic basis of these appearances has been disputed. This is significant, since many of these patterns have also been seen with predominantly interstitial disease processes, including coalescence, and the presence of air-bronchograms.

To date, the role of CT in the evaluation of patients with air-space disease has gone unexplored. This is primarily because of the ease with which air-space disease is diagnosed from plain radiographs. In this section, patterns of air-space disease specifically definable with CT are discussed; the potential role of CT in evaluating patients with pulmonary consolidation is considered as well.

Acinar Lung Disease: The Acinar Nodule

The acinus is generally defined as all lung distal to a terminal bronchiole, and corresponds to a unit of lung with a diameter that varies from 6 to 10 mm. The role of the acinus as an anatomic unit in the configuration and pattern of lung disease has long been disputed. The sole exception is in the classifi-

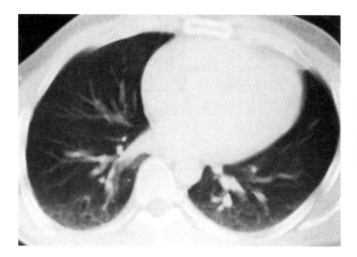

FIG. 7. Normal variant: pulmonary vascular prominence. Section through the lower lung fields imaged at end-expiration. There is an anteroposterior gradient in lung density due to crowding of the pulmonary vessels in the dependent portion of the lower lobes. This is a normal variant and should not be mistaken for pathology.

cation of emphysema, for which the acinus is accepted as the basic morphologic unit (14). The contribution of the acinus to other disease processes, however, is unclear.

According to Fraser and Pare (15), there are three reasons to consider the acinus as a roentgenologic unit. First, it is radiographically visible. Gamsu et al. (16) demonstrated the feasibility of roentgenographic visualization of individual acini by using a special tantalum suspension and progressively opacifying segments of normal excised lungs distal to a wedged catheter. They found that progressive filling of an acinus initially produced a rosette appearance, and over time, a poorly margi-

nated spherical lesion ranging in size from 6 to 10 mm.

Second, unlike secondary pulmonary lobules, acini are recognizable throughout the entire lung. Secondary pulmonary lobules are more variable, generally better defined as a unit in the lung periphery.

Finally, the acinus functionally constitutes the gas-exchange portion of the lung. The last exclusively air-conducting structure is the terminal bronchiole, from which an acinus subtends.

The notion of acinar-filling disease was first applied to lesions resulting from the endobronchial spread of tuberculosis, and was termed the "acinar-

8a,b

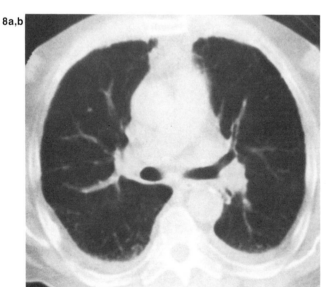 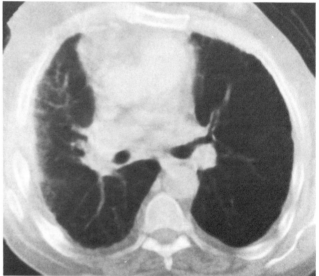

FIG. 8. Congestive heart failure: variations of lung density with patient positioning. **a:** Supine section in a patient with mild interstitial pulmonary edema. In addition to small bilateral effusions, there is a fine reticular pattern in the lungs. **b:** Same patient as in (a), scanned in the right lateral decubitus position at about the same level of the thorax. The effusions have layered. The vascular markings are quite prominent in the dependent portions of the right lung; there has been a corresponding decrease in the prominence of markings in the left lung.

nodose" lesion by Aschoff. Caseous foci in the respiratory bronchioles are common, and, as shown by Barrie (17), infection limited to acini can be defined pathologically in patients with endobronchial tuberculosis.

The notion of an acinar nodule has been further refined by Ziskind et al. (18), who found this pattern to be characteristic of three distinct groups of airspace diseases: diseases caused by aspiration, such as endobronchial spread of tuberculosis, and aspiration pneumonitis, including lipoid pneumonia; diseases in which infection produces acinar consolidation by mechanisms other than aspiration (including simple bacterial and viral pneumonias in which acinar nodules can be recognized along the periphery of larger areas of confluent consolidation, presumably involved by spread through collateral air channels); and diseases in which there is intraacinar transudation and/or hemorrhage, such as pulmonary edema, alveolar proteinosis, and idiopathic pulmonary hemosiderosis.

Despite this, the role of the acinus as a radiologic unit has been disputed. As pointed out by Heitzman (1), there never has been convincing anatomic–pathologic correlation to establish that the acinus is the basis of radiographically demonstrable alveolar disease.

Recavarren et al. (19), in their study of the pathology of acute alveolar lung disease, have shown that bronchopneumonia frequently first appears as an intraluminal, bronchiolar inflammatory exudate, which soon spreads via the canals of Lambert into peribronchiolar alveoli. The result is a small, poorly marginated inflammatory nodule, the "peribronchiolar nodule" (Fig. 9). Pathologically, these focal nodular areas of exudate are not confined to isolated acini, which casts doubt on the significance of the acinus *per se* as a pathologic and radiologic unit.

Itoh et al. (20), in a study of the radiology and pathology of small lung nodules, found that, in fact, there are two types of "acinar" or sublobular lung nodules. The first is the peribronchiolar nodule, as first described by Recavarren et al. (19), which represents a focus of inflammation around the smallest bronchioles. Peribronchiolar nodules are characteristic of bronchopneumonia, acinonodose tuberculosis, and simple pneumoconiosis, in which inhaled particles are found deposited in terminal airspaces adjacent to the respiratory bronchioles.

The second is an intra-acinar nodule in which there are focal or nodular densities in the alveolar spaces that have no definable relationship to airway structures. Instead, these nodules result from the outpouring of edema fluid and/or hemorrhage directly into the distal air-spaces. In this study, intra-acinar nodules were characteristic of pulmonary edema and Goodpasture's syndrome, and occasionally patients with peripheral bronchopneumonia. Interestingly, metastatic nodules were also shown pathologically to be primarily intra-acinar filling diseases, cancer cells either growing to fill alveoli with a solid mass or lining the alveolar walls. Unlike the nodules seen in patients with congestive heart failure, however, metastatic disease usually appears

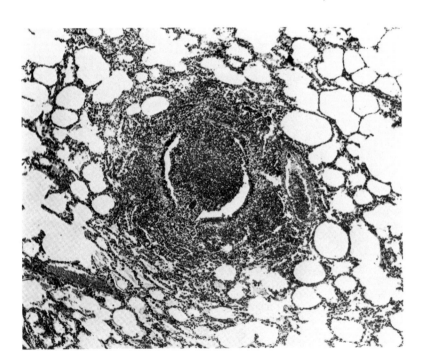

FIG. 9. Bronchopneumonia: the peribronchial nodule. Inflammatory exudate fills a bronchiole and extends through the walls, which are necrotic, to involve peribronchiolar alveoli. Alveoli peripheral to this zone are empty. A similar picture pathologically is characteristic of endobronchial tuberculosis. Radiographically, this lesion corresponds to an "acinar nodule," i.e., a poorly marginated lung nodule measuring 6–10 mm. (Reproduced with permission from ref. 19.)

to be sharply marginated, and hence is easily discriminated from other alveolar-filling diseases.

It is apparent that poorly defined or acinar nodules, as seen on chest radiographs, represent a variety of different pathologic processes affecting variable portions of the pulmonary air-spaces. Despite this pathologic variability, the fact remains that a distinctive radiologic pattern of poorly defined nodules up to 10 mm in size is frequently encountered. Because acinar nodules constitute a distinctive radiographic pattern, and, furthermore, because this pattern is helpful in differential diagnosis, the concept of "acinar" disease warrants retention, as long as it is understood that the acinar nodule represents a variety of configurations of airspace disease pathologically. Support for the value of the notion of acinar lung disease is provided by CT. This evidence is derived largely from examination of patients with endobronchial spread of tuberculosis.

Endobronchial Tuberculosis

Endobronchial tuberculosis occurs when a caseous focus ruptures through the wall of an adjacent bronchus, with subsequent discharge of its contents into the air passages (21). This results in the development of widespread pulmonary lesions.

The appearance on CT of endobronchial tuberculosis has been described recently (22). Cavitation is always present, although confirmation of the presence of cavities, especially when small, frequently necessitates CT. Foci of endobronchial tuberculosis are usually most prominent in the immediate vicinity of cavities, but they may be quite far removed, depending on the position of the patient at the time of aspiration. Characteristically, foci of endobronchial tuberculosis appear as ill-defined nodular densities that are markedly variable in size, including lesions as small as 2–3 mm (Fig. 10). These smaller nodules probably represent inflammatory foci in respiratory bronchioles, which also characteristically measure 2–3 mm in width.

Spread of disease may be extensive throughout both lungs. Usually, multiple, small, poorly defined nodules will be scattered throughout the lung. At individual sites, nodular lesions may become confluent and appear as small areas of patchy pneumonitis (Fig. 11).

As shown in Figs. 10 and 12, typical acinar nodules seen on chest radiographs correspond precisely to the poorly defined nodules seen on CT. While acinar nodules are generally easiest to identify along the periphery of areas of confluent pneumonitis, careful inspection within regions of confluence also reveals that discrete nodular foci can still be identified, suggesting that pneumonic infiltrates result from coalescence of individual nodules.

Progression of coalescence may result in a lobar distribution of disease, including the presence of air-bronchograms. Even in this setting, along the periphery, discrete nodular foci of air-space consolidation usually can be identified (Fig. 13).

Areas of pneumonic consolidation may be detected even when unsuspected on routine radio-

10a,b

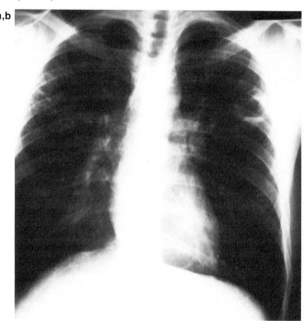

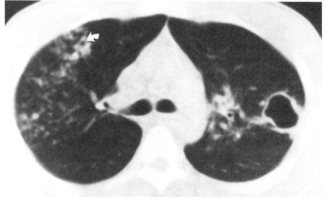

FIG. 10. Endobronchial tuberculosis. **a:** Posteroanterior (PA) radiograph. Subtle acinar nodules are present in the right upper lobe. **b:** Section through the upper thorax. A thin-walled cavity is present in the left upper lobe, within which there is a small air–fluid level. Scattered, ill-defined nodules are present in the lateral portion of the right upper lobe. These are of varable sizes, the smallest being 2–3 mm. These smaller nodules correspond in size to the approximate width of terminal bronchioles. Some of these nodules appear confluent; additionally, a very small cavity can be defined anteriorly (arrow).

11a

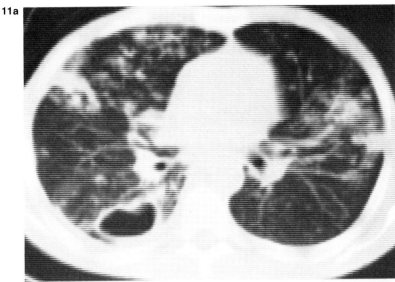

11b

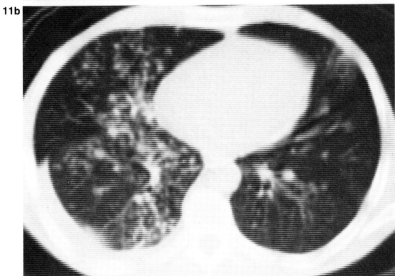

FIG. 11. Endobronchial tuberculosis. **a,b:** Sections through the mid and lower thorax, respectively. A large, thin-walled cavity is present in the superior segment of the right lower lobe, within which a small air-fluid level can be defined. Scattered throughout both lungs are innumerable nodules, ranging in size from 3 to 10 mm. In some areas, these nodules have coalesced to form ill-defined patches of tuberculous pneumonia.

graphs (Fig. 12). In a recent study, 25 patients with endobronchial tuberculosis were examined with standard radiography and CT (22). In 10 (40%), the only evidence that there were foci of endobronchial tuberculosis was provided by CT. As illustrated in Fig. 14, this has clear diagnostic implications. In this case, an area of consolidation and cavitation is present in the left upper lobe, extending to the left hilum. This initially suggested the presence of central tumor with postobstructive pneumonitis. The right lung appears normal. Sections through the area of consolidation confirmed the presence of cavitation, and, in addition, revealed patency of the bronchial tree. Additionally, small foci of nodular consolidation in both the right upper and lower lobes could be identified, which even in retrospect were not apparent on the plain radiograph (Fig. 14a). The pattern of disease as shown by CT suggested

the diagnosis of tuberculosis with endobronchial spread. Evaluation of serial sputums all proved negative. At bronchoscopy, absence of an endobronchial lesion was confirmed; biopsy and washings were not diagnostic. Because of the characteristic appearance of the CT scan, the patient underwent repeat bronchoscopy and biopsy, at which time the CT diagnosis of tuberculosis was confirmed.

Computed tomography can be of immeasurable value in elucidating the patterns of parenchymal disease, at times even allowing differentiation between diffuse air-space and interstitial disease. This is illustrated in Fig. 15. In this case, a diffuse bilateral pattern of pulmonary parenchymal disease is present, restricted to the midlung zones, with almost complete sparing of the apices and the lung bases. On the basis of the radiograph, it is difficult

12a,b

12c

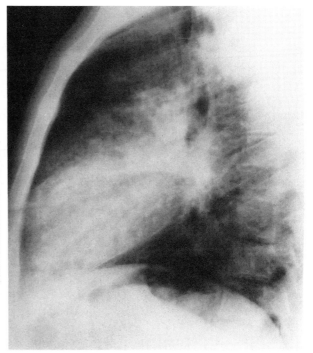

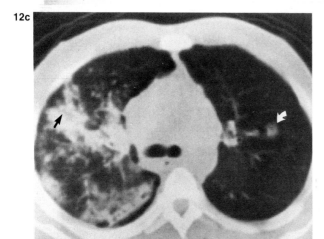

FIG. 12. Endobronchial tuberculosis. **a,b:** PA and lateral radiographs show a large, irregular cavity in the right upper lobe, associated with an ill-defined infiltrate throughout the right upper and middle lobes. Acinar nodules are also definable, best seen on the lateral radiograph. The left lung appears normal. **c:** Section at the level of the carina. Individual acinar nodules are present, best seen in the anterior portion of the right upper lobe. Even in areas of confluent pneumonitis, discrete nodular shadows can be defined *(arrow)*. In addition, focal pneumonitis is present in the midportion of the left lung *(curved arrow)*. Even in retrospect, this is not apparent in the accompanying chest film.

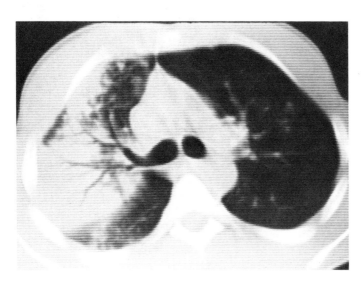

FIG. 13. Endobronchial tuberculosis. Section through the right upper lobe bronchus in a patient with a large cavity and extensive consolidation in the right upper lobe on routine radiographs (not shown). In this case, endobronchial spread had led to uniform consolidation of the right upper lobe, in which discrete air-bronchograms can be defined. Along the periphery of the infiltrate, both anteriorly and in the superior segment of the right lower lobe, acinar foci can be seen. As shown in this case, acinar nodules may be conceptualized as fundamental CT building blocks that, when coalescent, may account for virtually all conventional radiographic signs of air-space disease.

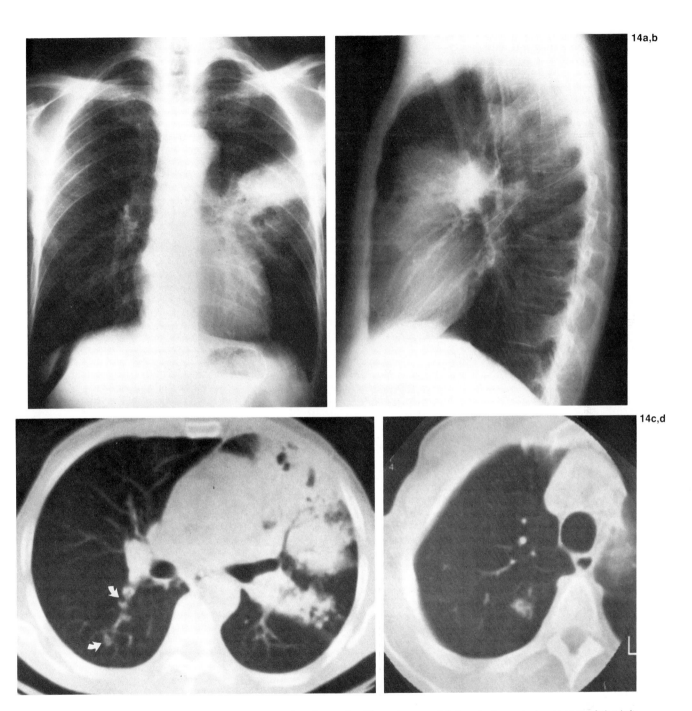

FIG. 14. Endobronchial tuberculosis. **a,b:** PA and lateral radiographs. There is consolidation in the anterior aspect of the left upper lobe, associated with cavitation. Disease extends to the left hilum, raising the possibility of a focal, endobronchial lesion. The right lung is normal. **c:** Section through the left upper lobe bronchus. There is no evidence of an endobronchial lesion. The left upper lobe is consolidated. Air-bronchograms and discrete areas of cavitation within the left upper lobe can be defined. A few discrete acinar nodules are present near the major fissure. Additionally, ill-defined acinar shadows are present in the superior segment of the right lower lobe *(arrows).* **d:** Enlargement of a section through the right upper lobe. There is a focal area of consolidation not seen on the plain films. This combination of findings suggested the diagnosis of tuberculosis, although sputum samples were negative and an initial biopsy at bronchoscopy was nondiagnostic. Repeat bronchoscopy and transbronchial biopsy in the left upper lobe confirmed the diagnosis.

15a

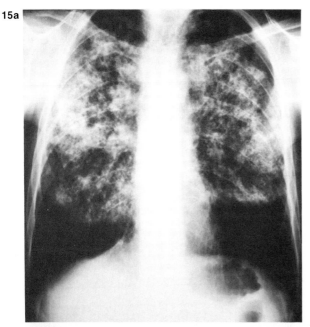

15b

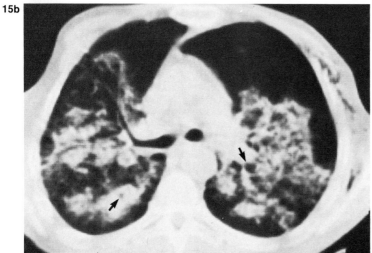

15c

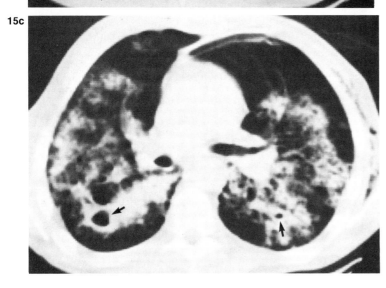

FIG. 15. Endobronchial tuberculosis. **a:** PA radiograph shows an unusual configuration of diffuse parenchymal disease involving the mid- and upper lung fields but sparing the lung apices and lower lung fields. Precise characterization of the nature of the parenchymal changes is difficult. **b,c:** Sequential sections through the midportion of the lung. There is a sharp line of demarcation between areas of normal and abnormal lung. Both sections show scattered cavities in both lungs *(arrows)*, associated with a distinctly acinar pattern of lung disease, which in many areas has progressed to confluent pneumonitis. Subcutaneous emphysema is present on the left, caused by a pleural tube inserted after an unsuccessful attempt at a thoracentesis.

to determine the exact nature of the disease process. Cross-sectional imaging, however, clarifies the radiograph. First, discrete areas of cavitation in both lungs are clearly present (Fig. 15b). Furthermore, careful analysis of the CT images shows that the remainder of the pathology is characterized by both individual and coalescent areas of poorly defined acinar nodules. The pattern on CT is that of diffuse air-space consolidation with cavitation; active cavitary tuberculosis was subsequently diagnosed.

From a study of the various patterns of parenchymal abnormalities encountered in this uniform population of patients with endobronchial tuberculosis, the following can be concluded: (a) CT is more sensitive than routine radiographs in detecting the presence of focal air-space pathology; (b) acinar nodules, as described, constitute the smallest visible units of air-space consolidation, and (c) acinar nodules are fundamental building blocks that, when coalescent, may account for virtually all conventional radiographic signs of air-space disease.

The applicability of the acinar nodule seen with CT in cases other than endobronchial tuberculosis has still to be explored. As suggested previously, acinar shadows may be encountered in patients with diverse diseases. Preliminary investigations suggest that acinar nodules play a crucial role in the development of all air-space disease, regardless of the etiology, although this remains speculative.

Acinar Nodules in Nontuberculous Pulmonary Disease

While the classic prototype of acinar lung disease is endobronchial tuberculosis, this same pattern can be seen in a diverse set of air-space diseases. Perhaps the most common etiology of air-space consolidation is congestive heart failure. As pointed out by Ziskind et al. (18), detection of individual acinar shadows in patients with severe congestive heart failure is difficult because of the diffuse and confluent nature of the disease process. This problem is obviated with CT. Figure 16 is an enlargement of a section through the right midlung in a patient with severe mitral stenosis and congestive heart failure with pulmonary edema. Distinct, poorly marginated nodules of varying sizes are present throughout the lung. Discrete air-bronchograms and areas of confluent air-space disease can be defined as well. The pattern is similar to that shown previously in examples of endobronchial tuberculosis, except for the absence of cavitation and the more widespread and uniform involvement of lung.

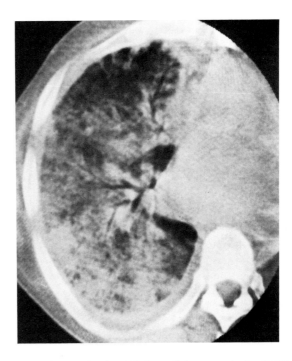

FIG. 16. Congestive heart failure. Enlargement of a section through the right midlung in a patient with severe congestive heart failure. Close scrutiny reveals innumerable small nodular (acinar) densities throughout the lung, which in some areas have become confluent. Air-bronchograms can be defined centrally. As may be anticipated, nodularity was not apparent on the plain radiographs (not shown).

A similar pattern of distinct nodular densities may also be defined in patients with a bat's-wing pattern of pulmonary edema. While the cause of this particular distribution of air-space consolida-

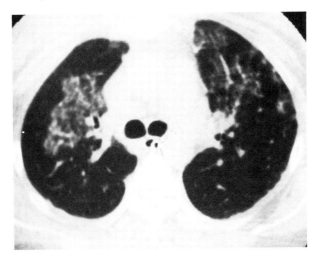

FIG. 17. Bat's-wing pulmonary edema. Section through the carina in a patient with chronic renal failure and recurrent episodes of pulmonary edema. There is perihilar consolidation, most prominent on the right side, with near complete sparing of the lung periphery. Within this area of consolidation, numerous discrete nodular (acinar) densities can be defined, similar in appearance to those in Fig. 16.

tion has never been adequately explained, the underlying pathologic changes are strikingly similar to the pattern seen in more widespread pulmonary edema (Fig. 17; compare with Fig. 16).

In addition to congestive heart failure and endobronchial tuberculosis, we have encountered acinar densities in diseases less commonly associated with diffuse air-space abnormalities. Foremost among these is sarcoidosis. Sarcoidosis is usually characterized by multiple, noncaseating granulomata located primarily in the pulmonary interstitium, as opposed to alveolar spaces. As shown by Solomon et al. (23), unsuspected pulmonary nodules can be defined in patients with sarcoidosis who were examined with CT; however, these are amost always sharply defined. Although the underlying pathology of acinar sarcoidosis is unknown, this form of the disease probably results from coalescence of small nodules, causing focal areas of parenchymal consolidation (Fig. 18).

Another unusual pattern of presentation of sarcoidosis is so-called "alveolar sarcoid." The radiologic hallmark of this form of the disease is poorly defined areas of parenchymal consolidation, frequently associated with air-bronchograms. Ra-

diologic–pathologic correlation to explain this pattern of the disease is conspicuously missing. As shown in Fig. 19, these poorly defined areas of consolidation in fact represent areas of confluent acinar nodules. Furthermore, it appears that the disease process has a predilection for air-spaces adjacent to the central airways. Despite the similarity in appearance to interstitial disease (centered as it is around the central bronchi), focal acinar shadows can still be defined along the periphery of larger areas of confluence. We have recently seen a similar pattern of parenchymal disease in a patient with far-advanced rheumatoid lung, with necrobiotic pulmonary nodules.

Another entity not usually associated with air-space consolidation is metastatic disease. As has already been discussed, Itoh et al. (20) have shown that metastatic nodules are primarily intra-acinar-filling diseases. Although generally well-defined, on occasion, poorly defined nodules will be encountered in patients with metastatic disease (Figs. 20 and 21). It is probable that some of these cases represent endobronchial spread of tumor. The appearance is not dissimilar to that exemplifying acinar sarcoid. Primary neoplastic lung disease may also

18a,b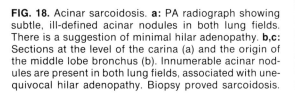

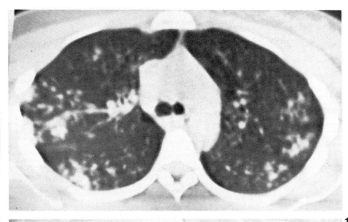

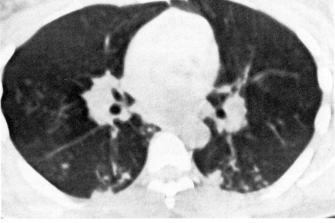
18c

FIG. 18. Acinar sarcoidosis. a: PA radiograph showing subtle, ill-defined acinar nodules in both lung fields. There is a suggestion of minimal hilar adenopathy. b,c: Sections at the level of the carina (a) and the origin of the middle lobe bronchus (b). Innumerable acinar nodules are present in both lung fields, associated with unequivocal hilar adenopathy. Biopsy proved sarcoidosis.

19a

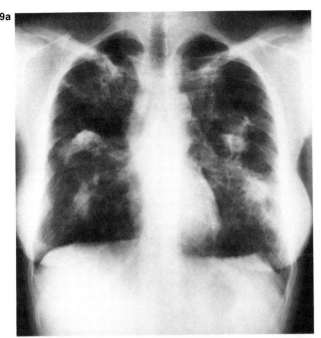

FIG. 19. Alveolar sarcoid. PA radiograph shows pattern characteristic of alveolar sarcoid with ill-defined infiltrates in both lungs associated with air-bronchograms, best seen in the right upper lobe, and diffuse adenopathy. **b,c:** Enlargements of sections through the middle lobe (b) and left upper lobe bronchus (c). The pattern of pulmonary disease is strikingly peribronchial in configuration. It is apparent why air-bronchograms would be visualized on routine films. Despite the confluent nature of this disease, individual, poorly defined nodules can be seen immediately adjacent to areas of confluence *(arrows)*.

19b,c

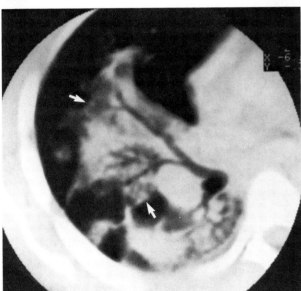 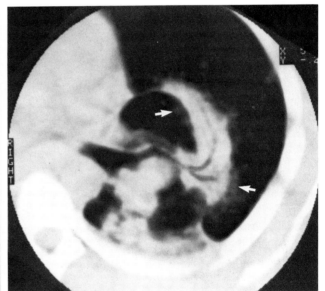

have an acinar configuration, as shown in Fig. 22, a scan of a patient with leukemic lung infiltrates.

Both inflammatory and neoplastic disease may be strikingly similar in appearance when seen in cross section. This is illustrated in Figs. 23 and 24, cases of endobronchial tuberculosis and bronchiolo-alveolar cell carcinoma, respectively.

Metzger et al. (24) have shown that CT plays a significant role in the evaluation of patients with bronchiolo-alveolar cell carcinoma by disclosing areas of parenchymal involvement otherwise unsuspected on routine radiographs. This is important, since the staging, therapy, and prognosis will vary depending on whether there is a solitary focus of disease or diffusion of diseases. It is generally accepted that bronchiolo-alveolar cell carcinoma starts as a unifocal disease that later spreads to the ipsilateral and contralateral lung. Of all primary lung tumors, bronchiolo-alveolar cell carcinoma is most prone to aerogenous spread. It is not surpris-

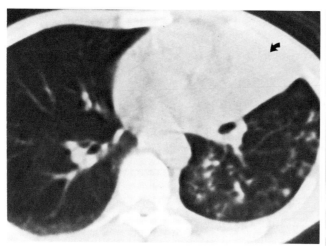

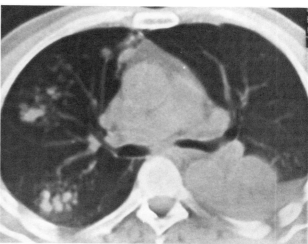

FIG. 20. Metastatic lung carcinoma. Section through the lower lobes and the lingula, which is airless and collapsed *(arrow)*. An endobronchial tumor occluded the left upper lobe bronchus proximally (not shown). Ill-defined acinar nodules are present throughout the left lower lobe, compatible with aspirated tumor (unproved).

FIG. 21. Metastatic lung carcinoma. Section through the left upper lobe bronchus in a patient with total collapse of the left lower lobe due to squamous cell carcinoma. Scattered throughout the right lung are innumerable, variably sized nodules, some of which have a typical acinar configuration (especially in the right upper lobe). Metastatic disease was confirmed by biopsy. The pattern suggests aspiration of necrotic tumor (compare with Fig. 20).

ing, therefore, that the appearance on CT of the disease may closely mimic endobronchial tuberculosis. As shown in Figs. 23 and 24, despite the confluent, segmental pattern of the disease, in both cases individual acinar shadows can be defined, accounting for the diseases' similarity in appearance.

While much work remains to be done to further clarify the nature of air-space disease, it is suggested from the material in this section that CT is a potentially important tool for evaluating parenchymal consolidation. The key to recognition of air-space disease on CT appears to be identification of diffuse, poorly marginated nodules ranging in size from 3 to 10 mm. These are present in most if not all

diseases that cause consolidation of the lung. When confluent, these nodules cause a spectrum of abnormalities that run the gamut of traditional radiologic patterns of air-space disease, as discussed and illustrated throughout this section. We have chosen to retain the notion of acinar disease to describe these air-space nodules, even though many of these probably represent subacinar, or peribronchiolar disease pathologically. The concept of acinar disease is worth retaining because it reinforces the important role played by nodules in the apparent pathogenesis of pulmonary consolidation. Furthermore, acini are

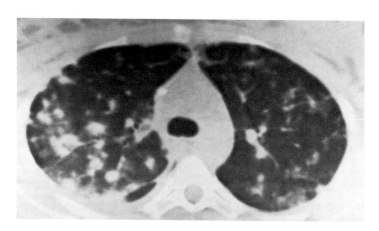

FIG. 22. Leukemic infiltrates. Section at the level of the carina shows numerous, variably sized, poorly defined nodules in both lungs, not dissimilar in appearance to the acinar sarcoid in Fig. 18 and examples of metastatic lung carcinoma in Figs. 20 and 21 (biopsy-proven).

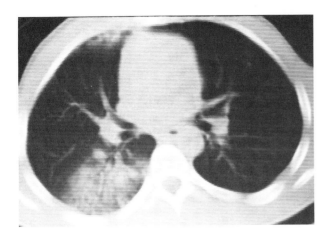

FIG. 23. Endobronchial tuberculosis. Section through the middle lobe bronchus and superior segmental bronchus on the right. There is extensive consolidation of the superior segment; typical acinar nodules can be defined throughout (compare with Fig. 24).

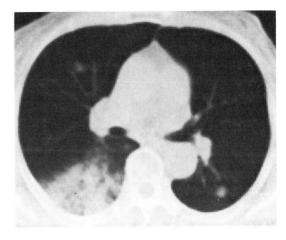

FIG. 24. Alveolar cell carcinoma. Section through the bronchus intermedius. There is extensive consolidation of the superior segment of the right lower lobe. Individual, discrete acinar shadows can be defined throughout, in a pattern strikingly similar to that shown in Fig. 23. Nodules are also present anteriorly on the right and in the left lower lobe (biopsy-proven).

the anatomic unit closest in size to most air-space nodules, and, undoubtedly, some of these nodules represent true consolidation of individual pulmonary acini.

INTERSTITIAL DISEASE

Many pulmonary diseases are characterized by predominant involvement of the interstitial tissues, with diffuse alteration of the lung architecture. A few of these diseases have distinctive roentgenographic patterns, but the majority appear similar and are difficult to distinguish.

As stated earlier, the radiographic-pattern approach to diffuse pulmonary diseases remains the main radiologic tool in the investigation of the abnormal interstitium. However, the radiographic interpretation of interstitial diseases is still associated with uncertainty. As pointed out by Felson (25), radiographic prediction of pathology in diffuse pulmonary disease is so inconsistent that it probably should be abandoned altogether, and more realistic, purely descriptive approaches adopted. Furthermore, intra- and extra-observer variability in pattern recognition with chest radiographs is significant.

Simple, precise, and consistent guidelines for the recognition of the various patterns seem difficult to define, compounding the problem of observer variations inherently associated with the visual interpretation of nonfocal and complex abnormalities. Fraser and Paré (26) underline the lack of accurate roentgenologic–pathologic correlative studies that

would be essential to the establishment of reliable criteria for pattern recognition. They emphasize that even the broadest correlation, such as the morphologic basis for the so-called reticular, nodular, or granular patterns is not known.

Conceptually, the chest radiograph can be considered to be the two-dimensional projectional sum of the equivalent of several thousand "histologic" slices. The question of the influence of such superimposition on the resultant images and on the ability to predict pathology is still unresolved. Some reticulonodular patterns are due to the "criss-crossing" effect of superimposed, thickened interstitial lines variously oriented in space, as suggested by Trapnell (27). How does one separate cases in which true nodules are present from the others?

Why are the tiny nodules of miliary tuberculosis, theoretically below the threshold of radiographic visibility, detected on plain radiographs? The mechanism of summation of several nodules to make a larger, visible one is generally invoked to answer this question. In the 1940s, Resink suggested that, in such cases, individual shadows became visible only when not summed. More recent, ingenious experiments by Heitzman (29), with implantation of subliminal lesions such as resected metastases and 3-mm polyethylene spheres into resected lung specimens, strongly indicate that alignment of subliminal structures parallel to the X-ray beam is the main factor in their visualization.

Since summation appears to be the mechanism by which subliminal abnormalities become visible, there must be a stage at which only a few of these abnormalities are present but are invisible because their small number does not permit significant alignment, and their size and contrast fall outside the dynamic range of standard radiography. Could CT be of value in this "invisible" phase by (a) detecting diffuse interstitial diseases before they produce radiographic abnormalities by summation, (b) improving definition and understanding of radiographic patterns, and (c) improving prediction of the pathology of diffuse pulmonary abnormalities?

Current Role of CT

As stated earlier, the application of CT in parenchymal diseases, in general and diffuse pulmonary abnormalities in particular, has been limited. Global assessment of density with CT demonstrates a correlation between lung density and the presence of diffuse lung disease. Decreased density is seen with processes which increase the air volume of the lung, such as emphysema (30). Increased density is seen with processes that increase the interstitial tissue volume, such as sarcoidosis (31). The use of quantitative information to characterize diffuse lung diseases is hampered by a host of technical as well as physiological factors. Numerous variables affect CT numbers, making absolute determinations of CT density unreliable. Global lung density represents the sum of blood, air, lung tissue, and extravascular fluid densities. Methods to automatically exclude blood vessels from lung-density measurements, as devised by Hedlund et al. (7), are certainly necessary. Air-volume change remains a poorly controlled variable, even though Robinson and Kreel (4) suggest that a correlation between chest wall expansion and air volume can be drawn, thereby allowing corrected measurements independent of inspiration–expiration differences in lung density. Despite all the potential sources of error, it appears that lung-density assessments with CT are more sensitive than plain radiography in the early detection of diffuse lung disease.

Lung density on CT represents the summation of component densities over the entire thickness of the CT slice. When abnormal, we can assume that increased or decreased amounts of one (or several) of the basic components of density (air, blood, lung tissue, and extravascular fluids) is responsible for the density change. CT would be more effective if it could visualize the abnormality itself rather than inferring it by the global average density change it produces. Goddard et al, (32), in a study of pulmonary emphysema, determined the percentage of

destroyed lung by visually analyzing areas of emphysema on CT scans; they found a good correlation between pulmonary function tests and CT. Could CT be used to visualize parenchymal processes other than emphysema? Would it be possible to see directly the abnormal interstitium?

As discussed and illustrated previously, CT provides an exquisite *in vivo* look at the various patterns of air-space consolidation and appears to support the concept of the acinus being the basic anatomicopathologic unit of the lung in air-space disease. Fluid-filled acini, like nodules, can easily be recognized with routine 8–10 mm CT sections by virtue of the high density gradient between the surrounding lung and this type of pathology, as pointed out in Chapter 1. However, early interstitial processes may not be detectable with thick CT sections since they may cause only subtle differences in density from the normal surrounding lung parenchyma and as a result, excessive partial volume averaging may render them invisible. Thin-section CT, therefore, may be more appropriate to characterize diffuse non-air-space processes (Fig. 25). Sections of 1–2 mm commonly available on modern scanners, may allow visualization of the lung architecture in cross section and with a much lower degree of superimposition than what occurs on plain films. Current scanners can achieve submillimeter spatial resolutions of 0.5–0.8 mm. Obviously, this degree of resolution is attainable only in anatomical parts with intrinsically high contrast, such as the inner ear. The lung, too, is an ideal organ for high-resolution CT studies because of its high natural contrast. If one considers the size of the pulmonary architectural elements (secondary lobule, 15–20 mm; acinus, 7 mm; respiratory bronchioles, 1–2 mm); it would appear that current spatial resolution with CT is adequate to analyze the fine details of the lung parenchyma. With appropriate techniques, maximal CT resolution can be obtained in the lungs. To that end, pixel size would have to be smaller than the effective resolution of the scanner, which, on current equipment, requires the use of the total matrix to reconstruct limited lung areas such as in the "targeted" reconstructions used for inner ear and lumbar spine studies.

The above considerations form the basis of a technique we have used over the past 2 years to test the concept of direct visualization of the pulmonary architecture with CT by virtue of (a) the cross-sectional plane of imaging, (b) the reduction of the problem of superimposition by using very thin CT sections, (c) the high spatial resolution that can be

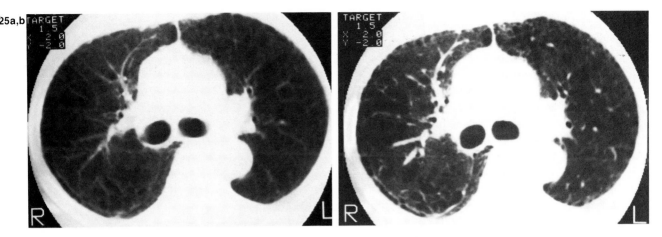

FIG. 25. Advantages of thin slices. **a:** 10-mm section. **b:** 1.5-mm section. The areas of emphysema and the thickened septa are better recognized in (b). Sharper margins for all visualized structures can be appreciated.

achieved in the lungs with current scanners, and (d) the inherently high contrast resolution of CT. Our preliminary results and conclusions are presented here (33).

High-Resolution CT of the Lung Parenchyma

Technique

The patients described here have all been studied on a General Electric 8800 scanner. The same results are achievable on any modern scanner with very thin sections and retrospective reconstruction capabilities. The essentials of the technique are as follows:

1. Very thin sections (1.5 mm).
2. High exposure factors to decrease noise (384–512 mAs).
3. Three to four representative sections located in the upper, mid- and lower lung zones obtained in suspended inspiration and expiration successively.
4. Targeted reconstructions over selected areas in each lung field, magnified with zoom factors of 1.7 to 3. This degree of magnification is necessary to match the resolution of the scanner with the smallest available pixel size.
5. Studies interpreted at the display console in order to analyze the scans at multiple window settings.

Normal Lung

Correlative CT and pathologic data for the lung parenchyma are limited. Coddington et al. (34) performed such a study using 13-mm sections, and could resolve vessels of 1 mm in diameter but could not visualize the septa between areas of emphysema. As suggested by Fig. 25, thinner sections are probably necessary to demonstrate the septa. As illustrated in Fig. 26, many minute structures besides vessels are seen on thinner sections, but are not appreciated on thicker sections. The precise interpretation of these structures would require accurate correlative lung specimen studies, which have not yet been completed. Based on current knowledge, we presume that some of these structures represent normal interstitial connective tissue septa.

Normal bronchi are difficult to see beyond their proximal portions. Sometimes, areas of lucency can be noted near vessels and may represent normal bronchi, which usually run parallel to pulmonary arteries. Except for clearly definable vessels and less visible septa and bronchi, the normal lung appears homogeneous in density on high-resolution CT.

Abnormal Lung

An understanding of normal lung architecture is necessary to interpret abnormal high-resolution CT studies of the pulmonary interstitium. The reader is referred to the authoritative works of Heitzman (29) and Weibel (35) for thorough reviews of the subject. We will highlight only the architectural features necessary to our discussion.

The pulmonary interstitium is best conceived of as the framework of tissue supporting the pulmonary vasculature and airways. As demonstrated by Weibel (35), the fibrous skeleton of the lung can be divided into a peripheral and an axial system. The

26a,b

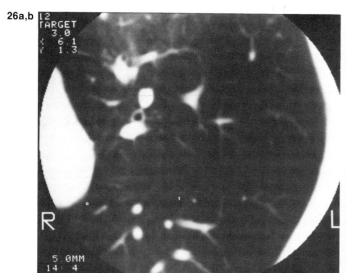
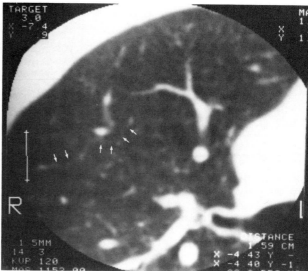

FIG. 26. The normal lung with high-resolution CT: effect of varying slice thickness on visualization of anatomic structures (30-year-old normal volunteer). **a:** Targeted 5-mm section of the midportion of the left lung, utilizing a target factor of 3 (pixel size of 0.364 mm). Branching vessels are seen throughout the slice. Two proximal bronchi are visualized in cross section; smaller bronchi are not visible. The major fissure can be identified as a faint line in the midportion of the image. The lung parenchyma is of a homogeneous, uniform density. **b:** Targeted 1.5-mm section of the right upper lobe, utilizing the same target factors as in (a). Vessels are more difficult to recognize because they cannot be visualized over a long distance in a 1.5-mm section. As a consequence, their branching, tapering nature is not appreciated. However, many more structures can be seen on this section than in (a), and the pulmonary background is not totally uniform and homogeneous. This suggests that we probably are visualizing some of the normal interstitial framework of the lung. For instance, the linear, nontapering densities *(arrows)* connecting several round structures cannot represent vessels, which normally have a binary branching pattern. Instead, this most probably represents the septa of a secondary lobule, joining several venules, seen here in cross section as round densities. Small areas of lucencies near vessels probably represent bronchioles. Clearly, precise anatomic–pathologic correlative studies are needed to better understand the normal anatomic structures visualized with this technique.

peripheral system envelops the lung and the pleura, and penetrates deep into the parenchyma as incomplete septa between acini, lobules, subsegments, and segments. These fibers are located at the periphery of airway units and are associated with branches of the pulmonary veins and lymphatics. The axial system of fibers originates at the hilus and fans out into the lung parenchyma along the central airways and pulmonary arteries to reach to the center of acini. These fibers then connect with the peripheral fiber system.

As a result of these interconnecting systems, lung tissue—from alveolar walls to acini to primary and secondary lobules to subsegments and segments—is supported by a fibrous skeleton that follows an "axial–peripheral" architectural design, with "core" structures including the airways and pulmonary arteries and "shell" structures including the veins and lymphatics within the connective tissue septa. The septa are best formed at the periphery of the lung, since this is where the peripheral fibrous system is anchored. The secondary lobule exemplifies the core–shell design of the lung parenchyma, with central bronchioles and arterioles supplying a few primary pulmonary lobules formed of several acini.

The secondary lobule is limited by septa containing the draining veins and lymphatics. The secondary lobule septa are well-formed on the anterolateral aspects of the lung bases and are generally oriented perpendicularly to the pleural surface. In the experience of Heitzman (29), the septa of the secondary lobules are also well-formed on the posterior aspect of the lung bases. When abnormally thick, these septa can be recognized as "Kerley B" lines on radiographs. In the most central portions and apices of the lungs, lobular septa are oriented in various directions and are not always complete.

It follows from the preceding discussion that the ability to recognize abnormal septa would be the first test of validity for CT of the lung utilizing a high-resolution technique. We will illustrate our findings in several conditions.

Interstitial Pulmonary Edema

The prototype of all interstitial processes is interstitial pulmonary edema. Accumulating interstitial fluid thickens the septa and engorges the lymphatics within the septa. As illustrated in Fig. 27, these phenomena are clearly demonstrated with CT. The sep-

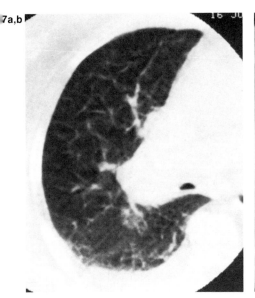

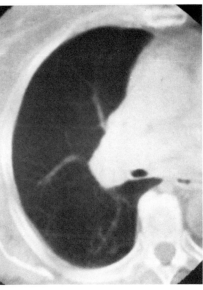

FIG. 27. Acute interstitial pulmonary edema. **a:** CT scan during the acute phase. **b:** CT scan after therapy. Numerous linear structures can be appreciated along with a small pleural effusion. The pattern is reticular, with more prominent lines noted in the dependent portions of the lung.

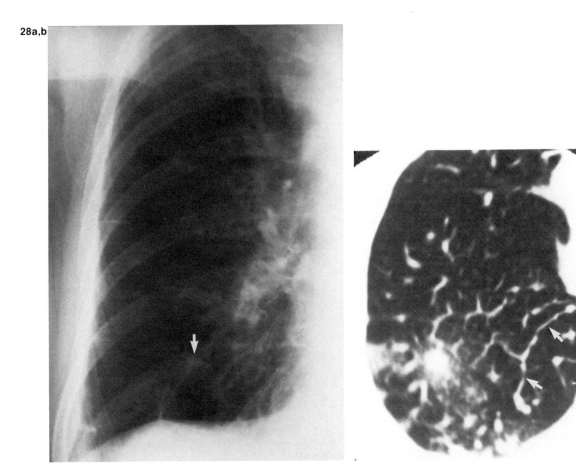

FIG. 28. Lymphangitic carcinomatosis (59-year-old female with breast carcinoma).**a:** Cone-down view of a PA radiograph. A reticular pattern can be seen, especially in the lower portion of the thorax. Also note a small nodule *(arrow)*. **b:** High-resolution CT scan with a target factor of 1.7 obtained at the same level as the nodule seen in (a). Lines are seen around the nodule, which geometrically appear polyhedral and are reminiscent of pulmonary lobules. A longer, linear structure, with areas of focal thickening connected to the mediastinal pleural surface, can also be appreciated *(arrows)*. Whether these lines represent thickened septa due to tumor infiltration or lymphatics *per se* is not known, but this pattern of thickened, knotty lines distributed in a polyhedral pattern more prominent toward the central portions of the lungs has been quite consistent in our limited experience with cases of lymphangitic spread of tumor.

ta are diffusely thickened, with smooth margins, and can be visualized in all portions of the lung (most prominently in the dependent portions).

Lymphangitic Carcinomatosis

Lymphatic invasion by metastatic disease can be considered to be a prototypical interstitial process. Lymphatics lie in the interlobular septa and enlarge when they are involved by tumor. With high-resolution CT, a very suggestive pattern of irregularly thickened lines is seen, arranged in a polyhedral pattern reminiscent of the boundaries of secondary lobules (Fig. 28). Some of these linear structures are connected to the pleural surface of the mediastinum and exhibit knot-like thickenings along their course. We do not know whether these linear structures represent thickened lymphatics or septa, but their orientation is suggestive of lymphatics, with either small tumoral deposits or possibly thickened valves or crossing lymphatics explaining their knotty appearance. Early on, lymphangitic carcinomatosis presents a "reticular" pattern, which probably corresponds to the reticular pattern seen on chest radiographs. As the disease progresses, a more nodular appearance can be observed, with individual nodules identified but with preservation of the underlying pattern of a polyhedral network of thickened lines (Fig. 29). Particularly interesting is the

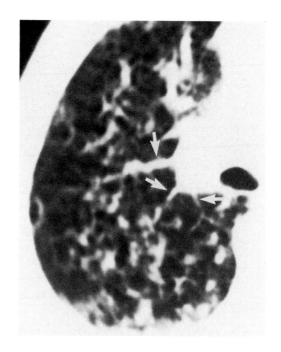

FIG. 29. Lymphangitic carcinomatosis. Section through the midportion of the right lung in a patient with carcinoma of the stomach and lymphangitic spread. Again note a reticular pattern of lines distributed centrally in a polyhedral fashion. Additionally, nodules can be defined that appear to be connected to the network of thickened lines. Note also the three linear structures directly connected to the mediastinal pleura *(arrows)*. This pattern is very suggestive of lymphangitic spread (compare with Fig. 28).

30a,b

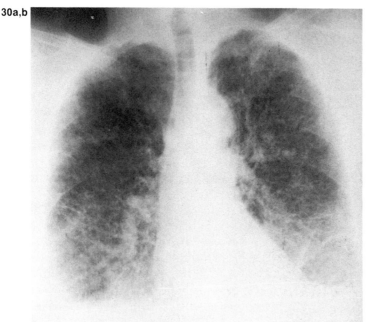

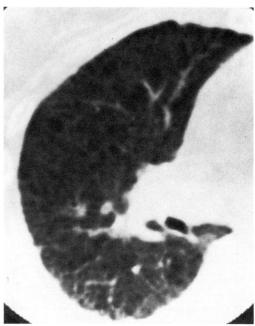

FIG. 30. A 35-year-old female with proven biopsy lymphangioleiomyomatosis. **a:** PA radiograph. There is diffuse, bilateral reticular lung disease. **b:** Section through the midportion of the right lung. Multiple, small air-cysts with a coarse reticular pattern can be noted throughout the lung. This pattern is different from that illustrated in Figs. 28 and 29, and is due to diffuse hypertrophy of the interstitium secondary to proliferation of muscle tissue. The air-cysts are areas of focal emphysema due to bronchial obstruction resulting from interstitial muscle hypertrophy.

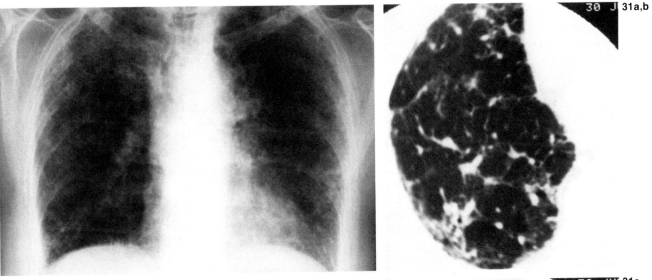

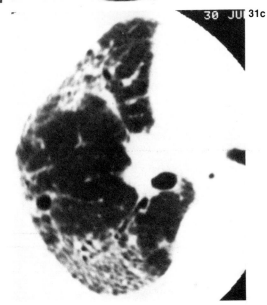

FIG. 31. Idiopathic interstitial fibrosis (52-year-old female with biopsy-proven diffuse interstitial fibrosis). **a:** PA radiograph. A diffuse reticular-nodular pattern is present. There are no apparent emphysematous changes. **b:** Representative high-resolution CT section through the right lower lobe. The caliber of vessels is diminished. A fine network of thickened septal lines can be seen, which is homogeneously distributed throughout the parenchyma. The lungs are not emphysematous. Additionally, a polyhedral pattern can be recognized, which probably represents the boundaries of secondary lobules. **c:** Section through the bronchus intermedius. Massive fibrosis is present, and differentiation from an early alveolar process is difficult. Two areas of increased density, with a stippled pattern, are noted on the posterior and anterolateral aspect of the section. Early pneumonia can have a similar appearance.

distribution of lymphangitic spread, with thickened lines seen in the central portion of the lungs near the mediastinum and hila and very little involvement of the subpleural areas of the lungs. This distribution is a distinctive feature, compared to the pattern of change seen in patients with interstitial edema, and is ideally visualized with CT because of the cross-sectional plane of imaging. The number of cases we have examined is limited, and definite conclusions regarding typical patterns are speculative.

Lymphangioleiomyomatosis is characterized by a proliferation of normal pulmonary tissue elements, of muscle fibers in particular. A diffuse reticular pattern, pleural effusions, and pneumothoraces are the most common roentgenographic findings in this disease. Air-cysts are almost always present, pre-sumably due to mechanical emphysema secondary to muscle hypertrophy, which causes partial bronchiolar obstruction. In the only case we have examined with CT, the cystic changes were readily apparent, and diffuse coarse thickening of the lung tissue around the air spaces was noted. The appearance of a linear polyhedral pattern, such as is seen with lymphangitic carcinomatosis, was not appreciated, suggesting that the reticular pattern seen on plain films is probably not due to lymphatic enlargement alone but mostly to interstitial hypertrophy (Fig. 30).

Interstitial Fibrosis

Fibrosis is an obligatory end-stage in the majority of diffuse pulmonary diseases. In most cases, a combination of cystic air-space and interstitial changes is seen. In rare instances, pure fibrosis is identified, as illustrated in Fig. 31. With fibrosis, the skeleton of the lung becomes very apparent, with thickening of the pleural surfaces. In our limited experience, the pattern on CT of fibrosis appears different from that of pulmonary edema and lymphangitic spread of tumor. The vessels appear diminished in caliber. The septa are irregularly distributed. A polyhedral distribution of thickened septa can be seen, but the lines have irregular margins.

Areas of massive fibrosis can closely resemble alveolar diseases such as early pneumonia (Fig. 31c). The pattern seen with interstitial fibrosis does not appear to be specific, and we have encountered it in cases of interstitial pneumonitis (Fig. 32).

Sarcoidosis

Sarcoidosis can increase global lung density, presumably because of the deposition of gran-ulomatous lesions in the lung interstitium. With high-resolution CT, the areas of interstitial thickening can be visualized directly (Fig. 33). Surprisingly, we have not seen a large number of thickened septal lines in patients with sarcoidosis. Small patches of increased density have been the most common finding, suggesting a multifocal distribution of disease rather than a truly diffuse interstitial process. When confluent, these focal areas of increased density become indistinguishable from alveolar-filling processes (see Figs. 18 and 19).

High-Resolution CT and Standard Radiographic Correlations

Marked discrepancies between the appearance of the lung on plain films and the degree of functional impairment are commonly observed. Perhaps the most important potential use of high-resolution CT is to achieve a better understanding of the reasons for such discrepancies. Some patients may demonstrate marked reticular changes on chest roentgeno-

32a,b

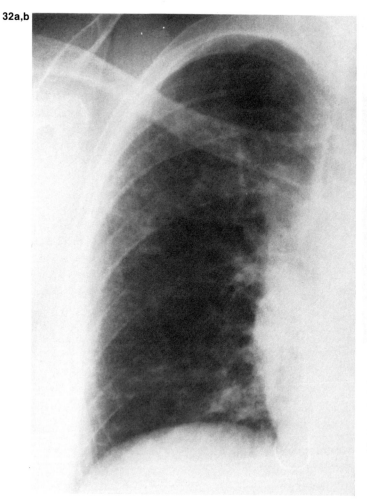

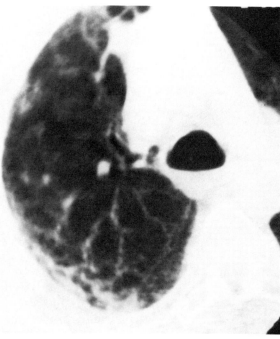

FIG. 32. Interstitial pneumonitis (62-year-old patient with lymphoma undergoing chemotherapy). This patient acutely developed a diffuse reticular pattern throughout both lung fields. **a:** PA radiograph. **b:** Representative section at the level of the carina. Thickened lines are again seen throughout the lungs, best appreciated in the posterior aspect of the section. These were interpreted to represent thickened septa. Biopsy showed nonspecific interstitial pneumonitis.

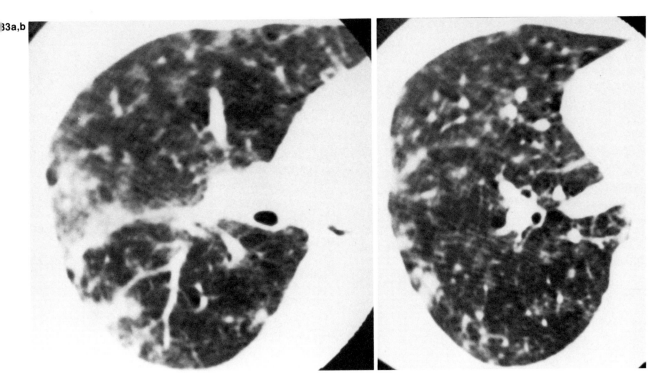

FIG. 33. Sarcoidosis. **a:** Section at the level of the bronchus intermedius. Scattered patches of increased density are seen throughout the section, most prominent anteriorly. These have a somewhat nodular configuration. Laterally, there is a presumed confluence of interstitial disease, which creates an appearance indistinguishable from an early alveolar infiltrate. Note the absence of thickened septal lines. **b:** Section at a lower level again demonstrates scattered patches of increased density, without a definite reticular pattern. Fine nodularity is present diffusely.

grams and yet have near-normal functional studies. Conversely, some patients may have near-normal radiographs and markedly altered pulmonary function. With CT, it is apparent that the *distribution* of abnormalities determines in great part whether or not they can be visualized on chest radiographs. When thickening of the interstitium occurs at the periphery of the lung, marked chest X-ray film abnormalities with a reticular pattern are seen (Fig. 34). When the abnormalities are centrally located and spare the periphery, very few radiographic abnormalities are apparent unless the changes are quite prominent (Fig. 35).

The occurrence of cases such as those illustrated in Figs. 34 and 35, in which exclusively central or exclusively peripheral changes are noted, lends some credibility to the concept of a lung organized into a medulla and cortex, and illustrates the potential of CT as a tool in the investigation of pulmonary parenchymal processes.

To date, we have not shown that CT can reliably demonstrate interstitial disease before it is apparent on chest radiographs because most of our patients have been selected on the basis of radiographic abnormalities, except for a few individuals in whom

markedly abnormal pulmonary function studies with normal radiographs prompted a CT study.

Analysis of Inspiration–Expiration High-Resolution CT Scans

Analysis of the lung architecture at inspiration and expiration can provide dynamic information on the status of the pulmonary parenchyma. Regional ventilation can easily be assessed, as illustrated in Fig. 5. The presence or absence of variation with diffuse abnormalities is a reflection of the compliance of the lung (Fig. 36). High-resolution CT, coupled with the dynamic structural information of inspiration–expiration scans, can become a valuable clinical tool in selected groups of patients, such as those with large bullae in whom resection is contemplated and information on the status of the underlying compressed lung is difficult to obtain by traditional means.

Preliminary Conclusions

The interstitium of the lung can be analyzed morphologically with CT if the proper technique is

34a,b

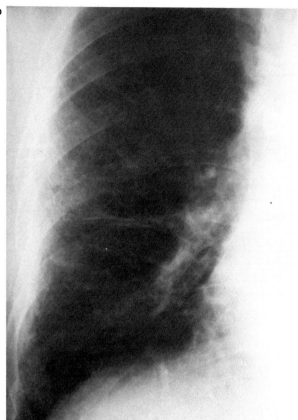
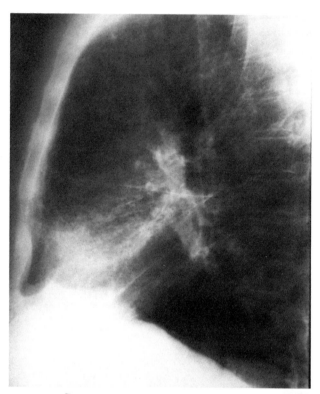

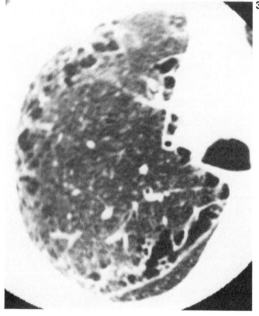

34c

FIG. 34. CT–plain film correlation: peripheral or "cortical" distribution. **a,b:** Cone-down view of the right lung (a) and a lateral radiograph (b). A diffuse reticular pattern is present. **c:** Representative CT section at the level of the carina. Cystic air-spaces lined by markedly thickened septa are noted at the periphery of the lung. The central or "medullary" portion of the lung is spared. This patient had very minimal pulmonary functional abnormalities. We presume that the marked reticular pattern seen on chest X-ray films is due to the location of the disease at the periphery of the lungs, where septa are perpendicular to the pleural surface and are more likely to be seen, giving the impression of extensive disease even though only the periphery of the lung is involved.

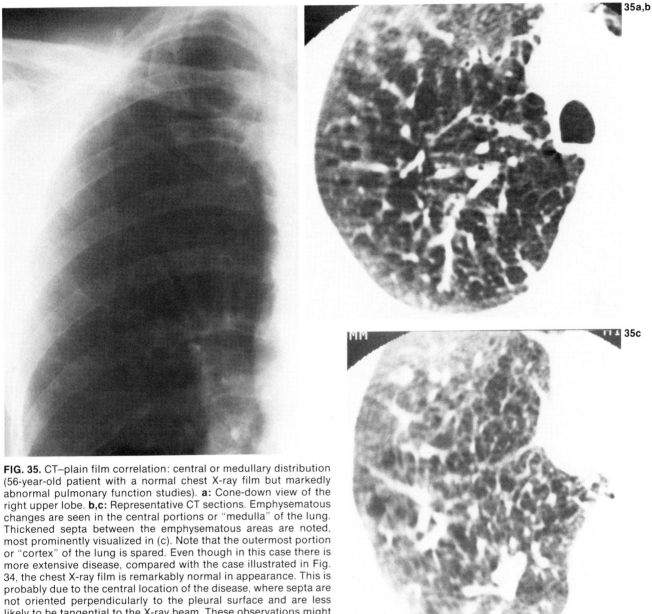

FIG. 35. CT–plain film correlation: central or medullary distribution (56-year-old patient with a normal chest X-ray film but markedly abnormal pulmonary function studies). **a:** Cone-down view of the right upper lobe. **b,c:** Representative CT sections. Emphysematous changes are seen in the central portions or "medulla" of the lung. Thickened septa between the emphysematous areas are noted, most prominently visualized in (c). Note that the outermost portion or "cortex" of the lung is spared. Even though in this case there is more extensive disease, compared with the case illustrated in Fig. 34, the chest X-ray film is remarkably normal in appearance. This is probably due to the central location of the disease, where septa are not oriented perpendicularly to the pleural surface and are less likely to be tangential to the X-ray beam. These observations might explain the discrepancies traditionally noted between chest X-ray films and pulmonary function studies.

36a,b

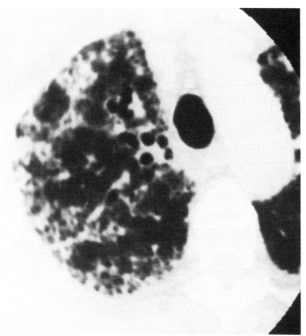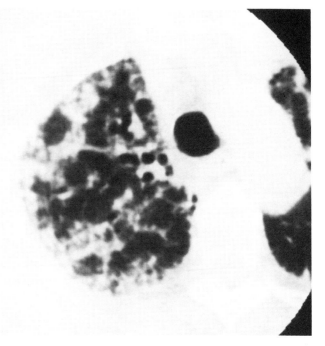

FIG. 36. Idiopathic interstitial fibrosis: the value of inspiration–expiration scans (patient with extensive idiopathic interstitial fibrosis and a marked restrictive defect on pulmonary function studies). **a:** CT section at inspiration. **b:** CT section at expiration. The two sections have been obtained at the same level. The lung increases slightly in density at expiration. Normally, a much larger increase in density should be noted. Some tiny air-spaces noted within the areas of fibrosis are not apparent on the expiration views, suggesting that they have collapsed. The minimal change in size of the visible structures probably indicates a marked decrease in compliance.

used. Visualization of the small details of the lung architecture are within the capabilities of current scanners. Normal and abnormal patterns can be defined and help in understanding the chest X-ray films. Cross-sectional analysis of the lung parenchyma, as well as inspiration–expiration comparisons, provides information not otherwise available. At present, CT of the lung interstitium is still experimental, and the definition of clinical applications awaits further research and experience.

CAVITARY–CYSTIC LUNG DISEASE

A wide range of pathologic conditions, both benign and malignant, are manifested by pulmonary cysts or cavities. As reviewed by Godwin et al. (36), differential diagnosis includes infectious diseases, congenital diseases (for example, cystic adenomatoid malformations), airway diseases (emphysema and bronchiectasis), embolic disease, autoimmune disease, diseases of unknown etiology (including sarcoidosis), as well as a variety of neoplasms. The semiology of cavitation, and to a lesser extent of pulmonary cysts, includes localization and characterization (specifically of size, wall thickness, and regularity), the presence of air–fluid lev-

els, intracavitary filling defects, and the nature of the surrounding pulmonary parenchyma (normal or abnormal). Despite this wide range of variables, histologic and/or bacteriologic specificity is rare, and correlation with presenting symptomatology and clinical history is crucial.

Computed tomography has several critical roles in the evaluation of patients with cavitary or cystic lung disease. It is efficacious in detecting the presence of otherwise unsuspected pathology. As shown by Kruglik and Wayne (37), CT can define the presence of otherwise occult cavities. The transverse orientation of CT sections avoids superimposition of vascular and bony shadows, and hence is most useful in areas that are generally difficult to define, specifically, the lung apices, lung adjacent to the mediastinum, the retrocardiac portions of the left lower lobe, and the inferior, posterior recesses of the lung (Fig. 37).

Of equal significance, but generally unrecognized, is the fact that CT can also disclose discrete cavities in areas of extensive pulmonary consolidation and/or fibrosis. In this setting, superimposition of abnormal lung densities limits detection and delineation of small cavities on routine radiographs (Fig. 15).

Finally, CT can be employed to differentiate con-

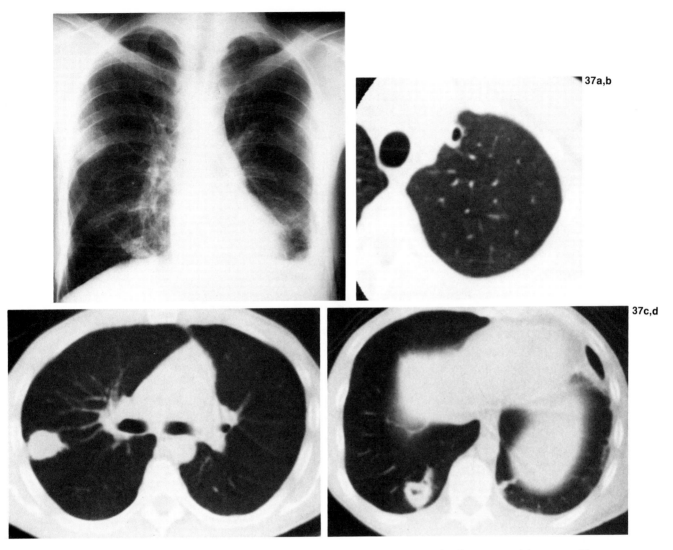

FIG. 37. Occult cavitation: septic pulmonary emboli. **a:** PA radiograph shows scattered pulmonary nodules, one with a suggestion of cavitation near the right hemidiaphragm. Pleural disease is present as well. **b:** Enlargement of a section through the left upper lobe. A small, thin-walled cavity is present adjacent to the mediastinal pleura, in which there is a small air–fluid level. It is apparent why cross-sectional imaging is more accurate in detecting small abscesses than are conventional radiographs. **c,d:** Sections through the mid- and lower lung fields. A focal, peripheral nodular density is present in (c); a similar nodule is present in the lower lobe (d), in which central cavitation can be defined. This range of abnormalities—from a solid-appearing nodule to a thick-walled cavity and finally to a thin-walled cavity—is typical of the sequence of events encountered in patients with septic pulmonary emboli, including the simultaneous appearance of all stages of evolution in the same study.

ditions that mimic pulmonary cavitation, such as empyema with a bronchopleural fistula, or herniation of bowel into the thorax secondary to a diaphragmatic defect. CT is less specific in differentiating among the various causes of parenchymal cavitation, although, as will be discussed, certain conditions such as emphysema do have characteristic appearances on CT.

Lung Abscesses

Lung abscesses result from a wide variety of etiologic agents, including bacteria, fungi, and para-sites. Over the last few years, there has been a change in the epidemiology of lung abscesses; these are now most commonly caused by *Staphylococcus* and gram-negative bacteria.

Most lung abscesses do not require evaluation with CT. Specific indications for CT include a clinical history consistent with pulmonary infection and cavitation, otherwise not apparent on routine radiographs; equivocal radiographs, in which cavitation cannot be excluded or in which a cavity is present but it is not clear if it is within the pulmonary parenchyma; evaluation of cavities to exclude intracavitary pathology; and, finally, evaluation of cavitary lung disease thought to be secondary to central endobronchial obstruction.

Abscess cavities are variably shaped, although they tend to be rounded. Abscesses usually have irregular wall thickness, nodular inner margins, and are frequently surrounded by irregular zones of parenchymal consolidation (Fig. 38). Air within a lung cavity implies communication with a bronchus. If the communication is sufficiently large, the contents of the abscess cavity, following liquefaction, may drain into the airways. If complete, the result is a thin-walled cystic cavity (Fig. 39). This may occur from any infectious etiology.

Thin-walled cysts, or more properly pneumatoceles, also result from pulmonary infection, frequently without evidence of initial cavitation. It has been estimated that approximately 60% of patients with staphylococcal pneumonias in the early stages of resolution develop pneumatoceles (38). The same may occur with gram-negative pneumonias and fungal infections. The mechanism of formation of pneumatoceles is essentially the same as that described for the evolution of lung abscesses. That is, pneumatoceles are thought to form in areas of pulmonic consolidation in which peribronchial abscesses, not apparent at first with routine radiographs, erode into adjacent bronchioles. The result is a thin-walled cavity that is generally transient.

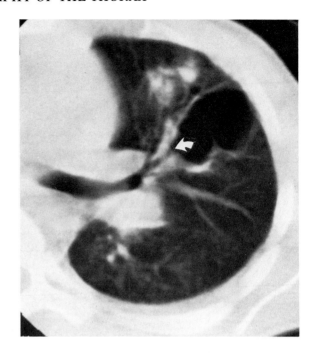

FIG. 39. Lung abscess: bronchial communication. Enlargement of a section through the left upper lobe. A thin-walled cystic abscess is present. There is clear communication between the abscess cavity and the anterior segmental bronchus of the left upper lobe (arrow). At bronchoscopy, this communication could be visualized, and the bronchoscope was actually passed into the cavity itself.

When they are chronic, abscess cavities may become superinfected, with resultant formation of a fungus ball, or mycetoma. This is especially common with *Aspergillus*. Traditionally, this diagosis has been made with plain radiographs, decubitus films, and conventional tomography. As reported by Breuer et al. (39), CT may disclose the presence of a mycetoma even when this is not apparent with other radiologic techniques. This is especially important in cases in which the cavity is small or in which the fungus ball fills most of the lumen of the cavity (Fig. 40). The presence of intracavitary filling defects, of course, is nonspecific, and could as well be secondary to intracavitary debris, tumor, or blood. The specific diagnosis of a fungus ball may first be suspected with CT, but the diagnosis requires corroborating clinical and laboratory evidence.

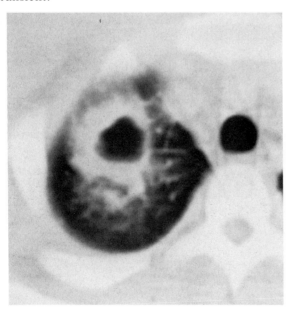

FIG. 38. Lung abscess. Enlargement of a section through an abscess in the right upper lobe. The wall of the abscess is thickened, and nodular, especially along its inner margin. The presence of air within the cavity means that the abscess communicates with an adjacent airway. Surrounding the abscess cavity is a poorly defined zone of pulmonary consolidation.

Neoplasia

Cavitation has been estimated to occur in up to 5% of pulmonary metastases, and is known to occur with primary lung tumors as well. Although this is most frequently seen with squamous cell carcinoma, it is not an infrequent complication of ade-

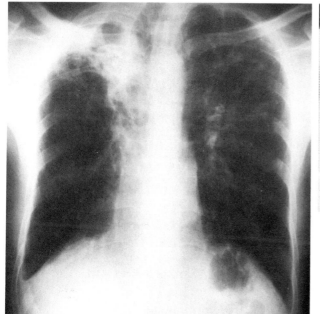

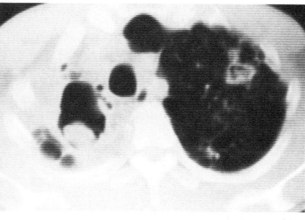

40a,b

FIG. 40. Intracavitary mycetomas: chronic tuberculosis. **a:** PA radiograph shows extensive cavitary and fibronodular changes in both lung apices. A large cavity is present in the right upper lobe, with a suggestion of an intracavitary filling defect. **b:** Section through the upper lobes. A thick-walled cavity can be defined in the right upper lobe, within which there is a well-defined circular filling defect. Prone CT sections revealed this defect to be free-moving (not shown). A smaller cavity is present in the left upper lobe as well, in which a filling defect can also be defined. This too was free-moving. Small cavities with intracavitary densities that fill most of the lumen of the cavity may be difficult to define unless seen in cross section.

nocarcinoma, or, in fact, of a wide range of metastatic lesions, especially sarcomas.

The pathogenesis of cavitation has been disputed. Ostensibly, cavitation occurs in squamous cell carcinoma as a result of extensive cornification of squamous epithelium in the center of these lesions, with subsequent liquefaction and evacuation into adjacent airways. A similar mechanism has been invoked for adenocarcinomas, in which mucin pro-duction and subsequent degeneration and evacuation produce central cavitation. More rarely, primary pulmonary lymphomas undergo cavitation, especially in patients with Hodgkin's disease. The pathogenesis of cavitation in these cases is uncertain. It is apparent that most cavitating neoplasms are similar in appearance, and may easily be confused with lung abscesses (Fig. 41; compare with Fig. 38).

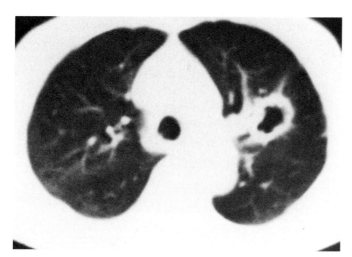

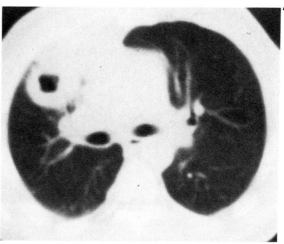

41a,b

FIG. 41. Cavitary neoplasia. **a:** Squamous cell carcinoma, left upper lobe. **b:** Primary Hodgkin's disease of the lung, right upper lobe. In this case, lung cavitation was the only abnormality. The similarities between these lesions are apparent. Differentiation among the various cavitary neoplasms is difficult, as is differentiation from lung abscesses (compare with Fig. 38). Finding a zone of poorly defined parenchymal consolidation around a thick-walled cavity is more common with lung abscesses, but should not be considered to be diagnostic.

Pulmonary cavitation may also occur in patients with pulmonary spread of laryngotracheal papillomatosis (40). This is a relatively frequent disease affecting infants and children. The condition is characterized by polypoid excrescences growing in the laryngeal and tracheal mucosa. These are sessile or papillary lesions composed of a vascular connective tissue stalk covered with a stratified, squamous epithelium. Pulmonary parenchymal involvement is rare, and there is generally a 10–15 year interval between presentation of laryngotracheal papillomas and involvement of the lung.

Characteristically, pulmonary lesions become evident following biopsies of central lesions and/or tracheostomies. Distal parenchymal involvement has been attributed to spread by aspiration after manipulation of central lesions. Lesions within the lung parenchyma vary from small, isolated clusters of squamous cells to large, cavitating lesions. Cavities are usually thin-walled (2–3 mm), and are lined with papillomas. Cavitation probably occurs as a result of necrosis and excavation of a solid nodular lesion, although airway obstruction with resultant emphysema, followed by ingrowth of papillomas along these distended air-spaces, has been described. The appearance can mimic that of cystic bronchiectasis (Fig. 42).

Pulmonary Infarction

Pulmonary thromboembolism with infarction is a rare cause of pulmonary cavitation. While cavitation has been reported at autopsy in approximately 3% of patients, McGoldrick et al. (41), in their series of 32 patients with 58 angiographically proven pulmonary infarcts followed serially with chest radiographs, failed to detect evidence of cavitation in any patient. In 50% of these patients, clearing was complete; in the remainder, linear pulmonary scars, pleural–diaphragmatic adhesions, and localized pleural thickening were the only sequelae. Occasionally, pulmonary cavitation following thromboembolism may result in large cavities. These may appear at some distance from the peripheral pleural surfaces (Fig. 43). Presumably, they are adjacent to the fissures.

More commonly, cavitation results from septic pulmonary emboli. These occur in patients with congenital heart disease, endocarditis, especially among abusers of intravenous drugs, or, more rarely, from surgery or infected in-dwelling catheters. The usual infecting organism is *Staphylococcus,* although various etiologic agents may be responsible. Characteristically, these lesions are multiple, and individual areas of septic infarction frequently progress and/or disappear as new lesions arise. As shown in Fig. 37, septic emboli will first appear as ill-defined nodular densities that undergo cavitation (with a resultant irregular, thickened wall) and finally progress to smooth-walled lesions, occasionally with air–fluid levels. The occurrence of all stages of evolution at the same time, while not pathognomonic, is sufficiently characteristic to suggest the specific diagnosis.

42a,b

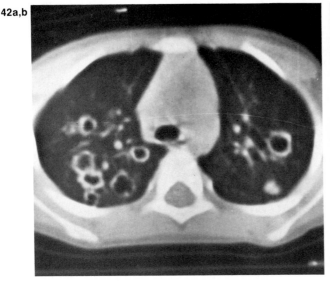 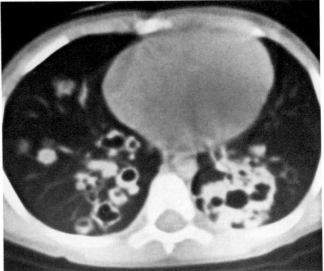

FIG. 42. Laryngotracheal papillomatosis. **a,b:** Images through the upper (a) and lower (b) lobes. Numerous thin- and thick-walled cavities are present in both lungs; the appearance is somewhat suggestive of cystic bronchiectasis, including the presence of air–fluid levels. While bronchiectasis may complicate this disease, in this case, all changes were due to neoplasia.

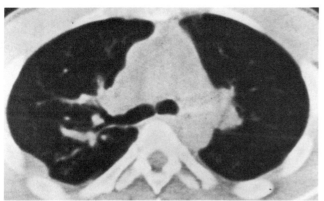
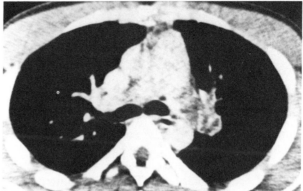

43a,b

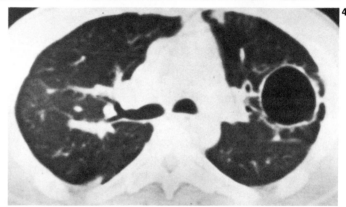

43c

FIG. 43. Pulmonary infarction. **a:** Section through the left main pulmonary artery, imaged with a wide window. The pulmonary parenchyma is normal. **b:** Same section imaged with narrow window following a bolus of intravenous contrast medium. A large filling defect is present in the left main pulmonary artery. Thrombus was confirmed by angiography (not shown). **c:** Section at approximately the same level as (a) several weeks later. A large thin-walled cavity is present in the left upper lobe. This sequence of events is unusual, since most cases of pulmonary thromboembolism resolve without resultant parenchymal cavitation. In this case, the cavity probably abuts the major fissure.

Airway Disease

Airway disease may be divided conveniently into two categories: emphysema and bronchiectasis. In both diseases, diffuse or focal cystic lung disease may result.

Emphysema

Emphysema has been defined as a condition characterized by a beyond-normal increase in the size of the air-spaces distal to the terminal bronchiole, either due to dilatation and/or destruction of their walls (14). Emphysema has been subdivided still further on the basis of its distribution within the pulmonary acinus into selective, nonselective, and irregular types. Pathologically, an emphysematous process that destroys all lung distal to a terminal bronchus is called pancinar, whereas selective destruction of lung distal to the terminal bronchus, especially when there is involvement predominantly affecting the respiratory bronchioles, is called centriacinar. Irregular emphysema is generally reserved for nonuniform involvement of an acinus, usually adjacent to pulmonary scars. Of

these, centriacinar emphysema is by far the most common (Fig. 1).

The terms bleb and bulla are also descriptive of emphysema. A bleb is a collection of air contained within the layers of the visceral pleura. A bulla is defined as an emphysematous space with a diameter greater than 1 cm. Bullae within the pulmonary parenchyma exist either as solitary spaces in otherwise normal lungs or as part of diffuse emphysema and chronic obstructive pulmonary disease.

Although controversial, it appears that the basic underlying pathologic process in diffuse emphysema is abnormalities of the distal airways, leading to obstruction and resultant air-trapping and overdistension. The ultimate result of protracted airtrapping is distension and then destruction of alveolar walls.

The plain radiographic findings of emphysema have been described (42). These include increased lucency of the lung secondary to air-trapping, changes involving the chest wall and diaphragms, and changes in the caliber of the pulmonary blood vessels, which become attenuated and widely spaced. As is well known, correlation between radiographic findings and gross pathologic findings is poor, especially when the disease process is mild.

Surprisingly little has been written concerning the use of CT in defining emphysema (32,43). Even as central a problem as the differentiation of panacinar from centriacinar emphysema has not been resolved. This is all the more surprising since CT is an exquisitely sensitive method of detecting increases in air-spaces with resultant decreases in density, both diffuse and focal, within the lung parenchyma (Fig. 1a).

While emphysematous changes usually arise *de novo*, air-trapping is also a concomitant of a large number of diffuse parenchymal diseases. Recognition of the presence of extensive air-trapping in this setting may aid in differential diagnosis. This is illustrated in Fig. 30, an example of pulmonary lymphangiomyomatosis (44). This rare disease generally affects women of child-bearing age. Symptoms include recurrent chylous effusions and/or spontaneous pneumothorax. Pathologically, there is an abnormal proliferation of smooth muscle in the interstitium as well as diffuse lymphangiectasis. Smooth muscle proliferation around the bronchioles leads to air-trapping, with resultant focal and/or bullous emphysema, and increased lung volume in the face of severe, diffuse interstitial disease.

While the diagnosis of air-trapping may be inferred from plain radiographs in a number of diffuse disease processes, CT is far superior in precisely defining and delimiting the extent of this process. In its most florid form, diffuse interstitial lung disease results in "honey-combing." This has been defined as replacement of normal lung parenchyma by small, rounded cyst-like spaces located amid areas of extensive pulmonary fibrosis. The cysts represent progressive confluence of distal air-spaces, together with thickening and condensation of the septa. Cysts generally measure 5 mm or more in diameter, and are lined by bronchiolar epithelium. Air-space dilatation found in honeycomb lung differs from the usual forms of emphysema or pulmonary myomatosis in that the cysts in these diseases are not entirely lined by bronchiolar epithelium, and fibrosis of the walls is slight or absent. In other respects, the underlying pathology of air-space dilatation is similar (Fig. 44).

As pointed out by Heitzman (1), the plain radiographic diagnosis of honeycombing may be difficult, especially when a reticular pattern is also present. CT is clearly of benefit in equivocal cases, since detection of thick-walled, dilated air-spaces is simplified when they are viewed in cross section.

Bullous emphysema may be defined in cross section as areas of abnormal pulmonary parenchyma in which all normal parenchymal markings, including

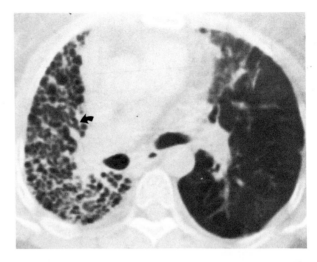

FIG. 44. Honeycomb lung. Section through the bronchus intermedius. The right lung is replaced by innumerable small cavities. Variability in the size of these cavities is present but not striking. In this case, the etiology of honeycombing was never confirmed. The presence of central bronchiectasis *(arrow)* and a history of previously treated tuberculosis suggested the probable etiology.

blood vessels, have disappeared (Fig. 45). These areas may not have definable walls. While bullae may occur in any location, generally they are found in subpleural locations. Strands, or septa, within these lesions are commonplace.

Fluid accumulation within bullae, infected or otherwise, is not infrequent. Confusion may arise in this setting and lead to misdiagnosis. Superficially, fluid accumulations in bullae, especially when they are subpleural in location, may be mistaken for loculated hydropneumothoraces (Fig. 46). The key to the differentiation of these is to recognize the characteristic strands or septa within the fluid-filled

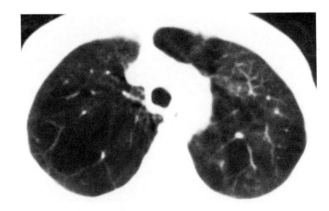

FIG. 45. Bullous emphysema. Section through the upper lung fields. There is marked diffuse bullous emphysema, characterized by a decrease in the overall density of the pulmonary parenchyma associated with a decrease in overall vascularity. Distinct walls cannot be defined, although bowing and stretching of vessels in both upper lobes suggests the presence of space-occupying lesions.

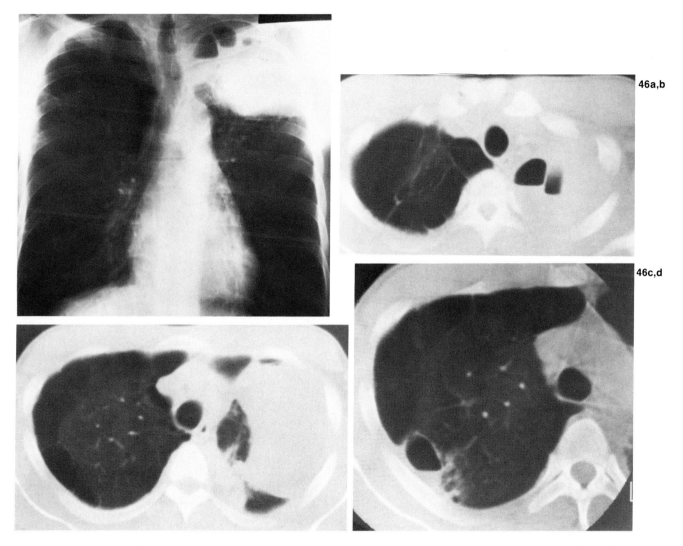

FIG. 46. Infected bullous emphysema. **a:** PA radiograph. There is considerable opacity in the left lung apex; in addition, air–fluid levels can be defined that have a stepladder configuration. The right lung apex is hyperinflated, suggestive of bullous emphysema. **b:** Section through the left lung apex. The stepladder configuration of the air–fluid levels seen in (a) is also apparent in cross section. Note that the inner margins of the cavities are exceedingly smooth. Separation of air–fluid levels is caused by fluid in separate locules, presumably caused by fibrous strands. These frequently may be defined in areas of bullous emphysema. **c:** Section through the midtrachea. A large fluid density is present laterally. The configuration of this lesion is unusual in that it is not clearly pulmonary in origin, yet it does not appear to conform to the shape of the chest wall and pleural cavity. Another smaller fluid-filled lesion is present posteromedially. This proved to be a long-standing infected bulla, which promptly drained with medical therapy. **d:** Enlargement of a section through the right upper lobe in the same patient, approximately 1 week after institution of medical therapy. The infected bulla on the left has spontaneously drained (not shown). A cavity with an air–fluid level is present on the right side. Comparison with the prior CT study shows that there was extensive peripheral bullous emphysema present in this same locale (compare with (c) on the right side). In this case, the patient aspirated fluid from the infected bulla on the left, which then filled a smaller bulla on the right side, thus illustrating graphically that peripheral bullae may still retain open communication with more central airways.

bullae. These may appear to have a "stepladder" configuration when individual locules within the bullae become fluid-filled.

As pointed out by Stark et al. (45) fluid accumulation in preexisting pulmonary air spaces generally has a benign natural course, adequately treated in most cases by conservative management. Inter-estingly, clearing of fluid in infected bullae in one part of the thorax may lead to aspiration and fluid accumulation in other bullae far removed from the original site of infection (Fig. 46).

Fluid within bullae may mimic lung abscesses. As shown in Fig. 47, apparent thickening of the walls may be secondary to compressed lung and/or par-

47a

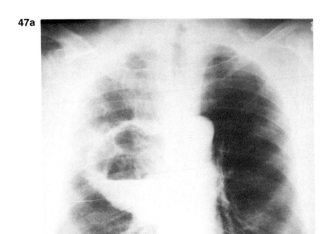

FIG. 47. Infected bullous emphysema. **a:** PA radiograph shows a large, apparently thick-walled cavity on the right side, initially thought to be a lung abscess. **b,c:** Enlargements of a section through this lesion imaged with wide (a) and narrow (b) windows. The lesion is peripheral, and there are numerous fine septa within. The outer or lateral wall of this cavity appears thickened; in fact, this represents compressed and consolidated parenchyma adjacent to the lesion. The actual wall thickness can be defined anteriorly with narrow windows, and is exceedingly thin *(arrow)* (surgically proven).

47b,c

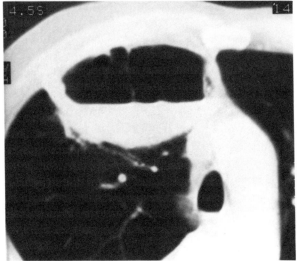
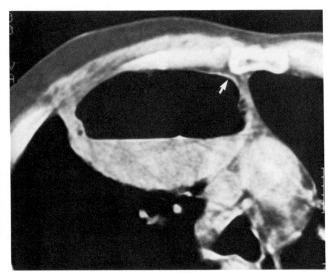

enchymal consolidation adjacent to enlarging infected bulla. Differential diagnosis is aided by CT when thin strands or septa can be defined in a thin-walled, subpleural cavity.

Bronchiectasis

This topic is covered in detail in Chapter 4. Unlike most cavitary lung disease, specific patterns of change within the pulmonary parenchyma allow precise characterization of this disease process on CT. Specifically, the finding of well-defined cavities adjacent to pulmonary arteries is characteristic (Fig. 48).

Miscellaneous Conditions

Any number of disease processes may be evidenced by cystic or cavitary lung disease. Most of them are not common. Certain categories, such as lung cavities caused by autoimmune diseases, rheumatoid arthritis, Wegener's granulomatosis, or polyarthritis nodosa, are generally accompanied by other, extrathoracic manifestations that help to establish the diagnosis. It has recently been suggested that cavitation in patients with lupus erythematosus or mixed connective tissue diseases may be the result of infection or pulmonary embolism, and that vasculitis with ischemic necrosis is unusual (46). It is doubtful that CT will have an important role in establishing the diagnosis in these diseases.

Computed tomography has been shown to be of value in the diagnosis of congenital cystic adenomatoid malformations of the lung (CCAM). This is an uncommon anomaly, generally showing up in infants who suffer from severe respiratory distress. Pathologically, CCAM is characterized by anomalous fetal development of terminal respiratory structures, resulting in an adenomatoid prolifera-

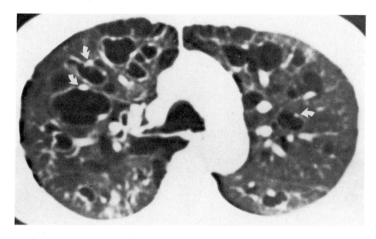

FIG. 48. Cystic bronchiectasis. Section through the right upper lobe bronchus in a patient with severe, diffuse cystic bronchiectasis. The key to the diagnosis is recognition that, despite the large size of these cavities, branches of the pulmonary artery can be defined eccentrically adjacent to each cavity—the signet-ring sign *(arrows).*

tion of bronchiolar elements and cyst formation. CCAM represents 25% of all congenital lung malformations. Blane et al. (47) showed that CT can be useful in differentiating CCAM from congenital lobar emphysema. Hulnick et al. (48) have reported the findings on CT of CCAM in adults. They found well-defined intrapulmonary masses composed of a combination of air-filled and fluid-filled spaces, as well as areas of solid tissue. CT best disclosed the complex nature of these lesions, especially the multiplicity and variability in the size of the cysts and the cyst walls.

Cystic lung disease is also known to frequently complicate diffuse parenchymal sarcoidosis (49). Usually, cystic changes in the lung accompany far-advanced, fibrotic lung changes, and can be demonstrated to represent blebs, bullae, and areas of cystic bronchiectasis. Airway disease probably occurs for a variety of reasons: the presence of endobronchial and peribronchial sarcoid nodules that compress and narrow the airways sufficiently to cause emphysema is frequently cited. Cavitation

also occurs from unrelated causes, such as microbacterial or mycotic infections.

Rarely, primary acute pulmonary cavitation occurs in sarcoidosis. Primary cavitation is easily distinguished pathologically from bullae, blebs, and bronchiectasis, although differentiation from other causes of cavitation may be difficult. Primary pulmonary cavitation has been attributed to ischemic necrosis within conglomerate areas of sarcoid granulomas. In one review (50), primary cavitating sarcoidosis typically occurred in young individuals with nodular disease elsewhere in the pulmonary parenchyma. Fibrosis was conspicuously absent. Cavities were generally noted to be thin-walled, and averaged 3–5 cm in diameter (Fig. 49).

Overview of Cavitary–Cystic Lung Disease

A wide array of disease processes causes cystic or cavitary lung disease, and differentiation among these entities may prove difficult. CT is of benefit in the following ways.

49a,b

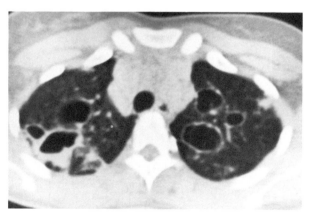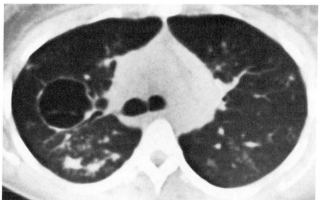

FIG. 49. Cavitary sarcoidosis. **a,b:** Sections through the upper and midlung fields in a patient with cavitary sarcoidosis. Numerous cavities, most thin-walled, are present in both lungs. One thicker-walled lesion with an air–fluid level is present in the right upper lobe. There is extensive mediastinal and bilateral hilar adenopathy. Additionally, scattered acinar nodules can be seen bilaterally (compare with Fig. 18). Cavitation in sarcoidosis usually is a complication of far-advanced disease, and represents blebs, bullae, and bronchiectasis. Primary cavitary sarcoidosis is rare, and is usually seen in association with acinar lung disease (biopsy-proven).

Computed tomography can help identify cavities and/or cysts that are not apparent on routine radiographs. Potentially, this is most applicable in defining the presence of otherwise unsuspected emphysema. While differentiation between the forms of emphysema (panacinar vs. centriacinar) may have little clinical significance, confirmation of the presence and extent of the disease process should prove clinically significant. Additionally, CT can be of value in determining the presence of cavitary disease in areas difficult to visualize with routine chest X-ray films, as has been illustrated (Figs. 15 and 37). In our experience, this has proven to be most clinically useful in patients suspected of having active cavitary tuberculosis.

Computed tomography can help in the analysis of cavitary–cystic lung disease. While there is considerable overlap among the appearances of most lung cavities, certain patterns seen in cross section are sufficiently distinct to suggest the correct diagnosis. This has been most clearly established with diffuse and/or focal pulmonary emphysema, but is also true of bronchiectasis and septic pulmonary infarcts (Fig. 37).

Of equal importance is the value of CT in confirming that a given cavity is, in fact, pulmonary in origin. This is most significant when attempting to differentiate lung abscesses from empyemas with associated bronchopleural fistulae. The characteristic appearance of lung abscesses has been discussed. Empyemas with bronchopleural fistulae may be differentiated in most cases because they conform to the shape of the pleural cavity and have smooth, thin walls. Differentiation is significant, since lung abscesses are generally treated conservatively, whereas empyemas require tube drainage (either open or closed).

Another potentially important use of CT is in precise characterization of lung cavities to differentiate benign from malignant disease. While it is usually acknowledged that absolute differentiation may be difficult, recent evidence suggests that accurate definition of wall thickness is of predictive value. Woodring et al. (51,52), in their studies of the significance of wall thickness in solitary cavities of the lung, found that by measuring the thickest portion of the cavity wall, 95% of all cavities with a maximum wall thickness of 4 mm proved to be benign. It is anticipated that accurate determination of true wall thickness will be more accurate with CT, as compared to other modalities. The clinical significance of this, however, remains to be determined.

CONCLUSIONS

There has been a significant delay in the evaluation of the role of CT in the diagnosis of pulmonary parenchymal disease. In part, this is due to the need for high-quality imaging, which necessitated the development of fast scanners. More important, delay has resulted from continued reliance on routine radiography as the standard for the detection and characterization of parenchymal abnormalities. Because of the naturally high contrast provided by aeration within the lung, chest radiography remains the mainstay of radiologic evaluation of lung disease. This should not obscure the important limitations that are encountered in interpreting pulmonary abnormalities with chest X-ray films.

Computed tomography, because of its tomographic, cross-sectional representation of the lung, allows visualization of extremely fine detail in the lung parenchyma. Avoidance of superimposition, not only of extrapulmonary structures, such as the ribs and chest wall, but of abnormal densities in the lung itself, provides insight into the nature of lung pathology previously unavailable.

We have attempted in this chapter to illustrate the potential of CT for augmenting our knowledge of pulmonary disease. Our material has been organized around the traditional approach of pattern recognition, largely because this is the time-honored means of characterizing parenchymal disease. Much of the material presented is necessarily speculative, since this type of detailed evaluation of the lung is in its earliest stages of development.

It is apparent that cross-sectional imaging has two significant advantages over routine radiologic evaluation of the lungs. First, CT is efficacious in the detection of focal and/or occult pulmonary disease. While this has been most thoroughly documented for the detection of pulmonary nodules, it is also true of the detection of subtle parenchymal consolidation and cavitation, as well as occasionally of diffuse pulmonary interstitial disease.

Second, and of even greater potential value, CT is superior to routine radiography in the precise characterization of the nature of parenchymal disease. As illustrated throughout this chapter, specific patterns of lung disease can be defined in cross section that are otherwise not apparent. Ultimately, this may lead to a redefinition of the basic categories of parenchymal disease. Documentation of medullary, as compared with cortical lung disease, is but one example. At the least, it should be anticipated that CT will further our understanding of the patterns of disease seen with chest X-ray films.

Finally, the question of CT densitometry still has to be resolved. Standardization of approach, interpretation, and technique will be mandatory before this type of evaluation becomes routine. It is to be expected, however, that, with time, these problems will be clarified.

REFERENCES

1. Heitzman ER. *The Lung: Radiologic–Pathologic Correlations.* Saint Louis, C.V. Mosby Company, 1973
2. Suchato C, Ostavanichvong K, Pekanan P. Double-exposure technique for computed tomographic imaging on x-ray film. *Radiology* 144:646, 1982
3. Borlaza GS, Seigel R, Fischer B, Kuhns LR. Double exposure technique for demonstration of osseous and pulmonary structure on a single CT film. *AJR* 130:375–376, 1978
4. Robinson PJ, Kreel L. Pulmonary tissue attenuation with computed tomography: Comparison of inspiration and expiration scans. *J Comput Assist Tomogr* 3:740–748, 1979
5. Rosenblum LJ, Mauceri RA, Wellenstein DE, Thomas FD, Bassano DA, Raasch BN, Chamberlain CC, Heitzman ER. Density patterns in the normal lung as determined by computed tomography. *Radiology* 137:409–416, 1980
6. Wegener OH, Oeser H. Measurement of lung density by computed tomography. *J Comput Assist Tomogr* 2:263–273, 1978
7. Hedlund LW, Anderson RF, Goulding PL, Beck JW, Effmann EL, Putnam CE. Two methods for isolating the lung area of a CT scan for density information. *Radiology* 144:353–357, 1982
8. Levi C, Gray JE, McCullough EC, Hattery RR. The unreliability of CT numbers as absolute values. *AJR* 139:443–447, 1982
9. Gur D, Drayer BP, Borovetz HS, Griffith BP, Hardesty RL, Wolfson SK. Dynamic computed tomography of the lung: Regional ventilation measurements. *J Comput Assist Tomogr* 3:749–753, 1979
10. Gur D, Shabason L, Borovetz HS, Herbert DL, Reece GJ, Kennedy WH, Serago C. Regional pulmonary ventilation measurements by xenon enhanced dynamic computed tomography: An update. *J Comput Assist Tomogr* 5:678–683, 1981
11. Robinson PJ, Jones KR. Improved control of respiration during computed tomography by feedback monitoring. *J Comput Assist Tomogr* 6:802–806, 1982
12. Ball WS, Wicks JD, Mettler FA. Prone supine change in organ position: CT demonstration. *AJR* 135:815–820, 1980
13. Spirt BA. Technical note: Value of the prone position in detecting pulmonary nodules by computed tomography. *J Comput Assist Tomogr* 4:871–873, 1980
14. Terminology, definitions, and classification of chronic pulmonary emphysema and related conditions. A report of the conclusions of a CIBA guest symposium. *Thorax* 14:286–299, 1959
15. Fraser RG, Paré JAP. *Diagnosis of Diseases of the Chest.* Philadelphia, W.B. Saunders, 1977
16. Gamsu G, Thurlbeck WM, Macklem PT, Fraser RG. Roentgenographic appearance of the human pulmonary acinus. *Invest Radiol* 6:171–175, 1971
17. Barrie, HJ. The architecture of caseous nodules in the lung and the place of the word "acinar" in describing tuberculous lesions. *Can Med Assoc J* 92:1149–1154, 1965
18. Ziskind MM, Weill H, Payzant AR. The recognition and significance of acinus-filling processes of the lung. *Am Rev Respir Dis* 87:551–559, 1963
19. Recavarren S, Benton C, Gall EA. The pathology of acute alveolar diseases of the lung. *Semin Roentgenol* 2:22–32, 1967
20. Itoh H, Tokunaga S, Asamoto H, Furuta M, Funamoto Y, Kitaichi M, Torizuka K. Radiologic-pathologic correlations of small lung nodules with special reference to peribronchiolar nodules. *AJR* 130:223–231, 1978
21. Dannenberg AM. Pathogenesis of tuberculosis. In: *Pulmonary Disease and Disorders*, ed. by A Fishman, New York, McGraw Hill, 1979
22. Naidich DP, McCauley DI, Leitman BS, Geneiser N, Hulnick DH. Computed tomography of pulmonary tuberculosis. *Contemporary Issues in CT*, vol. 4, 1984
23. Solomon A, Kreel L, McNichol M, Johnson N. Computed tomography in pulmonary sarcoidosis. *J Comput Assist Tomogr* 3:754–758, 1979
24. Metzger RA, Mulhearn CB, Arger PH, Coleman BG, Epstein DM, Geffer W. CT differentiation of solitary from diffuse bronchioloalveolar carcinoma. *J Comput Assist Tomogr* 5:830–833, 1981
25. Felson B. A new look at pattern recognition of diffuse pulmonary disease. *AJR* 133:183–189, 1979
26. Fraser RG, Paré JAP. *Diagnosis of Diseases of the Chest.* Philadelphia, W.B. Saunders, 1977, pp 423–424
27. Trapnell PH. Radiological appearances of lymphangitis carcinomatosa of the lung. *Thorax* 19:251–260, 1964
28. Resink JEJ. Is a roentgenogram of fine structures a summation image or a real picture? *Acta Radiol* 32:391–397, 1949
29. Heitzman ER. *The Lung: Radiologic–Pathologic Correlations.* St. Louis, C.V. Mosby, 1973, pp 64–70
30. Rosenblum LS, Mauceri RA, Wellenstein DE, Bassano DA, Cohen WN, Heitzman ER. Computed tomography of the lung. *Radiology* 129:521–524, 1978
31. Gilman MS, Laurens RG Jr, Somogyi JW, Honig EG. CT attenuation values of lung density in sarcoidosis. *J Comput Assist Tomogr* 7:407–410, 1983
32. Goddard PR, Nicholson EM, Laszlo G, Watt I. Computed tomography in pulmonary emphysema. *Clin Radiol* 33:379–387, 1982
33. Zerhouni EA. High resolution CT of the lung parenchyma—theory, technique and preliminary observations (submitted to *J Comput Assist Tomogr*)
34. Coddington R, Mera SL, Goddard PR, Bradfield JWB. Pathological evaluation of computed tomography images of lungs. *J Clin Pathol* 35:536–540, 1982
35. Weibel ER. Looking into the lung: What can it tell us? *AJR* 133:1021–1031, 1979
36. Godwin JD, Webb WR, Savoca CJ, Gamsu G, Goodman PC. Review: Multiple, thin-walled cystic lesions of the lung. *AJR* 135:593–604, 1980
37. Kruglik GD, Wayne KS. Case report: Occult lung cavity causing hemoptysis: Recognition by computed tomography. *J Comput Assist Tomogr* 4:407–408, 1980
38. Meyers HI, Jacobson G. Staphylococcal pneumonia in children and adults. *Radiology* 72:665–671, 1959
39. Breuer R, Baigelman W, Pugatch RD. Case report: Occult mycetoma. *J Comput Assist Tomogr* 6:166–168, 1982
40. Kramer SS, Wehunt WD, Stocker JT, Kashima H. Pulmonary manifestations of juvenile laryngotracheal papillomatosis. Paper presented at the 25th annual meeting of the Society for Pediatric Radiology, New Orleans, Louisiana, May, 1982
41. McGoldrick PJ, Rudd TG, Figley M, Wilhelm JP. What becomes of pulmonary infarcts. *AJR* 133:1039–1045, 1979
42. Thurlbeck WM, Simon G. Radiographic appearance of the chest in emphysema. *AJR* 130:429–440, 1978

43. Fiore D, Biondetti PR, Sartori F, Caiabro F. The role of computed tomography in the evaluation of bullous lung disease. *J Comput Assist Tomogr* 6:105–108, 1982

44. Berger JL, Shaff MI. Case report: Pulmonary lymphagioleiomyomatosis. *J Comput Assist Tomogr* 5:565–567, 1981

45. Stark, P, Gadziala N, Greene R. Fluid accumulation in pre-existing pulmonary air spaces. *AJR* 134:701–706, 1980

46. Webb WR, Gamsu G. Cavitary pulmonary nodules with systemic lupus erythematosis: Differential diagnosis. *AJR* 136:27–31, 1981

47. Blane C, Donne SM, Mori K. Case report: Congenital cystic adenomatoid malformation of the lung. *J Comput Assist Tomogr* 5:418–420, 1981

48. Hulnick DH, Naidich DP, McCauley DI, Feiner HD, Avitabile AM, Greco MA, Genieser NB. Late presentation of congenital cystic adenomatoid malformation of the lung. *Radiology*, 1983 (submitted)

49. Harden KA, Barthakor A. "Cavitary" lesions in sarcoidosis. *Dis Chest* 35:607–614, 1959

50. Rohatgi PK, Schwab LE. Primary acute pulmonary cavitation in sarcoidosis. *AJR* 134:1199–1203, 1980

51. Woodring JH, Fried AM, Chuang UP. Solitary cavities of the lung: Diagnostic implications of cavity wall thickness. *AJR* 135:1269–1271, 1980

52. Woodring JH, Fried AM. Significance of wall thickness in solitary cavities of the lung: A follow-up study. *AJR* 140:473–474, 1983

Chapter 9

Pleura and Chest Wall

There is great potential for the use of CT in the evaluation of the pleura and chest wall, reflecting in part the range of pathology that affects these areas (1). In this chapter, the value and limitations of CT in the assessment of diffuse and focal pleural disease, as well as chest wall lesions, will be discussed and illustrated.

TECHNIQUE

There is no standardized technique for the evaluation of the pleura and chest wall. Each case should be considered individually with regard to number of slices, thickness of sections, and use of intravenous contrast material. The shortest available scan times should be employed.

Posteroanterior (PA) and lateral radiographs are always obtained prior to the CT study. If the disease process to be examined is generalized, contiguous sections are unnecessary; a few additional sections through the region of greatest interest, however, should be obtained to further clarify pathology. Sections should also be obtained inferiorly through the posterior pleural recesses (see Chapter 11) to exclude occult pleural fluid collections.

If the disease process is localized, thorough examination of the entire chest may be unnecessary; in these cases, contiguous sections through the region of interest should be obtained from the start.

In our experience, the routine use of intravenous contrast medium is unnecessary. However, there should be no hesitation to use contrast medium in those cases in which it is indicated. Specifically, contrast enhancement aids in precise differentiation between tissue densities, such as, for example, in determining if a lesion is cystic or solid. It is also helpful in demonstrating areas of necrosis within a tumor mass and in identifying a hypervascular abscess wall. In these cases, whenever possible, sections should be obtained before intravenous contrast medium is administered to establish baseline densities in regions of interest.

GENERAL PRINCIPLES

Computed tomography is of greatest efficacy in (a) confirming the presence of a lesion and determining its precise location and extent, and (b) characterizing the tissue density within a lesion by means of attenuation coefficients (see Chapter 1).

Localization

Peripheral lesions are generally classified as extrapleural, pleural, or parenchymal, and are usually characterized radiographically by the angle (either acute or obtuse) formed by the interface between the lesion and the adjacent pleura. As shown in Fig. 1, there is considerable overlap in the cross-sectional appearance of these lesions.

FIG. 1. Schematic drawing of the cross-sectional appearance, typical and atypical, of extrapleural, pleural, and peripheral parenchymal lesions. *Extrapleural lesions* displace the overlying parietal and visceral pleura (a), resulting in an obtuse angle between the lesion and the chest wall. Associated chest wall pathology (for example, rib erosion) helps define the lesion as extrapleural. *Pleural lesions* generally remain confined between the layers of the pleura and cause obtuse angles between the lesion and the chest wall (b). Pleural lesions, however, may be pedunculated (c), in which case they may prolapse into the pulmonary parenchyma, resulting in acute angles between the lesion and the chest wall. Additionally, pleural fibrosis may result in fusion of the parietal and visceral pleura (d), leading to abnormal configurations of pleural lesions and/or loculation of pleural fluid. *Parenchymal lesions,* if subpleural, abut the pleura (e), resulting in acute angulation. If the pleura is infiltrated (f), the result is obtuse angulation with the chest wall. Clearly, while the mechanics vary, there is considerable overlap in the cross-sectional appearance of extrapleural, pleural, and parenchymal lesions. In practical terms, all peripheral soft-tissue lesions should be biopsied, regardless of site of origin.

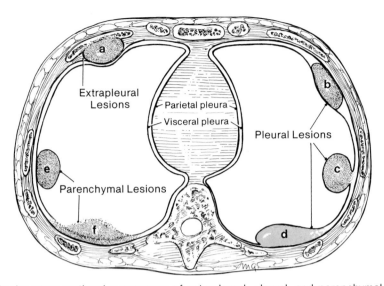

Extrapleural lesions usually displace the overlying parietal and visceral pleura, resulting in an obtuse angle between the lesion and the chest wall. Associated changes, such as, for example, rib destruction, help to confirm the site of origin as extrapleural, although these may be absent.

Pleural lesions, arising from the visceral or parietal pleura, usually remain confined to the pleural space and have a configuration similar to that of extrapleural lesions. Pedunculated pleural lesions, especially those arising from the visceral pleura, are an important exception (2,3). As shown in Fig. 1, these may prolapse or invaginate into the adjacent pulmonary parenchyma. If the lesion is small, the appearance will mimic a peripheral, subpleural parenchymal nodule (Fig. 2). If the lesion is larger and its base broad, the appearance of a pedunculated pleural lesion may mimic larger, intraparenchymal subpleural lesions (Fig. 3).

The cross-sectional appearance of pleural lesions, especially loculated pleural fluid collections, will also be affected by pleural adhesions along the margins of the lesion. Pleurodesis restricts the mobility of the pleural layers; the result may be acute angulation between the pleural lesion, and/or fluid, and the adjacent chest wall (Fig. 1).

Pulmonary parenchymal lesions, when peripheral, may abut the pleura; this results in acute angulation between the lesion and the chest wall. An important exception occurs when peripheral pulmonary masses infiltrate the adjacent pleura (Fig. 1). In this case, at the level of maximum infiltration, there may be obtuse angulation between the lesion and the adjacent chest wall (Fig. 4). In a report of 13 cases of peripheral lung cancer invading the adjacent pleura, Williford et al. (4) showed that, in each case, the result was obtuse angulation between the parenchymal mass and the adjacent chest

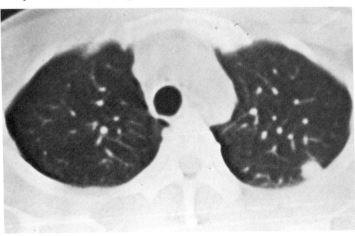

FIG. 2. Benign fibrous mesothelioma. Section through the left midlung. A well-defined tumor nodule can be identified, which, at surgery, proved to be a benign, pedunculated mesothelioma.

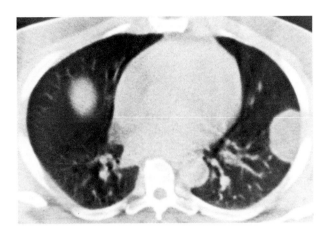

FIG. 3. Pleural lipoma. Section through the lower lobes. There is a sharply defined mass, the tissue density of which measures within the range of fat. Note the acute pleural–lung interfaces along the margins of the lesion.

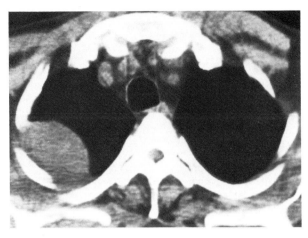

FIG. 4. Large cell undifferentiated carcinoma. A large, soft-tissue density mass is present posteriorly on the right side. The margins of this lesion are obtuse. At surgery, the lesion infiltrated both the pleura and adjacent chest wall. This appearance is indistinguishable from that of most pleural and extrapleural masses.

5a,b

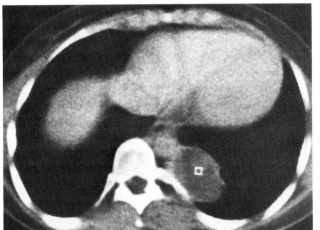

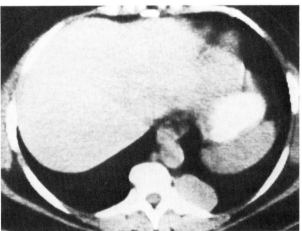

5c

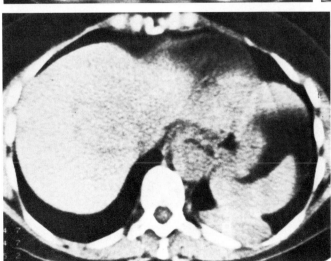

FIG. 5. Extralobar pulmonary sequestration–bronchogenic cyst–pleural fibroma. These three surgically proven cases illustrate how similar pleural-related masses may appear. **a:** Pulmonary sequestration situated between left lower lobe and diaphragm (not shown). The mass has a density slightly greater than water. **b:** Bronchogenic cyst. This is similar in appearance to the pulmonary sequestration shown in (a). Frequently, these cysts have a mean density greater than water, probably due to the presence of debris. **c:** Pleural fibroma. This appears as a non-descript, solid pleural mass. Note that in all three, despite differences in site of origin, the interface between the lesion and the chest wall is acute.

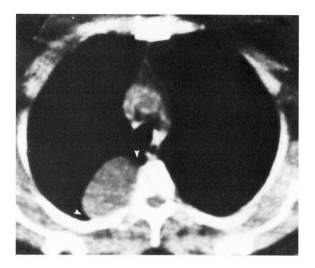

FIG. 6. Neurolemmoma. Section through the right upper lobe. Although this tumor is extrapleural, the pleural–lung interfaces are acute *(arrowheads).*

wall. It should not be assumed, however, that a peripheral lung lesion that simply abuts the pleura has not histologically invaded the pleura. Exclusion of tumor infiltration into the pleura requires biopsy.

It is apparent that, while the mechanics of pathology vary, the end result is that there is considerable overlap in the appearance of extrapleural, pleural, and peripheral subpleural parenchymal lesions when seen in cross section. The degree of difficulty that may be encountered in defining the site of origin of peripheral lesions is illustrated in Fig. 5, which shows examples of extralobar pulmonary sequestration (Fig. 5a), a peripheral bronchogenic cyst (Fig. 5b), and a pleural fibroma (Fig. 5c) (5–7). Despite differences in the sites of origin of these

lesions, their cross-sectional appearances (specifically, the angles formed by the lesions and the adjacent chest wall) are strikingly similar.

Finally, even extrapleural lesions occasionally can prolapse into the adjacent lung, resulting in acute angulation between the lesion and the chest wall. In the absence of underlying chest wall disease, the separation of these lesions from pleural or parenchymal lesions may be impossible (Fig. 6).

It should not be assumed from the preceding discussion that CT does not provide exquisite anatomic localization. If differentiation between extrapleural, pleural, and parenchymal lesions is difficult, CT still provides precise delineation of the extent of pathology (Fig. 7). This is of special significance in patients with peripheral lung cancer extending into the chest wall. While it was previously thought that chest wall extension precluded resection, with advances in plastic reconstructive surgery, large portions of the chest wall can now be resected, especially in patients with squamous cell carcinoma. Preoperative planning requires detailed evaluation of the extent of chest wall tumor infiltration. As shown in Fig. 7, as compared with routine techniques, CT is far superior in localizing and delineating the exact extent of pathology.

Tissue Density Characteristics

Computed tomography can reliably differentiate between air, fat, fluid, soft tissue, and calcium. This has obvious diagnostic significance, for example, in differentiating a pleural lipoma from a soft-tissue mass or cyst (Fig. 8a). CT is rarely this specific, however, a fact which is particularly pertinent in

7a,b

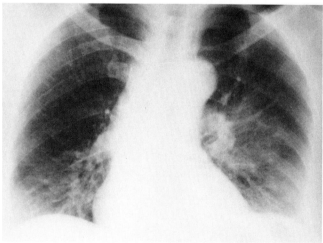
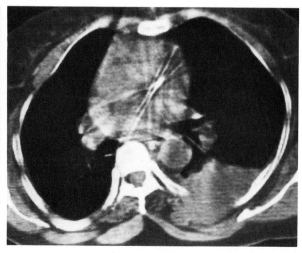

FIG. 7. Localization—bronchogenic carcinoma invading the chest wall. **a:** PA radiograph shows ill-defined mass with adjacent rib erosion on the left side. **b:** Section through the mass shows extensive infiltration of the chest wall and erosion of adjacent ribs. This type of precise localization is critical for surgeons attempting resection of tumors invading the chest wall.

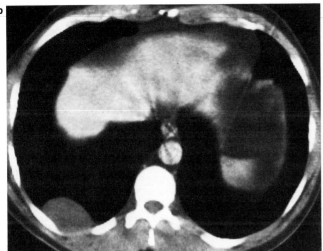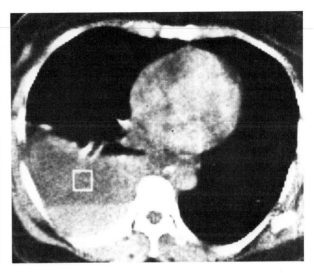

FIG. 8: **a:** Mesothelial cyst. A sharply defined mass is present on the right, with obtuse angles between the lesion and the chest wall. Measurements within this lesion indicated fluid (surgically proven). **b:** Hemorrhagic pleural fluid. Metastatic renal cell carcinoma. Section through the lower thorax. There is a large pleural fluid collection on the right in which a distinct fluid–fluid level can be identified. The fluid in the dependent portion of the pleural space measures approximately 90 Hounsfield units.

the evaluation of pleural fluid collections (8). In our judgment, CT will always define the presence of pleural fluid; however, CT cannot be used to differentiate between transudates and exudates, or be used to reliably detect chylous effusions (9). Sometimes, pleural hemorrhage, if acute, can be identified (Fig. 8b). These same limitations apply in the evaluation of soft-tissue masses, for which specific histologic diagnosis can be made only rarely.

From a practical standpoint, any peripheral soft-tissue mass, regardless of its probable site of origin, should be biopsied.

THE PLEURAL FISSURES

The normal appearance on CT of the pleural fissures has been described (10). In the series reported by Marks and Kuhns (11), pleural fissures could be identified in 84% of 23 consecutive CT scans. Frija et al. (12), in their report of 30 normal subjects, identified the fissures in 100% of cases. Delineation of the pleural fissures is important for the following reasons: (a) the fissures serve as major landmarks within the pulmonary parenchyma, allowing for accurate localization and staging of parenchymal disease; (b) lack of familiarity with the appearance of the pleural fissures may lead to erroneous interpretations; and (c) accurate identification of loculated fluid within the fissures and differentiation between loculated fluid and parenchymal disease presupposes knowledge of the normal location and appearance of the fissures.

The appearance on CT of the major fissures is

variable, depending on their axis relative to the plane of cross section. Most often, the major fissures can be identified as broad avascular bands within the pulmonary parenchyma (Fig. 9a). They appear to be "avascular" because of diminished blood flow to the peripheral portions of the lung.

Less frequently, the major fissures may be identified as linear structures. This occurs if the vertical axis of the major fissure is perpendicular to the plane of the CT section (Fig. 9b). Occasionally, the fissures appear as broad dense bands, especially on sections obtained through the uppermost portions of the fissures (Fig. 9c). The reason for this appearance is uncertain. Although partial volume averaging has been cited as an explanation, this seems unlikely, since the density always lies anterior to the line of the fissure, never posterior (11) (Fig. 9c). It is more likely that the density is caused by the effect of gravity with accumulation of fluid in the dependent portion of a lobe. The dense band usually is seen only on end-expiratory scans. Regardless of its cause, the dense-band appearance is a normal variant and should not be confused with pathology.

Unlike the major fissure, there is no significant variation in the appearance of the minor fissure. It can be identified as a broad, frequently triangular, avascular band in the anterior portion of the right lung at the level of the bronchus intermedius. The minor fissure is usually seen in only one section (Fig. 9d). Goodman et al. (13) labeled this the "right mid-lung window," and were able to identify this area of diminished vascularity in 92% of 50 pa-

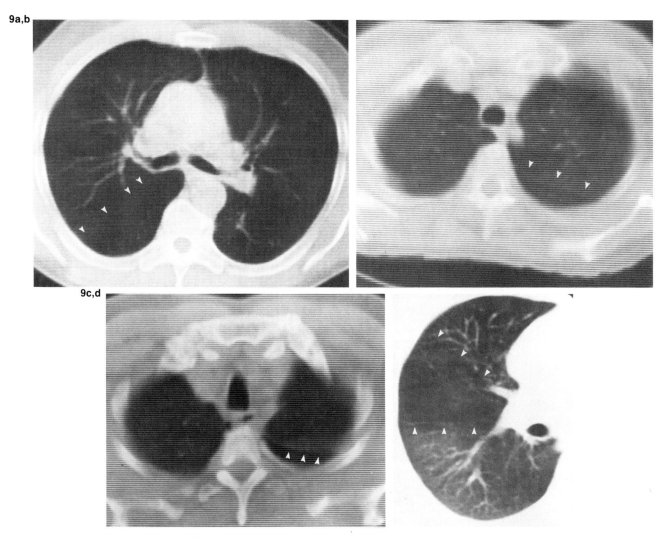

FIG. 9: Normal fissures. **a:** Section through avascular right oblique fissure *(arrowheads)*. Note the position and general angulation of the fissure at the level of the right upper lobe bronchus. The fissure divides the posterior segment of the right upper lobe from the superior segment of the right lower lobe. **b:** This section through the upper portion of the oblique fissure on the left is perpendicular to the plane of the CT scan; the fissure can be identified as a solid line *(arrowheads)*. **c:** The upper portion of the oblique fissure on the left is not quite perpendicular to the plane of the CT scan. The fissure appears as a broad band of increased density, sharply marginated posteriorly *(arrowheads)*. The increased density is probably due to crowded vascularity in the posterior portion of the left upper lobe (end-expiratory scan). **d:** Section through the minor fissure, which appears as a triangular wedge of decreased density in the anterior portion of the parenchyma at the level of the bronchus intermedius *(arrowheads)*. The fissure divides the anterior segment of the right upper lobe from the superior segment of the right lower lobe.

tients. Unlike the major fissures, the minor fissure is never seen as a line or broad band of increased density because the minor fissure always lies in approximately the same plane as the CT section.

In addition to normal fissures, accessory fissures—most commonly the azygous fissure—may be identified. Alterations in the normal appearance of the lung and mediastinum produced by an azygous lobe have been described (14). The azygous fissure limits the lateral margin of the

azygous lobe, which frequently extends well behind the trachea and even behind the esophagus (Fig. 10). The azygous fissure itself extends from the brachiocephalic vein anteriorly to a position alongside the right posterolateral aspect of the T4 or T5 vertebral body, and is usually identifiable as a thin, curved line on CT.

Another normal, frequently recognizable, anatomic feature of the pleura is the inferior pulmonary ligaments. These ligaments represent reflections of

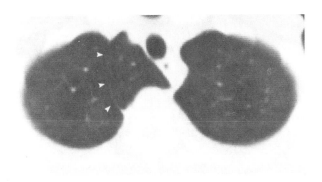

FIG. 10. Azygous fissure. The azygous fissure can be identified as a thin line marginating the lateral aspect of the azygous lobe *(arrowheads).*

the parietal pleura that extend from just below the inferior margins of the pulmonary hila caudally and posteriorly. On the right side, the inferior pulmonary ligament lies adjacent to the inferior vena cava; on the left side, it lies alongside the distal esophagus. The inferior margins of these ligaments are variable; in their most caudal extension they may assume a triangular configuration as they reflect onto the diaphragm (Fig. 11). The significance of the inferior pulmonary ligaments will be discussed more thoroughly in Chapter 11.

FREE PLEURAL FLUID

Free pleural fluid has a characteristic appearance when seen in cross section. Fluid typically looks "meniscoid," occupying the posterior pleural space

in patients scanned in the supine position. As effusions increase in size, they conform to the natural boundaries of the pleura; laterally, these boundaries are formed by the lateral chest wall and the lateral aspect of the oblique fissures, into which fluid may track; medially these boundaries are formed by the inferior pulmonary ligaments (Fig. 12). On occasion, small effusions may prove difficult to differentiate from pleural thickening and/or fibrosis. In these cases, scans obtained with the patient in the lateral decubitus position may be helpful.

FISSURAL PSEUDOTUMORS

Fissural pseudotumors are common and are usually secondary to congestive heart failure. Loculation of fluid within the fissures implies adherence of the pleural layers in the peripheral portions of the fissure, usually secondary to previous inflammatory disease. Identification of interlobar fluid is significant because its appearance on CT may be confused with that of an intrapulmonary lesion. The typical radiographic appearance of loculated fissural fluid has been described by Baron (15). Fissural fluid has the following characteristics: (a) the fluid collection lies in the expected region of the fissures and (b) unless the fissure lies exactly perpendicular to the plane of the radiograph, the margins of the fluid collection appear hazy or poorly defined. These principles also apply to the appearance of fluid within fissures on CT. An example of a small interlobar pleural fluid collection is shown in Fig. 13.

Fluid may collect in any portion of the fissures. If

11a,b

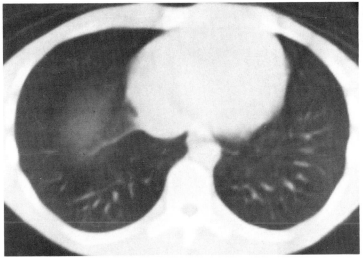

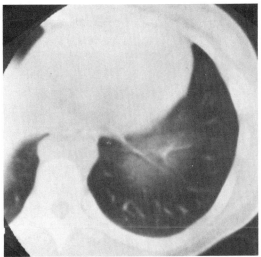

FIG. 11. Inferior pulmonary ligaments. **a:** Section through the lowest portion of the right inferior pulmonary ligament. The ligament can be identified as a solid line medially, in close proximity to the inferior vena cava; laterally, the ligament can be identified above the dome of the right hemidiaphragm, to which it is affixed. **b:** Magnified view of the left inferior pulmonary ligament.

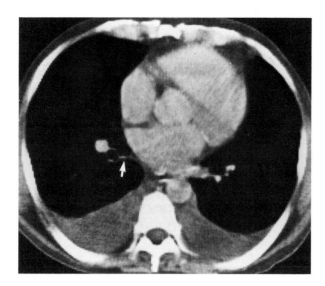

FIG. 12. Free-moving pleural fluid. Section shows typical "meniscoid" appearance of free pleural fluid. Note that the fluid is bounded medially by the inferior pulmonary ligament, clearly seen on the right side *(arrow)*.

the collection is sufficiently large, it will be seen on multiple sections (Fig. 14). If there is free communication between the lateral portion of the oblique fissure and the remainder of the pleural space, fluid will extend into the fissure and assume a characteristic triangular configuration, with the apex pointing toward the hilum (Fig. 15).

PARAPNEUMONIC EFFUSIONS–EMPYEMA

Infection within the pleural space most frequently follows primary infection in the lung, from acute bacterial pneumonias, septic pulmonary emboli, and/or lung abscesses (16,17). Less frequently, infection may spread to the pleura from contiguous extrapulmonary sites, for example, from osteomyelitis of the spine, infection in the subdiaphragmatic spaces, or the liver. Additionally, pleural infection may be iatrogenic, following needle aspiration and/or biopsy or thoracic surgery.

The incidence of parapneumonic effusions is dependent to some degree on the infecting organism, ranging from about 10% for pneumonias caused by *Streptococcus pneumoniae* to over 50% for those caused by *Staphylococcus pyogenes* (16). Regardless of the infecting organism, however, the natural history of empyemas may be predicted. As classified by the American Thoracic Society, three stages in the development of empyema can be described (18). These stages are pathophysiologically and therapeutically distinct, and can be distinguished with CT.

Exudative Stage

In the initial exudative stage, the underlying pneumonic process causes inflammation of the visceral pleura. This results in the accumulation of thin, uninfected pleural fluid, probably secondary to increased capillary permeability, with resultant protein loss. Differentiation between parenchymal consolidation and pleural fluid may initially be difficult with CT, even when narrow windows are used (Fig. 16). Such differentiation may not be critical, however, since most parapneumonic effusions at

13a,b

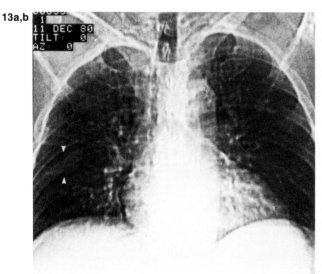

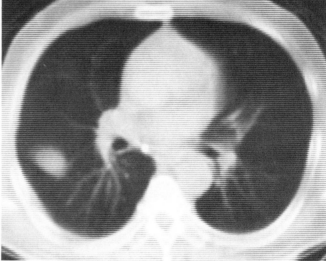

FIG. 13. Fissural pseudotumor—oblique fissure. **a:** Scanogram of the thorax shows an ill-defined density in the right midthorax *(arrowheads).* **b:** Fissural pseudotumor in the oblique fissure. Note that the margins of this lesion are not sharp. The "mass" measured within the range of water.

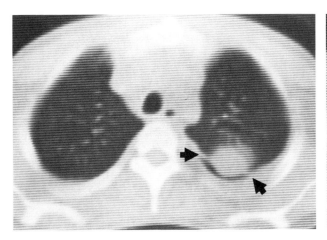
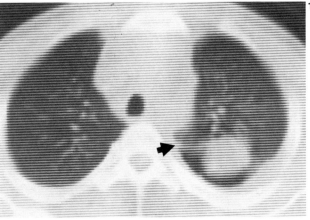

14a,b

FIG. 14. Fissural pseudotumor—oblique fissure. **a,b:** Sequential sections through a large fissural pseudotumor in the upper portion of the left oblique fissure. Thickening of the medial and lateral portions of the fissure can be seen *(arrows)*. The shape of the fluid collection corresponds to the configuration of the fissure; the margins of the fluid are hazy. This appearance should not be confused with an intraparenchymal tumor mass.

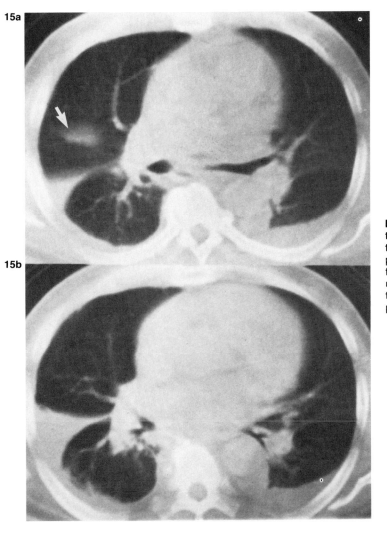

15a

15b

FIG. 15. Fissural fluid. **a,b:** Sequential images through the midthorax in a patient with bilateral effusions. On the right, there is free communication between the pleural space and the lateral margin of the oblique fissure; interfissural fluid assumes a triangular configuration, with the apex pointing toward the hilum. Note that, in (a), a small loculated fluid collection lies in the posterior portion of the minor fissure as well *(arrow)*.

16a,b

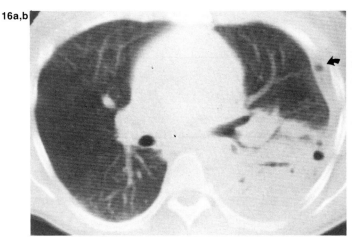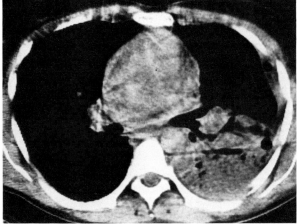

FIG. 16. Parapneumonic effusion—exudative phase. **a:** Section through the left midlung field. There is extensive consolidation of the left lower lobe. Pleural fluid can be recognized anterolaterally *(arrow).* **b:** Posteriorly, differentiation between infiltrate and pleural fluid is difficult, even when imaged with narrow windows.

this stage resolve without requiring tube drainage, even when the underlying etiology is tuberculous.

Fibrinopurulent Stage

In this stage, large numbers of polymorphonucle-ar leukocytes and bacteria accumulate in the pleural space, and sheets of fibrin are deposited over the visceral and parietal pleura. As a consequence, there is a progressive tendency toward fluid locula-tion; fluid resorption is impaired, presumably be-cause of decreased lymphatic drainage (Fig. 17). Proper therapy requires prompt use of closed tube drainage, for which CT may be particularly helpful in determining the best site(s) (Fig. 17).

If the initial presentation occurs during this stage,

differentiation between lung abscess and empyema (or loculated pleural fluid collections) may prove difficult, especially in the presence of a bron-chopleural fistula (19,20). While several criteria for differentiating lung abscesses from empyemas with bronchopleural fistula have been proposed, the fol-lowing are most useful:

1. Evaluation of the three-dimensional shape of the lesion. Because they originate within the pulmo-nary parenchyma, most lung abscesses retain a spherical shape. Empyemas, enclosed within the pleural cavity, conform to the shape of the chest wall. Accurate differentiation requires evaluation of sequential sections.

2. Evaluation of the walls of the lesion. Consid-eration must be given to wall thickness, uniformity, and smoothness, of both the interior and exterior

17a,b

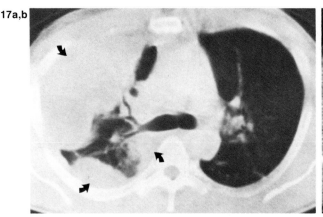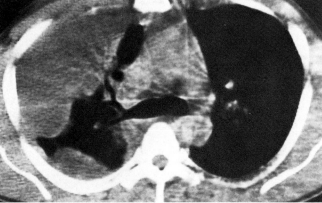

FIG. 17: Empyema—fibrinopurulent phase. Identical sections through the right upper lobe bronchus imaged with a wide window **(a)** and a narrow window **(b)** show three distinct areas of loculated pleural fluid *(arrows).* There is only minimal residual parenchymal consolidation. The right upper lobe bronchus is grossly normal in appearance, despite the large pleural fluid collections.

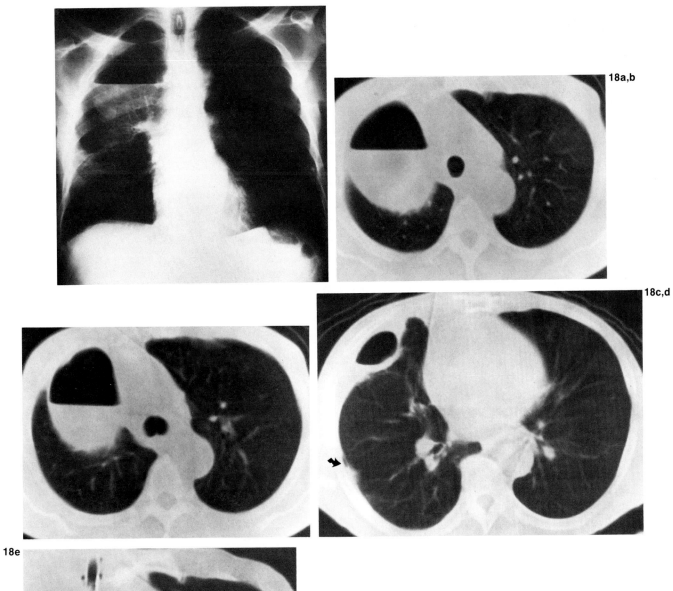

18a,b

18c,d

18e

FIG. 18. Empyema—bronchopleural fistula. **a:** PA radiograph shows a large air–fluid level in the right upper lung field. Precise localization is difficult. **b–d:** Sequential images show a large, smooth-walled cavity with an air–fluid level. The overall configuration of this lesion conforms to the shape of the pleural cavity, tapering inferiorly. A small focal collection of air in the lateral pleural space can be identified as well *(arrow).* **e:** Section obtained after insertion of a pleural tube, confirming this as an empyema.

margins. Most empyemas have thin, smooth walls, especially along their inner margins. Abscesses tend to have thickened, irregular walls and rough margins.

Application of these criteria is illustrated in Fig. 18. Ancillary criteria that have been proposed include the findings of compressed lung adjacent to the inner margins of an empyema, as well as displacement of vessels and bronchi by large pleural fluid collections (21). While these may prove helpful, these findings are seen with somewhat less regularity and are thus less reliable (Fig. 17). Overall, by use of the above criteria, CT can usually distinguish abscesses from empyemas. In this regard, Stark et al. (22) have reported accurate localization of 70 lesions (58 empyemas and 12 abscesses) in all but one of 63 cases.

Organizing Stage

In this stage, there is an ingrowth of fibroblasts along the fibrin sheets lining the visceral and parietal pleura. The end result is pleural fibrosis, which acts as an inelastic membrane trapping the adjacent lung (17,18). Progression from the fibrinopurulent to the organizing stage may be quite rapid, occasionally occurring in the course of therapy with closed pleural tube drainage. This is illustrated in Fig. 19. Once the pleura has fibrosed, effective therapy requires surgical intervention, either with open pleural drainage or an Eloeser skin flap if there is residual loculated fluid, or pleural decortication (17).

Although, as illustrated in Fig. 19, progression to the organizing stage may be extremely rapid, in most cases, the ingrowth of fibroblasts occurs over a more prolonged period, and the result is a well-defined, thick-walled, loculated pleural fluid collection (Fig. 20). There is a tendency for this to occur particularly with tuberculous pleural disease. Eventually, the pleura calcifies, which initially appears as small, punctate foci involving both the visceral and parietal pleura (Fig. 20) and eventually progresses to form a calcified rind of pleura (Fig. 21). In these cases, there is contraction of the involved hemithorax and, perhaps as a compensating mechanism, an increase in the amount of extrapleural fat.

Although pleural calcification and fibrosis are the end result of long-standing pleural infection, they do not necessarily indicate quiescent disease. As shown by Hulnick et al. (23), CT plays an important role in evaluating pleural calcifications, especially in patients with a prior history of pneumothorax therapy for tuberculosis. In this setting, the potential for reactivation has been documented (24). Unlike plain radiography, CT can disclose focal areas of residual or recurrent fluid loculation in association with pleural calcification (Fig. 22); in the series reported by Hulnick et al. (23), this was evidence of ongoing, active tuberculous infection. CT can also demonstrate otherwise unsuspected complications of chronic tuberculous empyema, specifically, bronchopleural fistulae (Fig. 23) and empyema necessitatis (Fig. 24).

In summary, at each stage in the development of an empyema, the radiologic manifestations of the disease will vary. As has been illustrated throughout this section, CT offers a distinct advantage over traditional radiologic modalities as long as the information it provides is correlated with knowledge of

19a,b

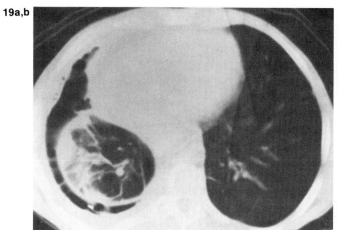
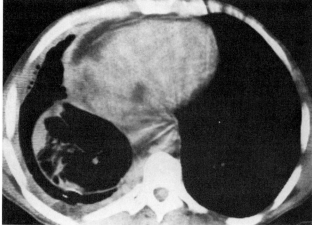

FIG. 19. Empyema—organizing phase. **a,b:** Identical images through the right lower lobe, imaged with wide and narrow windows. A pleural tube can be identified posteriorly. There is marked thickening of the visceral and parietal pleura, with only minimal residual pleural fluid. Strands can be seen in (a) bridging the pleural space. The right lower lobe is entrapped.

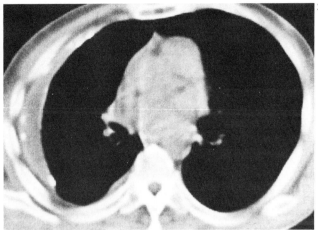

FIG. 20. Chronic empyema. **a:** Large, lenticular fluid collection is present on the left side. Both the visceral and parietal pleura are thickened. **b:** Similar appearance to that shown in (a), but in a different patient. Note the punctate calcifications involving the parietal and visceral pleura.

the natural history and pathophysiology of pleural infection.

ASBESTOSIS

The features on CT of asbestos-related pleural disease have been described (25,26). Pleural plaques at first appear as focal areas of soft-tissue thickening, usually most prominent at the lung bases. Calcification of plaques is generally a late manifestation of the disease; calcified and non-calcified plaques frequently coexist.

The pattern of pleural fibrosis and calcification resulting from asbestos exposure in most patients is specific. Initially, the disease process is discontinuous and plaques are seen as "skip lesions" (Fig. 25). Asbestos plaques are normally of uniform density. Calcifications may be punctate, linear, or, occasionally, "cake-like"; the latter are most frequently found along the diaphragmatic surfaces. Calcified plaques may be pedunculated, in which case they may be mistaken for intraparenchymal nodules (Fig. 25). Rarely, asbestosis may cause circumferential pleural thickening.

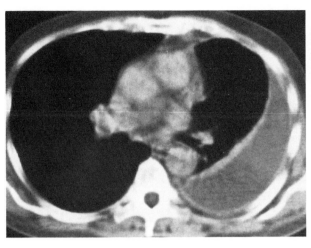

FIG. 21. Calcified fibrothorax. Section through the lower lobe shows the appearance of a typical calcified fibrothorax. The region in the *cursor* measured fat.

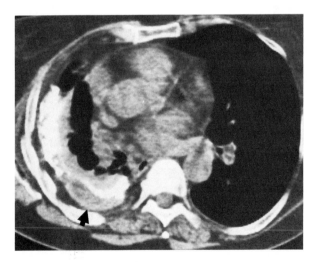

FIG. 22. Calcified tuberculous empyema. Section through a calcified tuberculous empyema. There is a small collection of residual fluid in the pleural space, easily differentiated from adjacent pleural fibrosis and calcification *(arrow);* it is evidence of ongoing, active tuberculous infection.

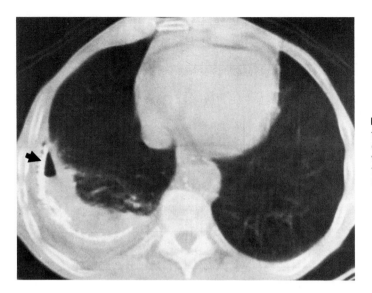

FIG. 23. Tuberculous bronchopleural fistula. Scan through the right lower lobe. There is a rind of pleural calcification with a focal air–fluid collection medially within the pleural space *(arrow)*. Without a history of thoracentesis, air in the pleural space indicates a bronchopleural fistula.

Katz and Kreel (27) have shown CT to be significantly more sensitive than plain radiographs in the detection of asbestos-related pleural disease. In their series of 36 patients with known asbestos exposure, 27 (75%) were found to have abnormal pleural thickening on CT, whereas 24 (66%) were interpreted to have abnormalities on chest radiographs. In this same series, CT was 50% more sensitive in detecting pleural calcifications than were conventional radiographs. The increased sensitivity of CT reflects in part an enhanced capability to detect disease in areas that are difficult to visualize with PA and lateral chest films—the most inferior portions of the diaphragms and the paravertebral and mediastinal pleura (Fig. 25).

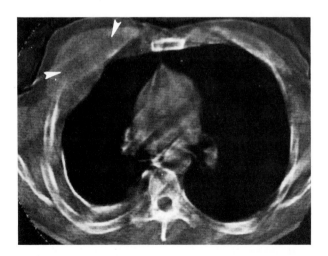

FIG. 24. Empyema necessitatas. Section through the right midthorax in a patient with a calcified fibrothorax. A soft-tissue mass is present, deforming the right anterior chest wall *(arrowheads)*. At surgery, this proved to be a "cold" tuberculous chest wall abscess.

ATELECTATIC PULMONARY AND PLEURAL ASBESTOTIC PSEUDOTUMOR

Another manifestation of asbestosis is a distinctive, complex lesion encountered with increasing frequency that has been called atelectatic pulmonary and pleural asbestotic pseudotumor (APA-PAP) (28). The condition consists of an area of pleural thickening with an irregular zone of peripheral lung atelectasis immediately adjacent (29). As indicated by its name, APAPAP is seen most often in individuals with a history of asbestos exposure (29,30). The lesion has also been called rounded atelectasis (31) and pleuroma (30). Two typical cases are illustrated in Fig. 26.

MALIGNANT PLEURAL DISEASE

Evaluation of patients with suspected pleural malignancy represents an important potential use of CT. This is largely a reflection of the frequency of malignant pleural disease. Leff et al. (32) have noted that approximately 25% of all pleural effusions in older patients in the general hospital setting are malignant in origin. In their series of 96 patients with carcinomatous involvement of the pleura, Chernow and Sahr (33) showed that an effusion provided the basis for the first diagnosis of cancer in 44 of 96 patients (46%).

Conventional radiography is limited in its usefulness for differentiating among various etiologies of pleural effusions; definitive diagnosis of malignant pleural disease usually requires pleural fluid cytology, pleural biopsy, or even exploratory thoracotomy. While statistics vary, a final diagnosis of

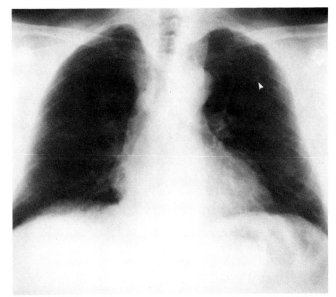

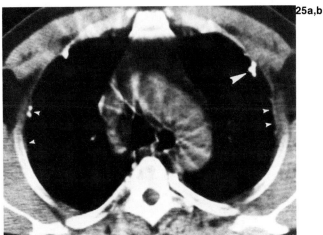

25a,b

25c

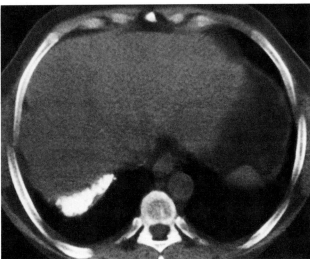

FIG. 25. Asbestosis. a: PA radiograph shows an ill-defined nodule in the left upper lobe *(arrowhead)*. b: CT section at the level of the aortic arch. There are bilateral, scattered calcified and noncalcified pleural plaques *(small arrowheads)*. The "nodule" seen in the PA film proved to be a pedunculated calcified pleural plaque *(large arrowhead)*. c: Section through the right diaphragm in the same patient. Focal, cake-like calcification can be seen in the diaphragm on the right side.

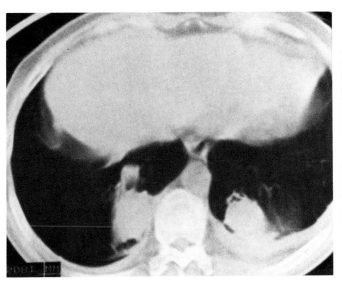

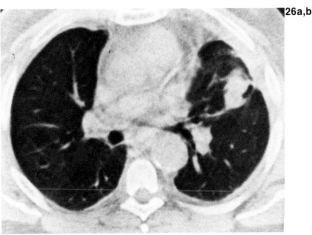

26a,b

FIG. 26. Atelectatic pulmonary and pleural asbestotic pseudotumor. a: 54-year old male with bilateral parenchymal–pleural abnormalities noted on routine chest roentgenogram. CT scan shows bilateral, organized parenchymal consolidation adjacent to thickened pleura. Percutaneous needle biopsies of lesions showed reactive fibrosis. The patient is alive and well, with no change in appearance of chest roentgenogram 4 years after scan. b: 55-year-old male with CT scan showing parenchymal consolidation adjacent to area of pleural thickening. Percutaneous needle biopsy showed dense fibrosis. Follow-up CT 3 years later showed no change.

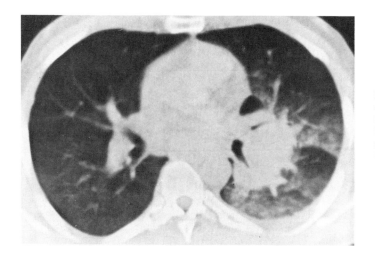

FIG. 27. Bronchogenic carcinoma—central lymphatic obstruction. Section through the left hilum shows a large central tumor mass. There are linear infiltrates in both the left upper and lower lobes, and a small associated pleural fluid collection. Changes are compatible with central venous and lymphatic obstruction. Pleural fluid cytology was positive.

malignancy can be made in 80–90% of patients by combined pleural cytology and biopsy (34,35). That this diagnosis may be elusive, however, was shown by Ryan et al. (36), who emphasized that pleural effusions caused by malignancy may go undiagnosed even with careful examination of the pleura, lungs, and mediastinum at thoracotomy. In their retrospective study of the outcome of 51 patients with pleural effusions of indeterminate cause at thoracotomy, 25% were found later to have malignant pleural disease.

Bronchogenic Carcinoma

The most frequent cause of pleural malignancy is bronchogenic carcinoma; it constitutes 35–50% of cases in most series (35,37). Evidence of involvement of the pleura significantly alters the staging, prognosis, and therapy of these tumors. The pathways by which the pleura becomes involved with tumor have been described by Heitzman et al. (37).

Tumor may extend to the pleura secondary to reversal of the centripetal flow of lymph (commonly caused by primary central tumors) or tumorous involvement of hilar nodes. Central venous obstruction may also be present. This pattern of malignant spread of central bronchogenic tumor is illustrated in Fig. 27.

Alternatively, peripheral tumors may directly invade the adjacent pleura, either by tumor growth along peripheral perivascular–lymphatic sheaths (Fig. 28) or by frank invasion of the adjacent pleura with subsequent pleural seeding (Fig. 29). Evidence of pleural seeding may be discovered in sites far removed from the primary tumor, including the mediastinal pleura. Tumor may involve the pleura, without producing pleural fluid; these tumors may

also involve the chest wall. This is frequently demonstrated only by CT (38) (Fig. 30).

Assessment of pleural involvement is limited when tumors, both peripheral and central, abut the pleura but do not appear to directly invade either the chest wall or mediastinum. In these cases, accurate staging is difficult. As shown by Williford et al. (4), invasion of the pleura by adjacent lung tumors usually results in obtuse angulation between the lesion and the adjacent chest wall (Figs. 1 and 4). In the absence of this sign, however, pleural invasion may be difficult to exclude (39).

Another problem is encountered in evaluating pa-

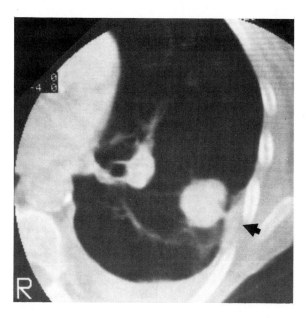

FIG. 28. Peripheral bronchogenic carcinoma—the CT "tail sign." Enlargement of a section through the left lower lobe. The tumor has extended peripherally by means of the perivascular sheaths and lymphatics to the adjacent pleura, which is markedly thickened *(arrow)*. A small pleural fluid collection is present as well.

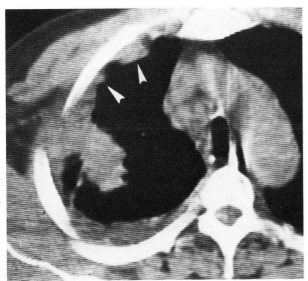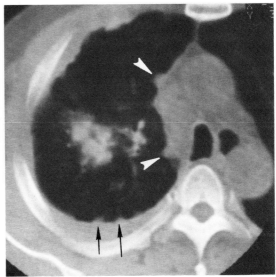

FIG. 29. Peripheral bronchogenic carcinoma. **a:** Section through the right upper lobe. Tumor directly invades the pleura and chest wall. Nodular tumor implants can be identified at some distance from the primary tumor *(arrowheads)*. A moderate sized pleural fluid collection is present posteriorly. Additionally, there is marked mediastinal adenopathy compressing the trachea. **b:** Section in same patient, slightly caudad to that shown in (a). Tumor nodules have implanted in the pleura *(arrows)*, overlying a small pleural fluid collection. Tumor implants can be identified along the mediastinal pleura as well *(arrowheads)*.

tients with central endobronchial lesions with secondary obstructive pneumonitis and/or apparent lobar collapse: differentiation of infiltrate from tumor may be difficult. On occasion, however, even in this setting, tumorous involvement of the chest wall and pleura will be apparent (see Fig. 29 in Chapter 5).

Mesothelioma

Although the appearance on CT of malignant mesothelioma has been extensively reviewed (40,41), the wide variation in these tumors has not been adequately stressed. Characteristically, mesothelioma permeates the pleural space, causing the pleura to become markedly thickened, irregular, and nodular. The tumor often encircles the lung, which may appear entrapped (Fig. 31).

Alternatively, mesotheliomas may present as massive unilateral pleural effusions, and, in these cases, the focus of malignancy may be difficult to identify, especially on routine radiographs (Fig. 32).

Intermediate between the appearances shown in Figs. 31 and 32 are the majority of cases, which typically show variable combinations of thickened, irregular pleura, entrapped lung, and focal, loculated pleural fluid (Fig. 33).

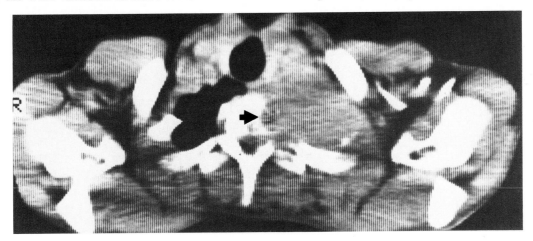

FIG. 30. Pancoast tumor. Section through the left lung apex discloses tumor infiltrating into the adjacent spine *(arrow)*. This was not appreciated on routine radiographs.

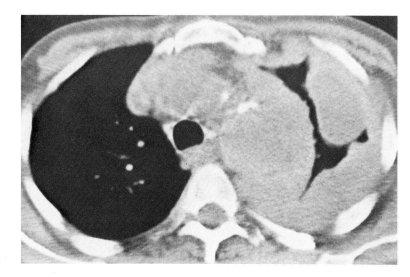

FIG. 31. Malignant mesothelioma. Section through the left midthorax reveals a thickened nodular rind of tumor encircling and trapping the left lung.

Despite the known association between asbestos exposure and malignant mesothelioma, calcification is rarely found in association with extensive tumor, probably because of tumor resorption of calcified plaques. Kreel (40) has reported finding evidence of calcified plaques in the contralateral thorax in one-third of cases; when present, they are diagnostic.

The diagnosis of malignant mesothelioma is complicated when discrete pulmonary nodules are discovered. While these may be manifestations of the primary neoplasm, the possibility of superimposed bronchogenic carcinoma cannot be excluded, especially in patients with known history of exposure to asbestos and a long history of smoking.

Computed tomography is most accurate in providing precise anatomic localization of tumor. Alexander et al. (41) have shown that plain radiographs, compared with CT, frequently underestimate the extent of disease. CT disclosed unexpected areas of involvement in each of their five cases. Extension into the contralateral chest was demonstrated in two cases, and extension into the abdomen and chest wall were each shown in one case. These findings have clear implications for both treatment planning and evaluation of response to therapy (see Fig. 35 in Chapter 11).

Rabinowitz et al. (42) have drawn attention to a variant of asbestos-related pleural fibrosis that closely mimics the appearance of malignant mesothelioma, as illustrated in Fig. 31. In their series of

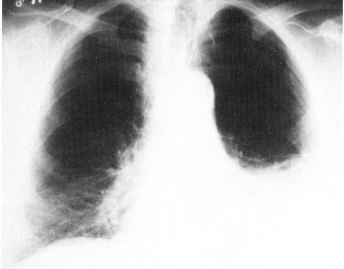

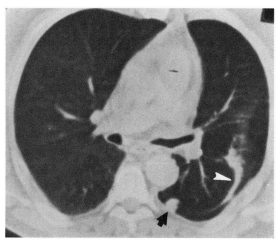

FIG. 32. Malignant mesothelioma. **a:** PA chest film shows a large, left pleural fluid collection. **b:** Section through the left upper lobe bronchus. A small tumor nodule is present posteromedially *(arrow)* in close relation to the oblique fissure. Fluid is present in the fissure *(arrowhead)* (surgically proven).

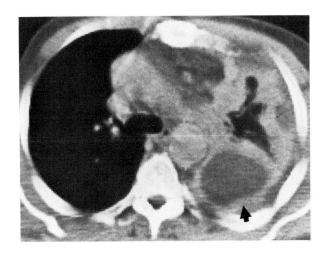

FIG. 33. Malignant mesothelioma. Section at the level of the aortic arch. Nodular, thickened pleura encircles the left upper lobe. A large loculated pleural fluid collection is present posteriorly *(arrow)*.

40 patients, 13 had "advanced asbestosis"; of these, 7 had a diffusely thickened, nodular pleura, indistinguishable from malignant mesotheliomas. However, none of these patients had evidence of malignant transformation detected by multiple biopsies or by surgery. These findings differ from other reports (40,41). The diagnosis of malignant mesothelioma may be fraught with difficulty; even thoracotomy may fail to establish the diagnosis. Among the 51 patients with indeterminate thoracotomies reported by Ryan et al. (36), four later proved to have malignant mesotheliomas at time intervals of up to 5 years post-thoracotomy. In our judgment, nodular thickening of the pleura, even when subtle (especially in a setting of known exposure to asbestos) correlates with malignancy with sufficient frequency to require at least numerous attempts at biopsy and careful long-term follow-up.

Metastatic Disease

Pleural metastases, apart from those due to bronchogenic carcinoma, occur most frequently from primary neoplasms of the breast, gastrointestinal tract (including pancreas), kidneys, and ovaries (43). Meyer (43), in an autopsy study of 52 patients with pleural metastases, showed that, in most cases, pleural metastases result from tumor emboli lodged in the distal branches of the pulmonary arteries.

Pleural fluid accumulates in metastatic pleural disease for a variety of reasons. These include increased permeability of the capillaries supplying tumor implants, as well as increased capillary

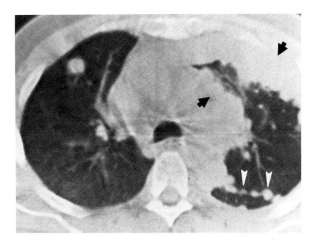

FIG. 34. Metastatic medullary carcinoma of the thyroid. Section through the carina. The pleura is markedly thickened and irregular, especially anteriorly *(arrows)*. Nodular implants can be recognized in the oblique fissure *(arrowheads)*. A discrete nodule is also present in the middle lobe. This appearance may be indistinguishable from that of mesothelioma (Fig. 31).

permeability due to pleuritis associated with obstructive pneumonitis if present; direct tumor erosion of pleural blood and lymphatic vessels; and decreased removal of pleural fluid due to mediastinal lymph node infiltration. The same wide variation in the appearance on CT described for mesotheliomas may be seen with metastatic pleural disease. Pleural metastases may cause marked thickening and nodularity of the pleura associated with only a small quantity of pleural fluid (Fig. 34;

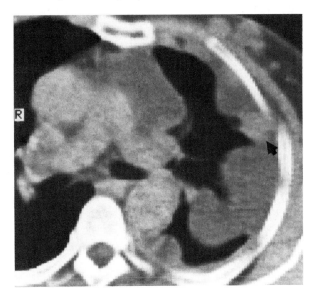

FIG. 35. Metastatic melanoma. Section through the left mainstem bronchus. There is evidence of loculated pleural fluid in which a well-defined metastatic pleural nodule can be identified *(arrow)*. Small metastatic nodules are also present anteriorly in the subcutaneous tissues (compare with Fig. 32).

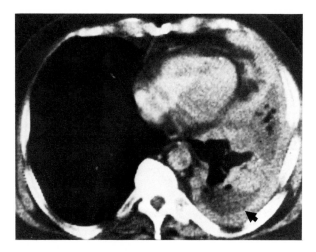

FIG. 36. Adenocarcinoma of unknown primary. Section through the lung base shows volume loss in the left lower lobe, a pocket of loculated fluid *(arrow),* and moderately thickened pleura on the left side. This appearance may be indistinguishable from that of mesothelioma (compare with Fig. 33).

compare with Fig. 31); alternatively, pleural metastases may cause large pleural effusions in which the foci of malignancy are difficult to identify (Fig. 35; compare with Fig. 32).

Not infrequently, pleural biopsy will reveal adenocarcinoma of the pleura of unknown primary. Many of these are presumed to be secondary to primary adenocarcinomas of the lung, although the primary tumor may be obscured by the extensive pleural disease. The appearance on CT of adenocarcinoma of the pleura may bear striking resemblance to malignant mesothelioma (Fig. 36; compare with

Fig. 33). Difficulties that may be encountered in differentiating adenocarcinoma from mesothelioma are, of course, familiar to pathologists (44).

Pleural Lymphoma

The mechanism by which pleural fluid accumulates in patients with lymphoma is still in dispute (45,46). Cases in which effusions occur secondary to gross hilar and/or mediastinal lymphadenopathy do not generally cause problems in recognition, although differentiation between lymphoma and other neoplastic diseases involving the hilum and mediastinum may be impossible.

Computed tomography is most advantageous in those cases in which pleural disease is secondary to direct pleural involvement. As pointed out by Burginer and Hamlin (47), pleural effusion may be the first manifestation of lymphoma. In their series of 112 cases of unselected patients with histiocytic lymphoma, pleural involvement was found in 20 cases (18%). They describe a characteristic presentation of localized, broad-based, lymphomatous pleural plaques, which are frequently hard to visualize with routine radiographs, especially in the presence of coexistent pleural fluid. It has been suggested that these lymphomatous pleural plaques originate in subpleural lymphatic tissue, and are likely to occur in non-Hodgkin lymphomas (Fig. 37). Lymphoma also may involve the pleura and chest wall by direct extension from the anterior mediastinum (Fig. 38).

37a,b

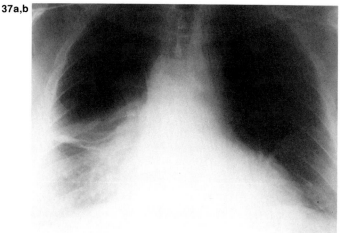
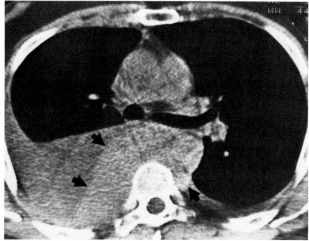

FIG. 37. Histiocytic lymphoma. Middle-aged male with undiagnosed recurrent pleural effusions. **a:** PA chest film reveals a large, nondescript pleural effusion on the right side. **b:** Section through the lower lobes reveals a large, loculated pleural fluid collection and a solid wedge of tumor crossing in front of the spine and involving the extrapleural space on the left *(arrows).* Needle biopsy of mass showed histiocytic lymphoma.

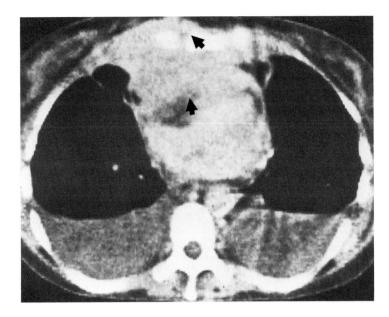

FIG. 38. Histiocytic lymphoma. There is a large, irregular, anterior mediastinal mass *(arrows)* invading the anterior chest wall and pleural space bilaterally. Bilateral, nondescript pleural fluid collections are present posteriorly.

Thymoma

Invasive thymoma characteristically involves the pleura by local invasion, contiguous spread, and, presumably, pleural seeding. CT has been shown to provide the most reliable assessment of the presence and extent of disease, and is discussed in detail in Chapter 3.

MALIGNANT PLEURAL DISEASE: OVERVIEW

It is apparent that CT represents a striking advance over routine radiography in the evaluation of patients with suspected pleural malignancy. This is largely due to the capability of CT to differentiate even subtle pleural thickening, nodularity, or masses from surrounding fluid. While specific histologic diagnosis may be impossible, the appearance of malignant pleural disease is sufficiently characteristic to suggest the diagnosis. This is significant in light of the difficulty frequently encountered in making the diagnosis by conventional means, including pleuroscopy and thoracotomy. Even in those cases in which evidence of pleural thickening, nodularity, or masses is lacking on CT, ancillary findings will suggest malignancy in a high percentage (Fig. 39).

While some overlap is anticipated, in our experience, malignant pleural disease usually can be distinguished from inflammatory pleural disease when scans are interpreted in light of the clinical history. This probably reflects differences in the pathophysiology and natural history of malignant, as compared to inflammatory, pleural disease. With malignant pleural disease, fluid accumulates primarily because of tumor extension or infiltration of the pleural surfaces. This results, in most cases, in irregularly sized pleural masses. Tumorous infiltration of the lymphatics also contributes to the formation of pleural fluid, and is generally easily identified when secondary to hilar and mediastinal nodal involvement. These patterns of spread of malignancy have been illustrated throughout this section.

Inflammatory pleural disease usually is a consequence of underlying parenchymal inflammation, either a bacterial pneumonia and/or lung abscess. Over time, there is a tendency toward restriction of the disease process within the pleural space by

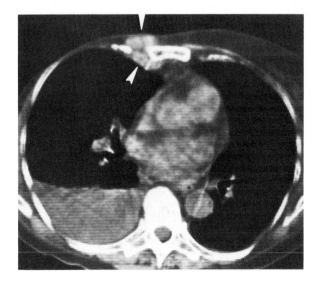

FIG. 39. Recurrent breast carcinoma. Section through the lower portion of the sternum reveals an area of chest wall recurrence *(arrowheads)* involving the internal mammary chain as well. Nondescript pleural fluid can be identified posteriorly.

40a,b

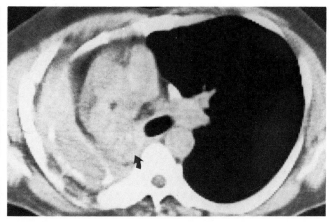

FIG. 40. Postpneumonectomy space—recurrent bronchogenic carcinoma. **a:** Section through carina. There is residual loculated fluid in the right pneumonectomy space, as well as a few areas of punctate calcification. The mediastinum is slightly rotated and shifted to the right; there is hyperinflation of the left lung. Adenopathy is present to the right of the trachea, posterior to the superior vena cava. **b:** Section 1 cm below that shown in (a). Recurrent tumor mass can be identified posterior to the right main pulmonary artery *(arrow)* (biopsy-proven).

means of fibrin deposition and, ultimately, fibrosis. The result is generally focal disease in which the pleural surfaces have become thickened, but are rarely nodular or irregular. This sequence of events was illustrated previously in the section on parapneumonic effusions and empyemas.

POSTPNEUMONECTOMY SPACE

Opacification of a hemithorax as a result of a previous pneumonectomy makes evaluation of this space difficult with plain radiographs. As shown by Biondetti et al. (48), CT is especially efficacious in this setting. A range of normal postoperative appearances may be anticipated, consequent to rotation and ipsilateral displacement of mediastinal and hilar structures, as well as hyperaeration of the contralateral lung. In a majority of cases, residual fluid will be present in the postpneumonectomy space. Recurrence of tumor can be identified in most cases, either in the mediastinum or hilum. Also, recurrent tumor masses within or adjacent to the postpneumonectomy space can be defined as they project into the lower-density fluid within the pneumonectomy space (Fig. 40).

THE CHEST WALL

Computed tomography plays an important role in the evaluation of patients with chest wall pathology (49–51). No other imaging modality provides such precise anatomic definition of chest wall lesions. Leitman et al. (52), in their report of 49 patients, showed that CT provided information beyond that

available by more conventional techniques. These data were of clinical importance for treatment planning in one-third of patients.

Examples of chest wall pathology have been illustrated (Figs. 7, 24, 29, 30, and 35). In specific cases, CT may provide precise histologic diagnosis (Fig. 41); more frequently, CT provides precise anatomic localization (Figs. 7 and 42). In patients with chest wall neoplasia, this may include visualization of previously unsuspected areas of involvement (Fig. 43).

Gouliamos et al. (49) have shown CT to be especially valuable in the assessment of patients with breast cancer. In their series of 110 cases of chest wall lesions examined with CT, 64 patients had

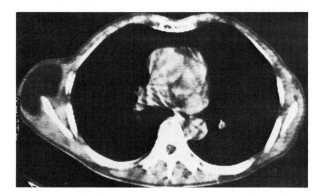

FIG. 41. Lipoma. Section through the midthorax shows a large, well-defined fatty mass on the right side, a portion of which is draped around the edge of the scapula. The presence of fine septations within the mass constitutes grounds for biopsy and/or excision to rule out a well-differentiated liposarcoma.

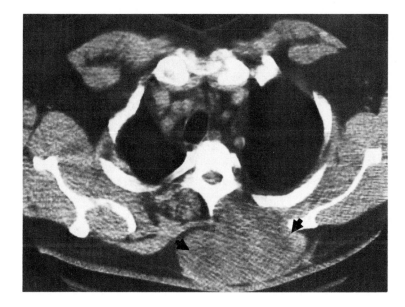

FIG. 42. Neurofibrosarcoma. Section through the midthorax. There is a large soft-tissue mass posteriorly *(arrows);* the tumor was present on multiple sections. At surgery, the tumor had invaded the periosteum of the spinous process shown in this section.

breast cancer; 21 of these patients were found to have axillary adenopathy, 9 showed internal mammary node enlargement, and 6 had local chest wall recurrence (Fig. 39).

Care must be taken to differentiate between chest wall tumor and infection, since these may have similar appearances (Fig. 44). In cases of suspected chest wall infection, the use of intravenous contrast medium, especially given as a bolus, may prove indispensable. This is because well-formed abscesses frequently have hypervascular walls due to surrounding inflammation and can easily be demonstrated with contrast-enhanced CT (Fig. 45).

Chest wall pathology may also occur secondary to inflammatory disease of the pleura or pulmonary parenchyma. Reactivation of pleural tuberculosis may result in a "cold" chest wall abscess (53) (Fig. 23). Actinomycosis may involve the chest wall secondary to a focus of infection within the pulmonary parenchyma (54) (Fig. 46).

CONCLUSIONS

Computed tomography plays a valuable role in assessment of patients with a wide variety of diseases of the pleura and chest wall. While the full

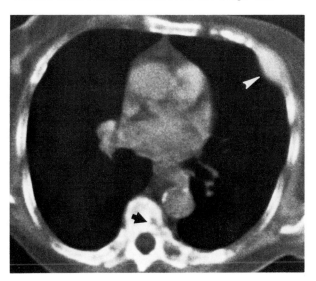

FIG. 43. Multiple myeloma. Section through the midthorax. The scan was obtained to evaluate a lytic lesion seen on routine radiographs *(arrowhead).* In addition, an unsuspected area of involvement in the thoracic spine is apparent *(arrow).*

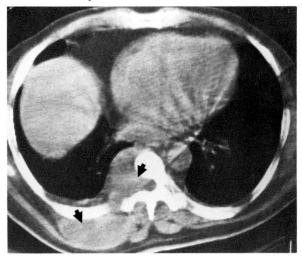

FIG. 44. Tuberculosis of the spine and chest wall. Section at the level of the right diaphragm. A large soft-tissue mass can be identified extending laterally from the spine, the posterior portion of which has been eroded *(arrows).* At surgery, this proved to be a "cold" tuberculous chest wall abscess. (Case courtesy of Dr. Margaret Whelan, New York University Medical Center, New York.)

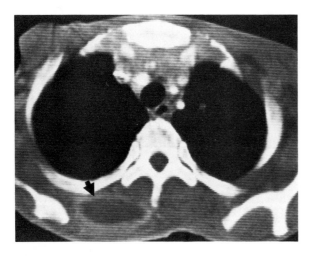

FIG. 45. Staph abscess. Section at the level of the great vessels. There is a well-defined soft-tissue mass which extended over many sections *(arrow)*. There is marked enhancement of the wall of this lesion, with no enhancement in the center, which measured just above fluid density.

range of indications for the use of CT has yet to be completely defined, the following generalizations can be made.

Despite some limitations, CT frequently provides precise anatomic localization of lesions of the pleura and chest wall. Of particular interest in this regard is the often-overlooked ability of CT to exclude the presence of significant disease. Leitman et al. (52) showed that, in their series of 49 patients referred for evaluation because of clinically palpable chest wall "masses," seven patients, in fact, had no mass. CT proved these apparent masses to be related to minimal scoliosis in three patients, asymmetry of the scapulae in one, and asymmetry of the

anterior chest wall muscles and costal cartilages in three other patients.

Computed tomography is also sensitive in differentiating between various tissue densities. In select cases, this allows for precise histologic diagnosis. Even in the majority of cases in which precise histologic characterization of tissue is impossible, CT still plays a vital role. This is most apparent in the workup of patients known to have pleural and/or chest wall disease of unknown etiology. Differentiation between benign and malignant effusions, for example, rests on the capability of CT to define small pleural nodules, plaques, or areas of pleural thickening apart from pleural fluid which are otherwise undetectable.

In summary, on the basis of these generalizations as illustrated throughout this chapter, we consider CT to be indicated as follows:

1. In the evaluation of any patient in whom PA and lateral chest radiographs are equivocally abnormal, or in the evaluation of abnormalities seen on PA and lateral chest films when the etiology is unknown.

2. In the evaluation of any patient with a known abnormality for whom surgery and/or radiotherapy is contemplated and in whom the precise extent of disease is unclear. In these cases, CT provides a roadmap, and frequently results in the alteration of the therapeutic approach.

3. In the follow-up evaluation of any patient receiving therapy for whom routine radiographs are insufficient to assess response.

Clearly, the range of indications is wide. Further, this list does not take into account the potential

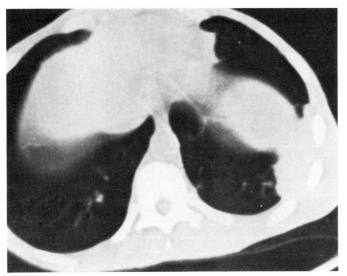

FIG. 46. Actinomycosis. Section through the base of the left lower lobe. Dense infiltrate is present in the lateral portion of the left lower lobe that extends through the pleura to involve the adjacent chest wall, which is markedly thickened (surgically proven).

value of CT in directing pleural and chest wall aspirations and biopsies. In this regard, CT has already been proven efficacious in guiding aspirations and biopsies of parenchymal lesions (55).

REFERENCES

1. Pugatch RD, Faling LJ, Robbins AH, Snider GL. Differentiation of pleural and pulmonary lesions using computed tomography. *J Comput Assist Tomogr* 2:601–606, 1978

2. Berne AS, Heitzman ER. The roentgenologic signs of pedunculated pleural tumors. *Am J Roentgenol Radium Ther Nucl Med* 87:892–895, 1962

3. Felson G. *Chest Roentgenology.* Philadelphia, W.B. Saunders, 1973

4. Williford ME, Hidalgo H, Putman CE, Korobkin M, Ram PC. Computed tomography of pleural disease. *AJR* 140:909–914, 1983

5. Baker EL, Gore RM, Moss AA. Retroperitoneal pulmonary sequestration: Computed tomographic findings. *AJR* 138:956–957, 1982

6. Thornhill VA, Cho KC, Morehouse HT. Gastric duplication associated with pulmonary sequestration: CT manifestations. *AJR* 138:1168–1171, 1982

7. Amendola MA, Shirazi KK, Brooks J, Agha FP, Dutz W. Transdiaphragmatic bronchopulmonary foregut anomaly: "Dumbbell" bronchogenic cyst. *AJR* 138:1165–1167, 1982

8. Levi C, Gray JE, McCullough E, Hattery RR. The unreliability of CT numbers as absolute values. *AJR* 139:443–447, 1982

9. Rawkin RN, Raval B, Finley R. Case report: Primary chylopericardium: Combined lymphangiographic and CT diagnosis. *J Comput Assist Tomogr* 4:869–870, 1980

10. Proto AV, Ball JB. Computed tomography of the major and minor fissures. *AJR* 140:439–448, 1983

11. Marks BW, Kuhns LR. Identification of the pleural fissures with computed tomography. *Radiology* 143:139–141, 1982

12. Friga J, Schmit P, Katz M, Vadrot D, Laval-Jeantet M. Computed tomography of the pleural fissures: Normal anatomy. *J Comput Assist Tomogr* 6:1069–1074, 1982

13. Goodman LR, Golkow RS, Steiner RM, Teplick SK, Haskin ME, Himmelstein E, Teplick JG. The right mid-lung window. *Radiology* 143:135–138, 1982

14. Speckman JM, Gamsu G, Webb WR. Alterations in CT mediastinal anatomy produced by an azygos lobe. *AJR* 137:47–50, 1981

15. Baron MG. Radiologic notes in cardiology: Interlobar effusion. *Circulation* 44:475–483, 1971

16. Light RW. Editorial: Management of parapneumonic effusions. *Chest* 70:3, 1976

17. Takaro T. The pleura and empyema. *Textbook of Surgery: The Biological Basis of Modern Surgical Practice,* 12th edition. ed. by DC Sabiston, Jr, Philadelphia, W.B. Saunders, 1981, pp 2079–2089

18. American Thoracic Society. Management of non-tuberculous empyemas. *Am Rev Respir Dis* 85:935, 1962

19. Baber CEJ, Hedlund LW, Oddson TA, Putman CE. Work in progress: Differentiating empyemas and peripheral pulmonary abscesses. The value of computed tomography. *Radiology* 135:755–758, 1980

20. Friedman PJ, Hellekant CAG. Radiologic recognition of bronchopleural fistula. *Radiology* 124:289–295, 1977

21. Merhar GL, Proto AV. Bronchial re-arrangement with large pleural collections: Plain film and CT findings. Presented at the Radiological Society of North America 68th Scientific Assembly and Annual Meeting, November 1982

22. Stark D, Federle MP, Podrasky AE, Goodman PC, Webb WR. CT in the diagnosis of lung abscess and empyema. Presented at the Radiological Society of North America 68th Scientific Assembly and Annual Meeting, November 1982

23. Hulnick D, Naidich DP, McCauley DI. CT of pleural tuberculosis. *Radiology* 1983 (in press)

24. McClement JH, Christianson LC. Clinical forms of tuberculosis. In: *Pulmonary Diseases and Disorders,* New York, McGraw-Hill Book Co., 1980

25. Kreel L. Computed tomography of the lung and pleura. *Semin Roentgenol* 13:213–225, 1978

26. Kreel L. Computer tomography in the evaluation of pulmonary asbestosis: Pulmonary experiences with the EMI general purpose scanner. *Acta Radiol [Diagn] (Stockh)* 17:4, 1976

27. Katz D, Kreel L. Computed tomography in pulmonary asbestosis. *Clin Radiol.* 30:207–213, 1979

28. Scott WW, Scott PP, Siegelman SS. Asbestos-related pleural disease emphasizing the asbestos plaque, asbestos pleural effusion and atelectatic pseudotumor. *Contemp Issues Comput Tomogr* 4 (in press)

29. Tylen U, Nilsson U. Computed tomography in pulmonary pseudotumors and their relation to asbestos exposure. *J Comput Assist Tomogr* 6:229–237, 1982

30. Sinner WN. Pleuroma—A cancer mimicking atelectatic pseudotumor of the lung. *Fortschr Geb Rontgenstr Nuklearmed Erganzungsband* 133:578–585, 1980

31. Mintzer RA, Gore RM, Vogelzang RL, Holz S. Rounded atelectasis and its association with asbestos-induced pleural disease. *Radiology* 139:567–570, 1981

32. Leff A, Hopewell PC, Costello J. Pleural effusion from malignancy. *Ann Intern Med* 88:532–537, 1978

33. Chernow B, Sahn SA. Carcinomatous involvement of the pleura: An analysis of 96 patients. *Am J Med* 63:695–702, 1977

34. Salyer WR, Eggelston JC, Erozan YS. The efficacy of pleural needle biopsy and pleural fluid cytology in the diagnosis of malignant neoplasm involving the pleura. *Chest* 67:5, 1975

35. Scerbo J, Keltz H, Stone DJ. A prospective study of closed pleural biopsies. *JAMA* 218:377–380, 1971

36. Ryan CJ, Rodgers RF, Unni KK, Hepper NGG. The outcome of patients with pleural effusion of indeterminate cause at thoracotomy. *Mayo Clin Proc* 56:145–149, 1981

37. Heitzman ER, Markarian B, Raasch GN, Carsky EW, Lane EJ, Berlow ME. Annual oration: Pathways of tumor spread through the lung: Radiologic correlations with anatomy and pathology. *Radiology* 144:3–14, 1982

38. Webb WR, Jeffrey RB, Godwin JD. Thoracic computed tomography in superior sulcus tumors. *J Comput Assist Tomogr* 5:361–365, 1981

39. Shevland JE, Chiu LC, Shapiro RL, Young JA, Rossi NP. The role of conventional tomography and computed tomography in assessing the resectability of primary lung cancer: A preliminary report. *CT* 2:1–19, 1978

40. Kreel L. Computed tomography in mesothelioma. *Semin Oncol* 8:302–312, 1981

41. Alexander E, Clark RA, Colley DP, Mitchell SE. CT of malignant pleural mesothelioma. *AJR* 137:287–291, 1981

42. Rabinowitz JG, Efremidis SC, Cohen B, Dan S, Efremidis A, Chakinian AP, Teirstein AS. A comparative study of mesothelioma and asbestosis using computed tomography and conventional chest radiography. *Radiology* 144:453–460, 1982

43. Meyer PC. Metastatic carcinoma of the pleura. *Thorax* 21:437–443, 1966

44. Suzuki Y. Pathology of human malignant mesothelioma. *Semin Oncol* 8:268–282, 1980

45. Fraser RG, Pare, JA. *Diagnosis of Diseases of the Chest,* vol. 3, 2nd edition, Philadelphia, W.B. Saunders, 1979

46. Black LF. Subject review: The pleural space and pleural fluid. *Mayo Clin Proc* 47:493–506, 1982

47. Burginer FA, Hamlin DJ. Intrathoracic histiocytic lymphoma. *AJR* 136:499–504, 1981
48. Biondetti PR, Fiore D, Sartori F, Colognato A, Ravaseni S. Evaluation of the post-pneumonectomy space by computed tomography. *J Comput Assist Tomogr* 6:238–242, 1982
49. Gouliamos AD, Carter BL, Emami B. Computed tomography of the chest wall. *Radiology* 134:433–436, 1980
50. Kirks DR, Korobkin M. Computed tomography of the chest wall, pleura, and pulmonary parenchyma in infants and children. *Radiol Clin North Am* 19:421–429, 1981
51. Toombs BD, Sandler LM, Lester RG. Computed tomography of chest trauma. *Radiology* 140:733–738, 1981
52. Leitman BS, Firooznia H, McCauley DI, Ettinger NA, Reede D, Golimbu CN, Rafii M, Naidich DP. The use of computed tomography in the evaluation of chest wall pathology. CT (submitted), 1983
53. Whalen MA, Naidich DP, Post JD, Chase NE. Computed tomography of spinal tuberculosis. *J Comput Assist Tomogr* 7:25–30, 1983
54. Webb WR, Sagel SS. Actinomycosis involving the chest wall: CT findings. *AJR* 139:1007–1009, 1982
55. Fink I, Gamsu G, Harter L. CT-guided aspiration biopsy of the thorax. *J Comput Assist Tomogr* 6:958–962, 1982

Pericardium

The pericardium may become involved by a large number of local or systemic diseases. Clinical manifestations of this involvement may be either difficult to detect or dramatically spectacular. Similarly, the hemodynamic alterations due to pericardial heart disease range from the clinically obvious to the very subtle.

During the last two decades, we have witnessed a quantum leap in our knowledge and understanding of the human pericardium and its role in health and disease. The mechanical, membranous, and ligamentous functions of the pericardium have been extensively reviewed (1–3). Advances in diagnostic instrumentation have contributed greatly to obtaining the morphologic–physiologic correlation that is so necessary in the imaging of the heart and pericardium. Echocardiography and CT are the diagnostic modalities that today allow a full view of the pericardium.

Before the advent of these two modalities, detection of pericardial heart disease was somewhat primitive and far more invasive. Historically, physicians have relied on fluoroscopy, chest roentgenograms, kymography, angiocardiography, capnoangiography, cardiac catheterization, nuclear medicine studies, pneumopericardiography, and diagnostic puncture and drainage of the pericardium (4). Since the arrival of echocardiography in the

mid-1960s, most of these procedures have been largely abandoned (5).

Echocardiography continues to be widely used for the diagnosis of pericardial heart disease, especially for diagnosing simple pericardial effusions, for which its sensitivity and specificity are well documented (6–8). Echocardiographic diagnosis of other pathologic alterations of the pericardium has been somewhat limited, however, although in a large retrospective study, two-dimensional echocardiography was able to diagnose pericardial thickening (9).

Until recently, the use of CT has been limited by the effects of biologic motion. Now, with newer scanners capable of 1–5 sec exposure times, image degradation has been greatly reduced. Motion still interferes with a well-defined image of the cardiac chambers to some degree, but the pericardium can be consistently visualized.

During the last 7 years, we have had the opportunity to use CT to diagnose and, in some cases, observe the natural history of more than 150 patients with pericardial heart disease. In addition, we have studied the normal pericardium in adult patients examined for noncardiac problems to determine the ability of CT to detect the normal pericardium, to learn if it is possible to identify the normal pericardial space and its fluid, and to identify the normal anatomic landmarks covered by the visceral pericardium. This chapter reviews the morphological basis of pericardial heart disease and our experience with CT in the evaluation of the pericardium.

INCIDENCE OF PERICARDIAL HEART DISEASE

The exact incidence of pericardial heart disease is unknown. Over a century ago, Osler (10) pointed out the discrepancy between the autopsy incidence and the clinical frequency of pericardial heart disease. In 1953, clinically diagnosed pericardial heart disease was reported in less than 1% of admissions to a large general hospital (11). However, these statistics were collected when fewer people were living into old age, and before the widespread use of cardiothoracic surgery, newer treatments for chronic renal failure, radiation therapy, and an array of drugs that can damage the pericardium (12–16). Thus, the prevalence of pericardial heart disease remains unknown. We are aware that the clinical incidence of pericardial heart disease is increasing. However, this is believed to be the result of modern therapeutic measures, combined with greater clinical awareness and immensely improved diagnostic methods.

TECHNIQUE

The referring physician's request for examination of the chest should be made directly to one of the radiologists in the imaging department. All options of examination can then be discussed, and all pertinent information, such as roentgenograms, electrocardiograms, cardiac catheterization data, echocardiography findings, and reports on any previous medical or surgical treatments, can be sent to the radiologist immediately. With this information in hand, the radiologist can tailor the examination to a specific problem (e.g., constrictive pericarditis versus restrictive cardiomyopathy).

The images printed in this chapter were obtained with the OMNI-6000 and the G.E. 8800 whole body scanners; both are third-generation machines capable of obtaining a good image with 140 Kvp-40 mA, a slice thickness of 1 cm, and a 5 sec exposure time. The images are obtained during suspended respiration.

Patients are examined in the supine position. Additional views with the patient in the lateral decubitus or prone position are occasionally of value when encapsulated effusions are suspected or in attempted gravity drainage of a pericardial diverticulum. A lesion bordering the diaphragm can sometimes best be demonstrated by sagittal and coronal reconstruction, although in the examination of the pericardium we have not needed to use these techniques.

A scanogram, an electronic digital image resembling a chest radiograph, is obtained routinely for determination of the upper and lower margins of the area to be examined. For the pericardium, we generally scan from the sternal notch to the xyphoid process, with 1-cm-thick sections taken 2 cm apart.

Computed tomography or ultrasound can be of great assistance in determining a site for percutaneous puncture of the pericardial sac. It helps in choosing the safest placement of the needle puncture, calculates the distance between skin and pericardial sac, evaluates volume and density of the remaining fluid, and guides the operator in avoiding a puncture of the lung. We find this method somewhat more prolonged but definitely the safest for drainage of the pericardium

USE OF CONTRAST MEDIA

Contrast enhancement of the heart is not routinely used in patients with suspected pericardial heart disease. Instead, we limit the use of contrast media to those patients suspected of constrictive pericarditis, encapsulated pericardial effusion, and cardiac or intrapericardial masses (17). We adhere to the recommended criteria and use all necessary precautions to prevent or diminish an adverse contrast media reaction. Renografin®-60, the contrast medium used for intravenous bolus injection, has an osmolality of 1,360 mOsmol/L. The contrast medium is administered through the basilic vein in the antecubital fossa, using a no. 19 butterfly needle with a rapid bolus (18), and we generally inject 25–40 ml. A dynamic study can sequentially demonstrate opacification of the right and left heart in a most elegant fashion, similar to conventional angiocardiography. A dynamic scan is, however, not necessary for a good study. It is possible to render an excellent enhanced scan of the right or left heart with a single slice if the exposure is timed appropriately. For opacification of the right chambers, we inject the radiopaque bolus simultaneous with the exposure, whereas we wait 6–9 sec after the injection for the left heart.

NORMAL PERICARDIUM

The pericardium is a double-layered, fibroserous sac enveloping and anchoring the heart and great vessels. The shiny, transparent, serous visceral layer or epicardium is closely adherent to the heart, while the fibrous parietal layer is free. The two layers have a continuous, common serosal lining. The smooth, moist, and glistening inner surface of the pericardium is lubricated by 20–25 ml of lymph fluid within the pericardial space. Recent electron microscopic studies of the pericardium have demonstrated that the serosal mesothelial cells have microvilli that act as friction-bearing surfaces and increase the surface area available for fluid transport (19).

The fibrous parietal pericardium forms a flask-like sac. Its narrowed upper segment attaches to the proximal portion of the great vessels. Its wide base is anchored to the central tendon of the diaphragm. Ventral insertions to the sternum are generally present, and some patients may have attachments to the dorsal spine (20).

Several investigators (21,22) have recently identified the normal parietal pericardium in virtually all patients. In general, the portion of the pericardium that is readily visualized is the caudal and ventral area that is surrounded by the mediastinal and epicardial fat pads. This epicardial fat layer is occasionally responsible for echo-free spaces, which may simulate an effusion (23). The parietal pericardium is seen as a pencil-thin, curvilinear, dense line, generally 1–2 mm thick (Fig. 1).

In a study of 100 patients who had an examination of the torso for noncardiovascular problems, a portion of the ventral parietal pericardium was visualized in each case. The dorsal aspect of the pericardium is regularly seen at its caudal insertion. At the level of the left heart, the dorsal aspect of the normal pericardium can be seen in fewer than 25% of cases. The cephalic portion of the parietal peri-

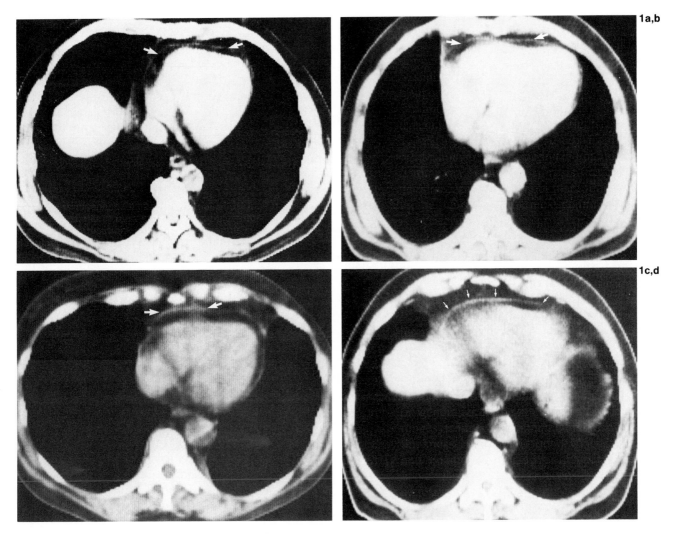

1a,b

1c,d

FIG. 1. Four examples of a normal parietal pericardium. **a,b:** Pencil-thin parietal pericardium in a background of abundant mediastinal and epicardial fat pads *(arrows).* **c:** Normal patchy thickening generally found ventral to the right ventricle *(arrows).* **d:** Normal thickening of the pericardium near its insertion in the central tendon of the diaphragm *(arrows).* (Fig. 1 reprinted with permission from ref. 24.)

cardium normally is not seen, due to the lack of fat in this area and the high degree of biologic motion. This part of the pericardium can only be seen when it becomes displaced by fluid or air in the pericardial sac or when it becomes thickened.

The parietal pericardium has a normal thickness of 1–2 mm. Patchy areas of slight pericardial thickening are normally found adjacent to the right ventricle, and are believed to be the result of stress from the transmitted pulsations of the ventricle (24). The caudal insertions onto the central tendon of the diaphragm may be thicker, sometimes measuring 3–4 mm. The visceral pericardium casts no shadow in the normal individual. Its surface is identified at the edge of the epicardial fat or the outer surface of the myocardium proper. Similarly, the pericardial space and its fluid are not visible on CT unless the space is increased by air or fluid.

INDICATIONS FOR CT IN THE DIAGNOSIS OF PERICARDIAL HEART DISEASE

Detection of pericardial heart disease has been a fascinating and formidable challenge since antiquity. Verification of pericardial pathology *in vivo* has now become an accessible goal with today's technology. This began in the mid-1960s with the advent of echocardiography as a diagnostic tool (25). This noninvasive method rapidly became the method of choice for detection of pericardial effusions, and, to a lesser degree, for demonstration of other types of pericardial pathology. Undoubtedly, echocardiography will continue to be the simplest and most widely used technique for imaging the pericardium.

The pitfalls and limitations of echocardiography have been extensively reviewed by Jacobs et al. (26) and others (23,27). Chest wall deformities with interposition of lung may preclude an adequate examination in some patients; failure to consistently demonstrate thickening of the pericardium and difficulty in reproducing comparable views on subsequent examinations represent some of the greatest drawbacks of the technique.

Computed tomography, on the other hand, has the disadvantage of using radiation, and, occasionally, administration of intravascular contrast media is required. The assets of CT, however, are formidable, since it allows detection of almost the whole gamut of diseases of the pericardium.

We have successfully used CT for diagnosis of pericardial heart disease. It readily identifies the normal pericardium and is of great value in the evaluation of congenital pericardial absence, pericardial cysts–diverticuli, effusion, calcific pericarditis, primary and metastatic neoplastic involvement, and postoperative changes. This diagnostic modality has opened new avenues for exploration of the pericardium, specifically in the demonstration of pericardial thickening and neoplastic involvement, which had traditionally been difficult to analyze by any other technique. In the case of pericardial effusion, we certainly expect echocardiography to be the primary diagnostic tool for initial diagnosis, but even in this apparently simple situation, CT can be of value in detecting encapsulated effusions or evaluating patients when there is disparity between clinical and echocardiographic findings.

CONGENITAL PERICARDIAL ANOMALIES

Congenital anomalies of the pericardium are rare. They have been classified by Edwards (28) as congenital absence of the pericardium, which can be partial or total, pericardial cyst or diverticulum, and benign teratoma of the pericardium. With standard radiographic techniques, these anomalies can mimic hilar, mediastinal, cardiac or pericardial tumors, a dilated pulmonary artery, or other masses in the anterior mediastinum or cardiophrenic angle. Even with angiography, ultrasound, and other modern diagnostic methods, many patients still require diagnostic thoracotomy. To highlight the special virtues of CT in resolving these diagnostic difficulties, we have selected patients who demonstrate various types of congenital anomalies.

Congenital Absence of the Pericardium

Moore (29) classified these anomalies into three groups: (a) left-sided absence, with the heart and left lung in a common cavity (60%); (b) a foramen-like defect, nearly always on the left between the pericardial space and pleural cavity (20%); and (c) total absence or only rudimentary development (20%). These anomalies occur more often in males (at a ratio to females of 3:1) and are found during autopsy in between 1 in 7,000 (30) and 1 in 13,000 (31) cases. The left-sided absence probably occurs because of premature closure of the duct of Çuvier, so that the vascular supply to the left pleuropericardial membrane is insufficient (32). The embryologic origin of the other anomalies is uncertain. Approximately one-third of patients also have anomalies of the heart, lungs, and mediastinum (33–36).

Computed tomography has proven to be successful in diagnosing these anomalies. Baim et al. (37) and others (24) have described the findings. Inability to identify the parietal pericardium, lack of continuity, a change in the axis of the heart and great vessels, levoposition of the heart, abnormal migration of the heart in a lateral decubitus position, and direct contact of the lung with the heart and great vessels are grounds for the diagnosis. In our experience, the last two signs are the most reliable.

Figures 2a–c are images from a CT study of a 48-year-old man with absence of the pericardium on the left side. This patient had a long history of chest pain and repeated bouts of premature ventricular contractions. His coronary angiography and cardiac catheterization proved to be normal. Note the levoposition of the heart, with rotation of its long axis toward the left, and lung tissue between the aorta and pulmonary artery. On turning the patient to the left lateral decubitus position, migration of the heart against the lateral thoracic rib cage is observed. This patient exemplifies the typical findings of absence of the left side of the pericardium.

While absence of the parietal pericardium was initially reported by Columbus (38) in 1559 and by Baille (39) in 1793, the first antemortem diagnosis was made incidentally during a thoracotomy by Ladd (40) in 1936. Although most patients without associated anomalies are asymptomatic, some have chest pain, dyspnea, dizziness, and syncope (41).

2a,b

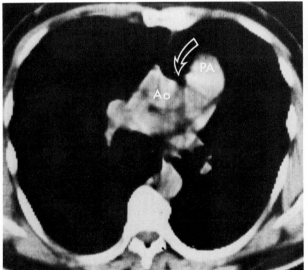
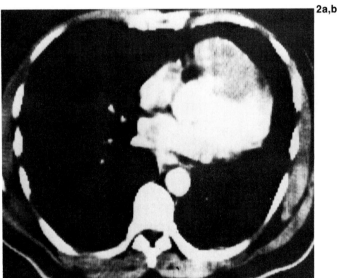

2c

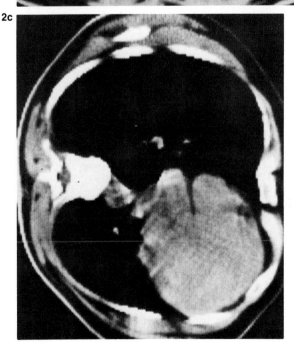

FIG. 2. Congenital absence of the left side of the pericardium. **a:** Air density of the lung tissue is in direct contact with the pulmonary artery (PA) and ascending aorta (Ao). **b:** The bulk of the heart is located in the left hemithorax; the long axis of the heart has rotated clockwise. **c:** The absence of pericardium allows migration of the heart, which comes in direct contact with the left rib cage in the lateral decubitus position.

Variable portions of the heart may herniate through the partial pericardial defect, including the atrial appendage (42) or atrium plus ventricle (43). The mechanical consequence may lead to compression of a coronary artery and even fatal cardiac incarceration and volvulus (45). Ellis et al. (46), in 1959, described the roentgenographic findings and recommended diagnostic pneumothorax for confirmation. These anomalies are often an unanticipated finding at autopsy (30). CT provides the best noninvasive method for detection of pericardial defects (24,37,47).

Pericardial Cysts and Diverticula

Congenital cysts of the pericardium occur more often in males than in females, at a ratio of 3:2. Most are found as asymptomatic lesions in middle-aged adults. Cysts are usually located in the costophrenic angles—most frequently on the right, but a few are more cephalad in the mediastinum. Most cysts are round or elliptoid and unilocular, sometimes exhibiting a pedicle. They usually weigh between 100 and 300 g and measure 3–8 cm in diameter. The cyst fluid is a transudate and usually is clear. Congenital pericardial cysts may also be lymphangiomatous or teratomatous in origin (28).

A pericardial diverticulum has an open communication with the pericardial sac and contains all the pericardial layers (48). A pericardial cyst results when a portion of the pericardium is pinched off during embryonic development and is thus disconnected from the pericardial sac. It is estimated that this anomaly occurs in 1 in 100,000 of the general population (49).

We present two asymptomatic patients in their 50s who underwent CT because of a suspected mediastinal mass detected by conventional roentgenograms. These two examples serve to give the reader an idea of the location and findings on CT of both common and rare sites of pericardial cysts. Figure 3a shows the classic appearance of a pericardial cyst. It is located at the cardiophrenic angle, has a low density comparable to water, and a wall so thin that it is not visible. Figure 3b is of a patient with coronary heart disease who eventually had to undergo a coronary artery revascularization procedure. The low-density mediastinal mass adjacent to the aorta proved to be a simple mediastinal cyst connected to the pericardium. The wall was composed of an outer layer of fibrous tissue and an inner layer of mesothelial cells.

It is important to point out that pericardial cysts, like other water-containing mediastinal cysts, may have attenuation higher than that of water, sometimes in the range of 20–40 Hounsfield units (HU). High attenuation in a cystic mediastinal mass or a mass of uneven density may alter the recommended conservative, nonsurgical management toward resection of the cyst for fear of overlooking a solid or a necrotic mass.

The differential diagnosis of a cardiophrenic angle mass generally includes benign mediastinal lipomatosis; masses of lung, pleural, diaphragmatic, or abdominal origin; ventricular aneurysm or diverticulum; and benign or malignant lesions of the peri-

3a,b
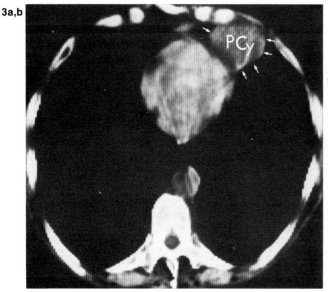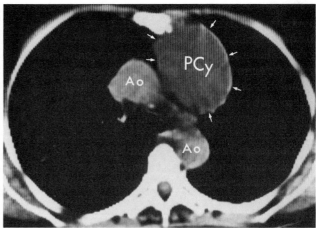

FIG. 3. a: Typical paracardiac position of a pericardial cyst (PCy) (arrows). b: Mediastinal low-density pericardial cyst (PCy) (arrows). Ao, aorta.

cardium. Plain roentgenograms of the thorax generally cannot discriminate among the densities of the various tissues that can comprise masses in the cardiophrenic angle. In contradistinction, CT is unmatched in its ability to consistently identify the water density of a pericardial cyst.

Pericardial cysts can be diagnosed easily when they are contiguous to the heart in either cardiophrenic angle and when the density of the mass is clearly within the range of water. The image of the low-density, cyst-like structure depicted in Fig. 3b was diagnosed as a thymic cyst because of its high and ventral position within the mediastinum. At surgery, a connection to the pericardium was found.

We firmly believe that conservative, nonsurgical management is the treatment of choice for the classic water-containing pericardial or mediastinal cyst. When the high density of the mass casts some doubt on the diagnosis or when significant symptoms exist, surgical removal of the cyst is the only option that can resolve the issue with certainty. Time and experience will eventually limit surgery to those patients with symptomatic large cysts or those cysts that could conceivably interfere with organ function (50,51).

Intrapericardial Teratoma

Intrapericardial teratoma is a rare and potentially lethal condition. Even though the lesion is histologically benign, its intrapericardial location may lead to compression of the right heart and a rather malignant clinical course. Most cases are diagnosed during the neonatal period or infancy. An isolated case reported in an adult has recently been published (52).

An intrapericardial teratoma frequently originates from the anterolateral surface of the root of the aorta. The mass grows caudally along the right atrioventricular groove, compressing the right atrium and ventricle dorsally and toward the left (Fig. 4). The tumor generally does not invade the surface of the right cardiac chambers or great vessels.

While thoracic teratomas are relatively common in the anterior mediastinum and are known to occasionally compress the heart and great vessels, the intrapericardial teratoma generally compresses and distorts the right cardiac chambers. This leads to high right atrial pressures, which are reflected clinically as systemic venous hypertension (edema, organomegaly, ascites, etc.), cyanosis from a right

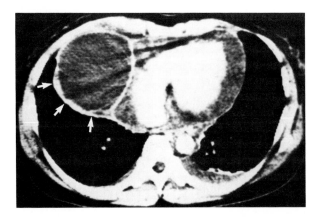

FIG. 4. Ruptured intrapericardial teratoma with pericardial effusion.

to left shunt through a patent foramen ovale, and deficit of the right cardiac output.

Intrapericardial teratoma in early infancy often causes critically severe cardiorespiratory distress, and often results in the death of the infant. Cardiorespiratory distress combined with an enlarged cardiothymic shadow should suggest the diagnosis (53–57). Echocardiography and CT can easily detect the intrapericardial position of the inhomogeneous tumor. Contrast enhancement studies serve to identify the mass and also to determine the degree of right heart compression. Early diagnosis and prompt surgical removal are the keys to a successful outcome.

PERICARDIAL EFFUSION

Echocardiography has proven to be highly reliable for the detection of pericardial effusion. Today, it continues to be the most popular and cost-effective method of diagnosis. Several prospective studies have demonstrated its sensitivity in detecting small quantities of fluid (6,7).

The advantages of echocardiography include ease of examination, absence of any known physical harm, relatively low cost, and the portability of the equipment. Despite the usefulness of this method, there remain technical limitations (58), difficulties in interpretation (23,26), and inability to perform studies when lung tissue between the heart and thoracic wall precludes appropriate transmission of ultrasound.

Because of the different absorption coefficients of the effusion and adjacent soft tissues on CT, a pericardial effusion is generally distinguished within the pericardial space. Manipulation of the window width setting is sometimes necessary to differenti-

5a,b

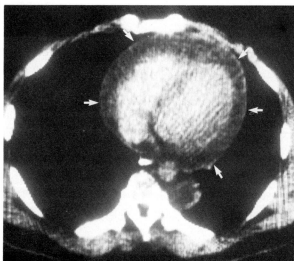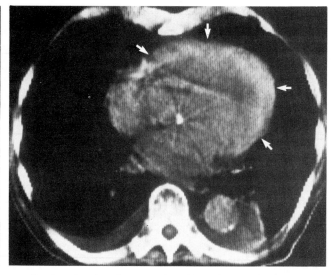

FIG. 5. Low- and high-density pericardial effusion. Note the contrasting low density of a transudate **(a)** and an exudate **(b)**; in the latter, the pericardial effusion is of greater density than the heart, whereas the contrary applies in the former. (Reprinted with permission from ref. 24.)

ate the fluid from the pericardium proper. Tomoda et al. (59) have measured the density of various types of pericardial effusions. In their experience, the HU density varied from 12 to 40, but no detailed description of the contents of the effusions, such as the hematocrit, cell count, or protein level, was given. We have encountered pericardial effusions with striking differences in density (Fig. 5). So far, we can only speculate that a high-density effusion represents hemopericardium or an exudate, and low-density fluid probably represents a transudate or chyle (59). The normal pericardium can be distended enormously with chronic effusions and still produce little or no hemodynamic alteration. How-

ever, small effusions (a few hundred milliliters) can lead to cardiac tamponade if the fluid accumulates rapidly. When increased thickness of the pericardium limits its distensibility, the volume of the fluid that can be accepted without hemodynamic effect is considerably smaller. Diagnosis of coexisting pericardial thickening and effusion can be accomplished by CT (24) (Fig. 6).

By observing the distribution of fluid in moderate-to-severe effusions, we learned that fluid accumulates in the most caudal portions of the pericardial sac, causing distention and change in the shape and axis of the sac to an extent proportional to the volume of the effusion. A small effusion usu-

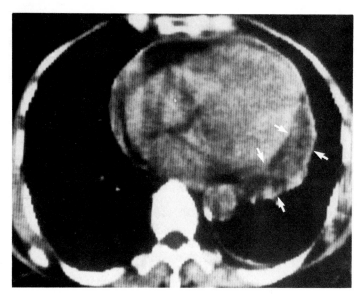

FIG. 6. Pericardial thickening and effusion. Mild universal thickening of the pericardium with coexisting effusion *(arrows).* Window manipulation is necessary to discriminate between fluid and thickened pericardium.

ally collects dorsal to the left ventricle as a thin, elliptical density. When the effusion is larger, the layer of fluid extends ventral to the right atrium and ventricle. Severe pericardial effusions form an asymmetric ring around the heart. Finally, in massive, long-standing effusions, the heart appears to float within the sac and its apex is tilted cephalad. The over-distended pericardium may then project caudally as a heavy water bag, compressing the diaphragm and abdominal organs (Fig. 7). Postoperatively, when the pericardium is left open, a pericardial effusion may extend into the mediastinum, resulting in a pericardial–mediastinal effusion (Fig. 8).

Adhesive pericardial heart disease can occasionally produce pericardial fluid encapsulation; fibrous adhesions sealing off at least two portions of the pericardial space are generally needed for fluid en-

capsulation. Fluid collections may occur in one or more isolated spaces; dorsal and right anterolateral loculations appear to be the most common. The volume and pressure exerted by encapsulated fluid may result in cardiac tamponade or produce constrictive pericarditis. Figure 9 shows the typical images of pericardial encapsulation; note that the encapsulated fluid bulges toward the heart. By manipulating the window width setting, it is possible to detect the fibrous strands that triggered the adhesive encapsulated effusion.

We feel that echocardiography is the primary modality for diagnosing pericardial effusion. CT complements it, particularly when there is coexisting pericardial thickening, a loculated effusion, primary or metastatic neoplasm, calcification, a mediastinal mass, or a need to evaluate the patient postoperatively.

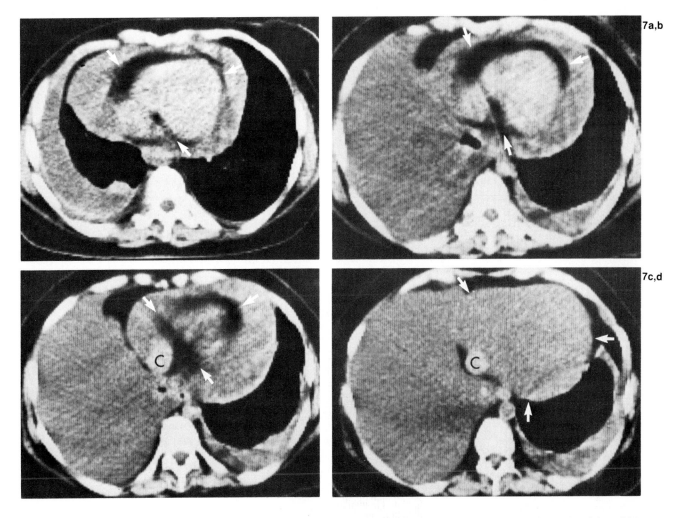

FIG. 7. Massive pericardial effusion. **a–c:** The curvilinear low-density areas represent the ventral epicardial fat pad and dorsal fat pads by the left atrioventricular groove and crus of the heart (*arrows* in a, b and c). **d:** In the most caudal image, the pericardial sac is over-distended with fluid (*arrows*), the cardiac apex has been tilted up and only the inferior vena cava (C) can be seen within the pericardium. A large right pleural effusion is also present.

8a,b

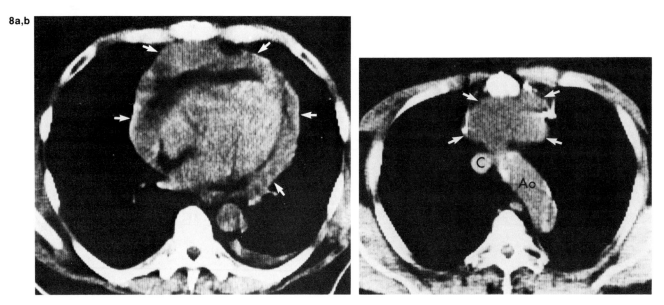

FIG. 8. Pericardial–mediastinal effusion. The pericardium was left open following aortocoronary revascularization. The ensuing pericardial effusion extended into the anterior mediastinum *(arrows).* Ao, aorta; C, superior vena cava.

9a

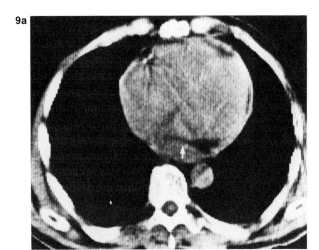

FIG. 9. a–c: Two examples of encapsulated pericardial effusion. The encapsulated fluid is usually at high pressure and bulges toward the heart *(arrows).* Identification of the fibrous strands responsible for the loculation can be accomplished by manipulating the window setting, as in (c). (Figs. 9b and c reproduced with permission from ref. 24.)

9b,c

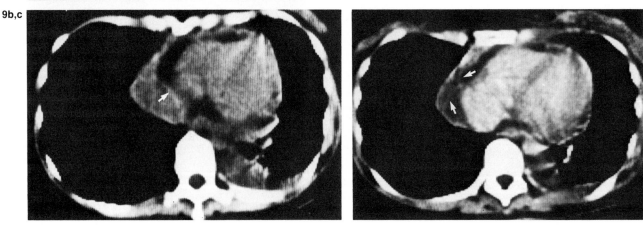

PERICARDIAL THICKENING

All organs have a finite number of ways of reacting to injury, and the pericardium is no exception. The normal pericardium reacts in three fashions: fluid exudation, fibrin production, and cellular proliferation. These may occur independently or concomitantly, and result in various morphologic alterations of the pericardial layers and their space (20). The etiology determines the type of effusion and cellular proliferation. Pericardial effusion, thickening, adhesions, calcification, and mass lesions may result from a local process or may be an expression of a systemic disease.

The unique ability of CT to demonstrate consistently and accurately the anatomic details of the normal and abnormal pericardium makes it valuable for the assessment and management of patients with pericardial thickening. As already stated, the normal parietal pericardium has a thickness of 1–2 mm, except in its most caudal portion where it inserts in the central tendon of the diaphragm. In this area, the pericardium thickens to 3–4 mm. Normal areas of slight pericardial thickening are found in the ventral pericardium adjacent to the right ventricle, presumably as a response to the stress from the transmitted pulsations of the right ventricle.

Pericardial thickening results from proliferation of fibrinous deposits, organized blood products, inflammatory reaction, fibrosis, calcification, and neoplastic invasion. In our institution, thickening of the pericardium is the most common manifestation of pericardial heart disease. For the inexperienced observer, it must be emphasized that, with the appropriate window width manipulations, one is able to differentiate pericardial effusion from the pericardium proper, thus avoiding confusion with pericardial thickening (Fig. 6).

Thickening of the pericardium has been encountered in a number of clinical conditions, including viral or bacterial pericarditis, uremia, radiation injury, as a component of a systemic disease, after pericardiotomy, and secondary to primary or secondary neoplastic involvement. Thickening may be patchy or generalized; the increase in pericardial width ranges from a few millimeters to 5 cm. Greater thickness is generally found ventrally. Thickening may be smooth, "bumpy," or nodular, particularly in neoplastic disease. Fibrous tissue may lead to adhesive pericarditis.

POSTPERICARDIOTOMY SYNDROME

The postpericardiotomy syndrome is characterized by malaise, myalgias, fever, and chest pain of variable degree and location following heart surgery (16,60–62). A similar syndrome, described by Dressler (63), may follow acute myocardial infarction. The pathogenesis of these clinical entities requires clarification, but the syndrome is believed to result from an autoimmune response to antigenic-injured myocardium. While the syndrome is associated with a rise in serum titer of anti-heart antibody, this antibody is neither heart nor species specific, is not cytotoxic to myocardial cells grown in cell culture, and elevated titers may even be found in some normal individuals (64).

Estimates of the frequency of the postpericardiotomy syndrome vary greatly, with an incidence of up to 45% following open heart surgery (16). Symptoms may appear as soon as 5 days after surgery, or may be delayed for more than 1 year. The postpericardiotomy syndrome is generally regarded as a benign condition that resolves spontaneously or responds to treatment with prednisone or other antiinflammatory agents.

The differential diagnosis encompasses inflammatory processes, congestive heart failure, pulmonary thromboembolic accidents, bone pain from the thoracotomy, drug-induced lupus-like polyserositis, and myocardial ischemia with or without thrombosis of the aortocoronary bypass grafts. A heavy load of cardiovascular surgery has resulted in our seeing a large number of patients suffering from this syndrome. Patchy or uniform thickening of the pericardium, ranging from a few millimeters to 2 cm, is the most common finding. Small effusions co-exist in about one-fourth of the cases.

Even though most patients with this syndrome will improve spontaneously or with medication, there are occasional patients who will go on to develop full clinical and hemodynamic constrictive pericarditis (Fig. 10).

We have had the opportunity to study a few patients serially—patients who had revascularization procedures and were otherwise asymptomatic. In these cases, we observed mild pericardial thickening ventrally and adjacent to the sites of actual surgical incision. The natural history of these postoperative findings is total clearance within a few days to 2 weeks after surgery. This is in contrast to the persistent and increasing degree of pericardial thickening seen in the postpericardiotomy syndrome.

NATURAL HISTORY OF PERICARDITIS

Clinical pericarditis may result from innumerable local and systemic processes (1,2). Over the years,

10a,b

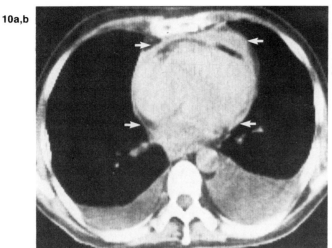 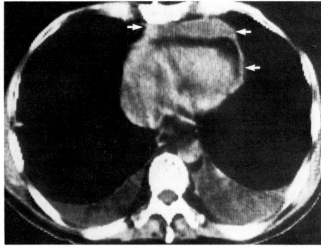

FIG. 10. a,b: Postpericardiotomy constrictive pericarditis. Universal thickening of the pericardium with patchy areas of greater thickening ventrally. Also, bilateral pleural effusion.

we have witnessed a diminution in certain forms of pericarditis, such as purulent pericarditis. Purulent pericarditis today is generally limited to children and immunocompromised patients. The qualitative and quantitative changes in the spectrum of pericarditis have also witnessed the appearance of new forms of pericardial heart disease. For example, dialysis resolves most uremic pericarditis, but it can be associated with both dialysis pericarditis and uremic constriction (65).

Certain etiologic factors, such as tuberculosis, have clearly decreased, while other etiologies, such as viral pericarditis, have become the most prevalent, community-acquired infections. Coxsackie-A viruses (types 4 and 16), echovirus types 9, 11, and 22, and poliovirus are the leading viral causes (66). Iatrogenic disease from surgery, medications, and radiation injury to the heart and pericardium are seen with increasing frequency (67).

Regardless of origin, we have, in the past, diagnosed and monitored the treatment of our patients clinically and in follow-up by echocardiography. Difficulties in consistently detecting pericardial thickening and the inability to faithfully reproduce the same information by subsequent examinations have been some of the traditional limitations of echocardiography. Today, a patient with pericarditis can easily be diagnosed by CT, since this instrument is capable of reproducibly depicting the altered morphology of the pericardium with a few transverse slices of the heart. The amount, density, and location of the existing pericardial fluid can be recorded; the thickened pericardium can be magnified and measured. Therefore, it permits the luxury of a true follow-up examination, with or without conventional medical or surgical treatment.

The natural history of a middle-aged patient with viral pericarditis is presented in Fig. 11. On initial hospital admission, a full-blown picture of a viral type of pericarditis was clinically evident. Note the presence of small bilateral pleural effusions and a small amount of fluid in the pericardial space. The parietal pericardium is moderately thickened. After 6 months of antiinflammatory agents, including corticosteroids, the patient is in frank recovery and the effusions have disappeared, although the parietal pericardium still remains mildly increased in width. A year later, the parietal pericardium is back to normal in appearance and dimensions. This patient represents an excellent example of the ability of CT to reconstruct fine anatomic detail of the inflamed pericardium throughout the natural history of a disorder.

Constrictive Pericarditis Versus Restrictive Cardiomyopathy

The clinical syndrome of constrictive pericarditis (Pick's disease) has been recognized for more than a century (68). The clinical differential diagnosis of constrictive pericarditis includes congestive cardiomyopathies, cardiac or pericardial neoplasm producing right heart obstruction, cardiac tamponade, tricuspid valvular disease, pulmonary hypertension, inferior vena cava webs or tumors, and cirrhosis of the liver. Echocardiography and cardiac catheterization eliminate some of these considerations. The principal problem remaining is the relative inability to distinguish between the manifestations of constrictive pericarditis and certain types of cardiomyopathies, such as restrictive (infiltrative) cardiomyopathy (69). Since the major pathophysio-

11a,b

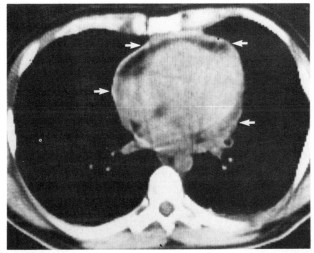

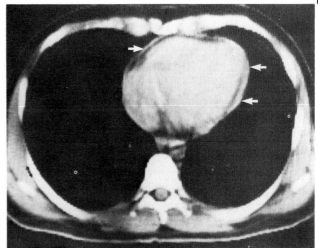

11c

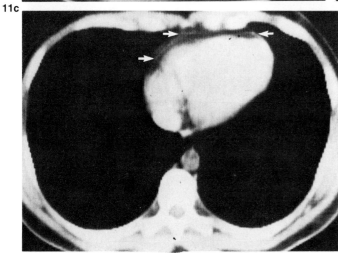

FIG. 11. Natural history of viral pericarditis. **a:** Initial examination shows universal thickening of the pericardium with a small amount of effusion dorsally *(arrows).* **b:** Mild thickening remains 6 months later *(arrow).* Effusion is no longer seen. **c:** Pericardium appears normal 1 year later *(arrows).*

logic disorder is identical in both—encumbered filling of the heart—patients often have similar clinical signs, symptoms, and hemodynamic characteristics (70).

The outstanding hemodynamic feature of constrictive pericarditis is elevation and equilibration of the diastolic pressure in all cardiac chambers, since diastolic expansion is abruptly limited by the quasi-unyielding hard shell of the constricting pericardium (71,72). Systolic function usually is well-preserved. Recently, differences in the pattern of diastolic left ventricular filling volume and filling rate were proposed to be features distinguishing restrictive amyloid cardiomyopathy and constrictive pericarditis (73). Similarly, Janos et al. (74) have used digitalized echocardiography to conclude that, in constrictive pericarditis, there is an increased maximal filling rate and shortened major filling period, whereas in restrictive cardiomyopathy, there is reduced maximal filling rate and prolonged major filling period. Even though the number of patients in these series is small, the findings appear strik-

ingly distinguishable, and perhaps further prospective data will support this contention.

Diagnosis sometimes is accomplished by angiography, but transvenous endomyocardial biopsy and exploratory thoracotomy often are required to distinguish surgically correctable constrictive pericarditis from the almost untreatable infiltrative cardiomyopathies.

In our institution, we have successfully utilized CT in 18 patients with constrictive pericarditis and in three patients with restrictive infiltrative amyloid cardiomyopathy. The accurate identification of a normal or thickened pericardium contributes greatly to the solution of this persistent clinical quandary. All patients with constrictive pericarditis had hemodynamic studies and, with surgery, proved to have constrictive pericarditis. The findings on CT of a thickened pericardium, ranging from 0.5 to 2.0 cm in width, plus external deformity of the right heart (22) with reflux of contrast media into the coronary sinus proved to be the most consistent and reliable findings. Secondary signs included systemic vein dilation, organomegaly, ascites, and, in some cases, pleural effusions (Fig. 12).

On the basis of our own clinical experience, we have arrived at the following conclusion: the finding of a normal pericardium by CT in patients with symptoms, signs, and hemodynamics suggestive of constrictive pericarditis virtually excludes the presence of constrictive pericarditis, thereby providing the diagnosis of restrictive cardiomyopathy, except on rare occasions when constrictive epicarditis is present with a normal parietal pericardium (75). If a thickened pericardium is detected by CT, a pericardiectomy is recommended for management. These guidelines have been successfully followed in the 21 patients described above. Recently, we had an opportunity to study a middle-aged patient with long-standing migraine headaches who received "standard" dosages of methysergide for a prolonged period. He was admitted with the classical symp-

toms and physical and hemodynamic findings of constrictive pericarditis. CT disclosed generalized, moderate thickening of the pericardium, consistent with the diagnosis of constrictive pericarditis. At the clinician's insistence, a transvenous endomyocardial biopsy was performed, which, surprisingly, showed extensive myocardial fibrosis. Since then, we have modified our position, and suggest that a percutaneous endomyocardial biopsy be performed in patients whose pericardium and myocardium might be simultaneously involved, as in the clinical example presented here, or with radiation injury, etc.

Calcific Pericarditis

Calcifications of the visceral and parietal pericardium are believed to represent the end stage of a previous pericardial insult, such as tuberculosis,

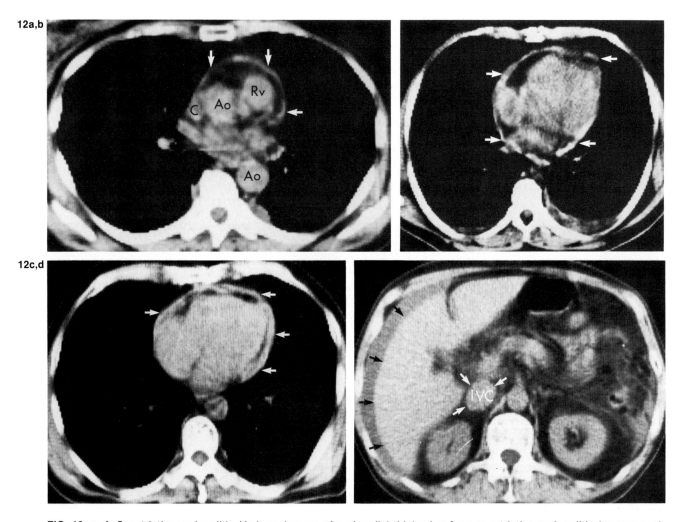

FIG. 12. a–d: Constrictive pericarditis. Various degrees of pericardial thickening from constrictive pericarditis (*arrows,* a–c). Ascites *(black arrows)* and inferior vena cava *(arrows)* dilatation are shown in (d). C, superior vena cava; Ao, aorta; Rv, right ventricle.

purulent pericarditis, hemopericardium, rheumatic fever, or idiopathic pericarditis (20). Pathologic examination of the calcified tissues rarely yields a clue about the duration or cause of the condition.

Calcifications in the visceral pericardium occur more often at the atrioventricular grooves, ventricular grooves, and the crus of the heart. The greatest deposits of calcification are generally noted at the crus of the heart. Calcifications in the parietal pericardium may be in patches or large uniform plaques, from a few millimeters to 2.0 cm in thickness (Fig. 13).

Large calcifications of the pericardium may be present in the absence of the clinical syndrome of constrictive pericarditis (76,77). Encasement of both ventricles by the calcific pericardium is generally necessary to produce constriction. Occasionally, an isolated band of strategically placed calcific tissue may result in hemodynamic dysfunction (78).

Postoperative Pericardium

Postoperative assessment of the mediastinum following pericardial fenestration or pericardial stripping has been extremely helpful in certain clinical settings. Recurrent clinical and hemodynamic constrictive pericarditis has been seen in a patient who developed constrictive pericarditis following a coronary revascularization procedure. One night prior to the pericardiectomy—and unknown to his physician—the patient ingested several aspirin tablets, thereby impairing platelet function. At surgery, persistent bleeding was eventually controlled and the patient was discharged without apparent complication. Several weeks after pericardiectomy, the pa-

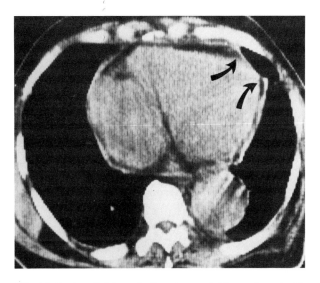

FIG. 14. Pericardial fenestration *(arrows).* (Reproduced with permission from ref. 24.)

tient was again admitted with recurrent signs of constriction (Fig. 10b). At his third surgical intervention, a thick core of fibrinous tissue measuring up to 1.5 cm in thickness was successfully removed, with relief of symptomatology.

Computed tomography is of value in determining the extent of pericardium removed (whether or not it extends to the phrenic nerves) and in defining the size of a pericardial window (Fig. 14). Postoperative retrosternal hematomas can be easily detected (Fig. 15). An additional complication following surgery of the pericardium is the development of an intrapericardial abscess. Detection of this abnormality is critically important, and yet it may be difficult to detect with routine radiographs. CT may be invaluable in this clinical setting (Fig. 16).

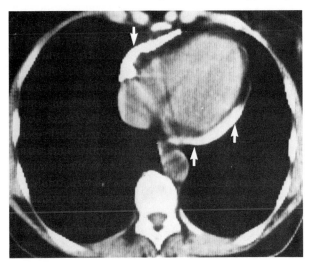

FIG. 13. Calcific pericarditis *(arrows).* (Reproduced with permission from ref. 24).

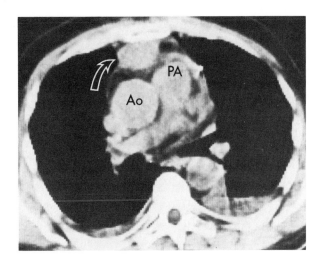

FIG. 15. Postoperative retrosternal hematoma *(arrow).* Ao, aorta; PA, pulmonary artery.

16a,b

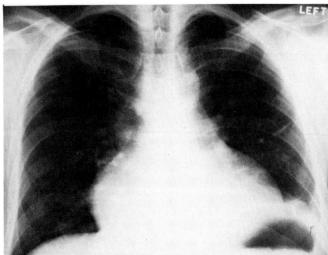
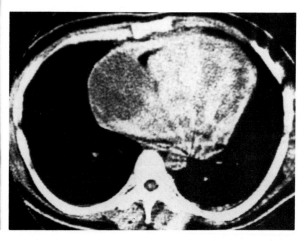

FIG. 16. Staphylococcal pericardial abscess. **a:** PA radiograph following placement of a pleuropericardial window in a patient with severe viral pericarditis. The heart is minimally enlarged. No other abnormalities are apparent. **b:** CT section at the level of surgery. A well-defined fluid collection is present within the pericardium on the right side. This proved to be a postoperative pericardial abscess. (Case courtesy of Dr. Dorothy McCauley, New York University Medical Center.)

NEOPLASTIC PERICARDIAL HEART DISEASE

Primary tumors of the heart are rare [1 in 60,000 (79) to 1 in 1,000 autopsies (80)] but they are seen more often than are primary tumors of the pericardium. Conversely, metastatic involvement of the pericardium is seen more frequently than is myocardial invasion. The ratio of malignant to benign primary neoplasms is 1:3 in the myocardium and 1:1 in the pericardium (81). Antemortem diagnosis of primary or metastatic pericardial heart disease continues to be a difficult task. With CT units accessible to most communities, we should logically expect a greater yield in the diagnosis and management of primary tumors of the heart.

Computed tomography is now used routinely to examine the thorax of patients with suspected or known thoracic malignancies, and is valuable in the evaluation of the pericardium. We present clinical examples of both benign and malignant primary pericardial tumors and metastatic involvement to highlight the advantages of CT over any other diagnostic modality.

Malignant Mesothelioma of the Pericardium

The association of asbestos disease with pleural mesothelioma is well-established (82). A similar association with peritoneal and pericardial mesothelioma has not been statistically validated by epidemiologic studies because of the relatively low number of reported cases (83), although some isolated cases clearly support a cause and effect relationship between asbestos disease and pericardial mesothelioma (84).

Pericardial mesothelioma appears at a median age of 44 years, but cases have been reported from age 1 to age 79. The male-to-female ratio is 1:1. The tumor may be a single mass, multicentric, or form diffuse plaques that involve the visceral and parietal pericardium, and can result in constrictive pericarditis. Pericardial mesotheliomas have been classified, according to the predominant tissue, as epithelioid, fibrous, or mixed (85); two-thirds are mixed and one-third epithelioid.

Unresponsive congestive heart failure, hemorrhagic pericardial and pleural effusions, pericardial constriction or tamponade, and cardiac arrhythmias are the most common clinical manifestations. Rapid clinical deterioration with ensuing death after 4–12 months is the natural history of these patients (86).

Diagnosis of mesothelioma by fluid cytology (87) is inconsistent and controversial (88). Pleural fluid with hyaluronic acid levels elevated above 0.8 mg/ml is a reliable indicator; however, mildly elevated levels of hyaluronic acid are found with metastatic disease (89).

The findings on CT of pleural and peritoneal mesotheliomas have recently been reported (90,91), whereas only isolated, single cases of pericardial mesotheliomas have been reported (24). Figure 17 shows the images of a middle-aged female with left lower lobe atelectasis and multiple visceral and parietal pericardial masses, ranging from a few mil-

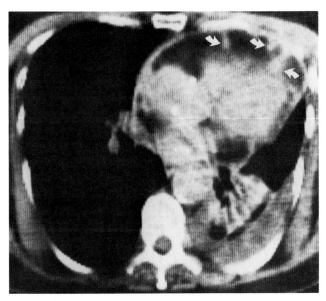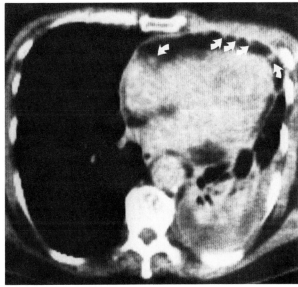

FIG. 17. a,b: Multicentric mesothelioma of the pericardium *(arrows)*. (Fig. 17a reproduced with permission from ref. 24.)

limeters to over 2.0 cm in diameter. Multiple metastatic foci or a multicentric mesothelioma should be the primary diagnostic consideration; an angiomatous lesion could conceivably be entertained as a possibility, but lack of intense enhancement after contrast medium administration excluded the latter. At surgery, a multicentric malignant mesothelioma was partially resected.

Intrapericardial Lipoma

Like their malignant counterparts, benign tumors of the pericardium are rare. We have had the opportunity to study two elderly male patients referred because of widening and distortion of the cardiomediastinal silhouette. Both had large intrapericardial masses of low density (-80 to -115 HU). Even though we lack surgical confirmation of these masses, our diagnosis is supported by the measurements of Mendez et al. (92) of the density of fat-containing masses. A lipoma generally has a density of -55 to -120 HU. Extreme care must be exercised in examining the fatty mass; nodular densities or strands within the fat may actually be an indication of a liposarcoma. Nonsurgical managemen was elected for these two patients. Re-examination at intervals during the ensuing year showed no change in the lipomas, nor any discernible clinical abnormality (Fig. 18).

Metastatic Neoplasm: Pericardial Involvement

Neoplastic involvement of the heart and pericardium by metastatic tumor is generally considered an

uncommon clinical condition. Autopsy series have demonstrated a frequency of pericardiac metastases that ranges from 1.5% to 21% of patients dying from a specific malignancy (85,93,94). DeLoach and Haynes (95) cited the first antemortem diagnosis of pericardial metastases in 1924. Since then, increasing numbers of cases have been recorded (95–101), with a wide variety of clinical manifestations (102–105). Clinical awareness, modern diagnostic methods (106–111) and therapeutic measures of surgical palliation and chemotherapy with prolonged survival are believed to be the reasons for the current apparent increase in the frequency of pericar-

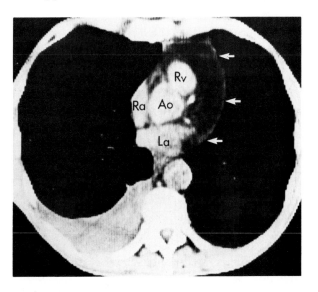

FIG. 18. Intrapericardial lipoma *(arrows)*. Ao, aorta; La, left atrium; Ra, right atrium; Rv, right ventricle. (Reproduced with permission from ref. 24.)

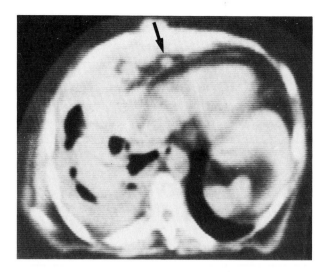

FIG. 19. Metastatic melanoma to the parietal pericardium *(arrow).*

dial metastases (85). The clinical differentiation of metastatic pericardial heart disease from the damage created by radiation injury to the heart and pericardium (112) remains a major challenge, not only at the bedside but also at the imaging console.

There are three known pathways by which neoplastic cells reach the heart and pericardium: direct invasion by a contiguous tumor (85), hematogenous spread (113), and lymphangitic spread (114,115). Carcinoma of the lung and breast are the two primary lesions that most commonly involve the heart and pericardium (85,103). Autopsy series have shown such metastases in as many as 22% of patients who have died of cancer of the lung (104). Lymphoproliferative (101–105) malignancies (113) and melanoma are the other two common etiologies of neoplastic pericarditis.

Like the Glisson fibrous capsule of the liver, the normal pericardium is a strong fibrous structure, generally resistant but not invulnerable to compression and direct invasion by adjacent mediastinal or pulmonary malignancies.

Normally, the lymph is transported from the endocardium toward the pericardium by a fine network of lymphatic capillaries. Once in the epicardium, the fluid is collected by several lymphatic vessels, which in turn drain toward the lymph nodes in the mediastinum (114). Lymphadenopathy is generally found in patients who have cardiac and pericardial metastases, and retrograde permeation in such an obstructed lymphatic system probably is the usual way in which tumor cells enter the heart and pericardium (115). Occasionally, certain tumors, such as melanoma, spread to the myocardium or pericardium without accompanying mediastinal lymphadenopathy. The hematogenous route probably is the pathway of spread in these patients (Fig. 19).

Metastatic involvement of the pericardium is most commonly reflected as a pericardial effusion. This fluid is generally considered exudative in type, with high protein and cellular content. When invaded by tumor, the pericardium usually becomes thickened (Fig. 20) in a plaque-like manner, with obliteration of the pericardial space in some areas. This thickening may be localized, patchy, or generalized. In some cases, discrete nodular masses attached to the pericardium have been reported (115).

Computed tomography has been of great value in the detection and follow-up of metastatic disease. The range of findings has been from minute thickening to masses of 5 cm in width. The nodular pattern is rarely seen.

We feel confident in recommending CT as the

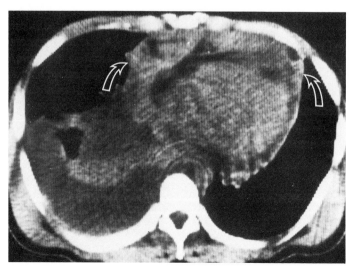

FIG. 20. Lymphomatous involvement of the pericardium *(arrows).*

best diagnostic method for neoplastic pericardial heart disease, as confidence is gained in the ability of CT to graphically contribute important morphologic information for its diagnosis and management. We expect the use of this method to increase, not only in primary diagnosis but also in the assessment of operative treatment, effectiveness of chemotherapy, and the effects of radiotherapy on the heart and pericardium.

REFERENCES

1. Spodick DH, ed. *Pericardial Diseases.* Philadelphia, F.A. Davis, 1976, pp 4–312
2. Spodick DH. The normal and diseased pericardium: Current concepts of pericardial physiology, diagnosis and treatment. *J Am Coll Cardiol* 1:240–251, 1983
3. Mangano DT. The effect of the pericardium on ventricular systolic function in man. *Circulation* 61:352–357, 1980
4. Hipona FA, Paredes S. The radiology of pericardial heart disease. *Cardiovasc Clin* 7:91–124, 1976
5. Feigenbaum H, Waldhausen JA, Hyde CP. Ultrasonic diagnosis of pericardial effusion. *JAMA* 191:711–714, 1965
6. Feigenbaum H. Echocardiographic diagnosis of pericardial effusion. *Am J Cardiol* 26:475–479, 1970
7. Martin RP, Rakowski H, French J, Popp RL. Localization of pericardial effusion with wide-angle phased-array echocardiography. *Am J Cardiol* 42:904–912, 1978
8. Teicholz LE. Echocardiographic evaluation of pericardial diseases. *Prog Cardiovasc Dis* 21:133–140, 1978
9. Schnittger I, Bowden RE, Abrams J, Popp RL. Echocardiography: Pericardial thickening and constrictive pericarditis. *Am J Cardiol* 42:388–395, 1978
10. Osler W. *The Principles and Practice of Medicine.* New York, D. Appleton Co. 1892, p 1079
11. Reeves RL. Cause of acute pericarditis. *Am J Med Sci* 255:34–38, 1953
12. Applefeld MM, Slawson RG, Hall-Craigs M, Green DC, Singleton RT, Wiernik PH. Delayed pericardial disease after radiotherapy. *Am J Cardiol* 47:210–213, 1981
13. Houston MC, McChesney JA, Chatterjee K. Pericardial effusion associated with minoxidil therapy. *Arch Intern Med* 14:69–71, 1981
14. Goldberg MJ, Husain M, Wajszczuk WJ, Rubenfire M. Procainamide-induced lupus erythematosus pericarditis encountered during coronary bypass surgery. *Am J Med* 69:159–162, 1980
15. Luft FC, Gilman JK, Weyman AE. Pericarditis in the patient with uremia. Clinical and echocardiographic evaluation. *Nephron* 25:160–166, 1980
16. Clapp SK, Garson A Jr, Gutgesell HP, Cooley DA, McNamara DG. Postoperative pericardial effusion and its relation to postpericardiotomy syndrome. *Pediatrics* 66:585–588, 1980
17. Gross BH, Glazer GM, Francis IR. CT of intracardiac and intrapericardial masses. *AJR* 140:903–907, 1983
18. Moncada R, Salinas M, Churchill R, Love L, Reynes C, Demos TC, Hale D, Schreiber R. Patency of saphenous aortocoronary bypass grafts demonstrated by computed tomography. *N Engl J Med* 303:503, 1980
19. Ishihara T, Ferrans VJ, Jones M, Boyce SW, Kawanami O, Roberts WG. Histologic and ultrastructural features of normal human parietal pericardium. *Am J Cardiol* 46:744–753, 1980
20. Roberts WC, Spray TL. Pericardial heart disease: A study of its causes, consequences, and morphologic features. *Cardiovasc Clin* 7:11–65, 1976
21. Houang MTW, Arozena X, Shaw DG. Demonstration of the pericardium and pericardial effusion by computed tomography. *J Comput Assist Tomogr* 3:601–603, 1979
22. Doppman JL, Reinmuller R, Lissner J, Cryan J, Bolte HD, Strauer BE, Hellwig H. Computed tomography in constrictive pericarditis. *J Comput Assist Tomogr* 5:1–11, 1981
23. Isner JM, Carter BL, Roberts WC, Bankoff MS. Subepicardial adipose tissue producing echocardiographic appearance of pericardial effusion. *Am J Cardiol* 51:565–569, 1983
24. Moncada R, Baker M, Salinas M, Demos TC, Churchill R, Love L, Reynes C, Hale D, Cardoso M, Pifarre R. Diagnostic role of computed tomography in pericardial heart disease: Congenital defects, thickening, neoplasms and effusions. *Am Heart J* 103:263–281, 1982
25. Feigenbaum H, Waldhausen JA, Hyde CP. Ultrasonic diagnosis of pericardial effusion. *JAMA* 191:711–714, 1965
26. Jacobs WR, Talano JV, Loeb HS. Echocardiographic interpretation of pericardial effusion. *Arch Intern Med* 138:622–625, 1978
27. Kronzon I, Cohen ML, Winer HE. Cardiac tamponade by loculated pericardial hematoma: Limitations of M-mode echocardiography. *J Am Coll Cardiol* 1:913–915, 1983
28. Edwards J. Congenital malformations of the heart and great vessels. F. malformations of the pericardium. In: *Pathology of the Heart and Great Vessels*, 3rd edition, ed. by SE Gould. Springfield, C.C. Thomas, 1968, pp 376–378
29. Moore RL. Congenital deficiencies of the pericardium. *Arch Surg* 11:765–777, 1925
30. Southworth H, Stevenson CS. Congenital defects of pericardium. *Arch Intern Med* 61:223–240, 1938
31. Verse M. Fall van kongenitalem defert des hertzbeutels. *Munch Med Wochenschr* 56:2665–2666, 1909
32. Perna G. Sopra un arresto di svillupo della sierosa pericardica nelluomo. *Anat Anz* 35:389–398, 1961
33. Schuster B, Alexjandrino S, Yavuz F, Imm CW. Congenital pericardial defect: Report of patient with associated ductus arteriosus. *Am J Dis Child* 110:199–202, 1965
34. Tabakin BS, Hanson JS, Tampas JP, Caldwell EJ. Congenital absence of left pericardium. *Am J Roentgenol* 94:122–128, 1965
35. Hipona FA, Crummy AB Jr. Congenital pericardial defect associated with tetralogy of Fallot: Herniation of normal lung into pericardial cavity. *Circulation* 29:132–135, 1964
36. Mukerjee S. Congenital partial left pericardial defect with bronchogenic cyst. *Thorax* 19:176–179, 1964
37. Baim RS, MacDonald II, Wise DJ, Lenkei SC. Computed tomography of absent left pericardium. *Radiology* 135:127–128, 1980
38. Columbus (Mattheaues Realdus) (1494–1559). De re anatomica libre XV, 3 p I, 269 pp I 1.4° Venetiis, Ex typong N. Beuilacquae 1559
39. Baille M. On the want of a pericardium in a human body. *Trans Soc Improve Med Cir Knowl* 1:91–102, 1793
40. Ladd WE. Congenital absence of pericardium, with report of a case. *N Engl J Med* 214:183–187, 1936
41. Fraser GR, Pare JAP. *Diagnosis of Diseases of the Chest.* Philadelphia, W.B. Saunders, 1970, p 1193
42. Rooge JD, Mishkin ME, Genovese PD. Congenital partial pericardial defect with herniation of left appendage. *Ann Intern Med* 64:137–141, 1966
43. Minocha GK, Falicov RE, Nijensohn E. Partial right-sided congenital pericardial defect with herniation of right atrium and right ventricle. *Chest* 76:484–486, 1979
44. Lajos TZ, Bunnell II, Colkathis BP, Schimert G. Coronary artery insufficiency secondary to congenital pericardial defect. *Chest* 58:73–76, 1970
45. Saito R, Hotta F. Congenital pericardial defect associated with cardiac incarceration: Case report. *Am Heart J* 100:866–870, 1980
46. Ellis K, Leeds NE, Himmelstein A. Congenital deficiencies in partial pericardium: Review with two new cases including successful diagnosis by plain roentgenography. *Am J Roentgenol* 82:125–137, 1959

47. Persigehl M, Erbel R. Congenital left-sided pericardial defects. *ROFO* 135:541–547, 1981
48. Nasser WK. Congenital diseases of the pericardium. *Cardiovasc Clin* 7:271–286, 1976
49. LeRoux BT. Pericardial coelomic cysts. *Thorax* 14:27–31, 1959
50. Engle DE, Tresch DD, Boncheck LI, Foley WD, Brooks HL. Misdiagnosis of pericardial cyst by echocardiography and computed tomography scanning. *Arch Intern Med* 143:351–352, 1983
51. Koch PC, Kronzon I, Winer HE, et al. Displacement of the heart by a giant mediastinal cyst. *Am J Cardiol* 40:445–448, 1977
52. Whitton ID, Mitha AS, Pillay SV. Intrapericardial teratoma: A case report. *S Afr Med J* 58:37–38, 1980
53. Pillay SV. Intrapericardial teratoma. A case report. *S Afr Med J* 54:982–984, 1978
54. Arciniegas E, Hakimi M, Farooki ZQ, Green EW. Intrapericardial teratoma in infancy. *J Thorac Cardiovasc Surg* 79:306–311, 1980
55. Sumner TE, Crowe JE, Klein A, McKone RC, Weaver RL. Intrapericardial teratoma in infancy. *Pediatr Radiol* 10:51–53, 1980
56. Banfield DF, Dick M, Behrendt DM, Rosenthal A, Pescheria A, Scott W. Intrapericardial teratoma: A new and treatable cause of hydrops fetalis. *Am J Dis Child* 134:1174–1175, 1980
57. Zerella JT, Halpe DC. Intrapericardial teratoma—neonatal cardiorespiratory distress amenable to surgery. *J Pediatr Surg* 15:961–963, 1980
58. Walinsky P. Pitfalls in the diagnosis of pericardial effusion. *Cardiovasc Clin* 9:111–122, 1978
59. Tomoda H, Hoshiai M, Furuya H, Oeda Y, Matsumoto S, Tanabe T, Tamachi H, Sasamoto H, Koide S, Kuribayashi S, Matsuyama S. Evaluation of pericardial effusion with computed tomography. *Am Heart J* 99:701–706, 1980
60. Janton OH, Glover RP, O'Neill TJE. Results of the surgical treatment for mitral stenosis. *Circulation* 6:321–333, 1952
61. Drusin LM, Engle MA, Hagstrom JWC, Schwartz MS. The postpericardiotomy syndrome. A six year epidemiologic study. *N Engl J Med* 272:597–602, 1965
62. Soloff LA, Zatuchni J, Janton OH, O'Neil TJE, Glover RP. Reactivation of rheumatic fever following mitral commissurotomy. *Circulation* 8:481–493, 1953
63. Dressler W. A post-myocardial infarction syndrome. Preliminary report of a complication resembling idiopathic, recurrent benign pericarditis. *JAMA* 160:1379–1383, 1956
64. Engle ME, Klein AA, Hepner S, Ehlers KH. The postpericardiotomy and similar syndromes. *Cardiovasc Clin* 7:211–217, 1976
65. Buselmeier TJ, Simmons RL, Natarian JS, Mauer SM, Matas AJ, Kjellstrand CM. Uremic pericardial effusion. Treatment by catheter drainage and local nonabsorbable steroid administration. *Nephron* 16:371–380, 1976
66. Johnson RA, Palacios I. Dilated cardiomyopathies of the adult (second of two parts). *N Engl J Med* 307:1119–1126, 1982
67. Stewart JR, Fajardo LF. Radiation induced heart disease. Clinical and experimental aspects. *Radiol Clin North Am* 9:511–531, 1971
68. Pick F. Uber chronischke unter dem bilde dem lerercirrhose verlairpende (ferikardische pseudolebercirrhose) (Curschman), Nebst bemerkungen ube die zuckerguss Leber. *Z Klin Med* 29:385–392, 1896
69. Meany E, Shabetai R, Bhargavia V. Cardial amyloidosis, constrictive pericarditis and restrictive cardiomyopathy. *Am J Cardiol* 38:547–556, 1976
70. Gunnar RM, Dillon RF, Wallyn RJ. The physiologic and clinical similarities between primary amyloid of the heart and constrictive pericarditis. *Circulation* 2:827–832, 1953
71. Shabetai R, Fowler NO, Guntheroth WG. The hemodynamics of cardiac tamponade and constrictive pericarditis. *Am J Cardiol* 26:480–489, 1970
72. Wood P. Chronic constrictive pericarditis. *Am J Cardiol* 7:48–61, 1961
73. Tyberg TI, Goodyer AVN, Hurst VW III, Alexander J, Langou RA. Left ventricular filling in differentiating restrictive amyloid cardiomyopathy and constrictive pericarditis. *Am J Cardiol* 47:791–796, 1981
74. Janos GG, Arjunan K, Meyer RE, Engel P, Kaplan S. Differentiation of constrictive pericarditis and restrictive cardiomyopathy using digitized echocardiography. *J Am Coll Cardiol* 1:541–549, 1983
75. Harken DE. Surgery of the pericardium. *Cardiovasc Clin* 7:287–290, 1976
76. Harvey RM, Ferrer MI, Cathcart RT, et al. Mechanical and myocardial factors in chronic constrictive pericarditis. *Circulation* 8:695–707, 1953
77. Mathewson FA. Calcifications of the pericardium in apparently healthy people. Electrocardiographic abnormalities found in tracings from apparently healthy persons with calcifications in the pericardium. *Circulation* 12:44–51, 1955
78. Shapiro JH, Jacobson HG, Rubinstein BM, et al. *Calcifications of the Heart.* Springfield, C.C. Thomas, 1963, p 198
79. Strauss R, Merliss R. Primary tumors of the heart. *Arch Pathol* 39:74–78, 1945
80. Dalgren S, Nordenstrom B. Primary fibrous hamartoma of the heart. *Acta Pathol Microbiol Scand* 63:355–360, 1965
81. Abrams HL, Sprio R, Goldstein N. Metastases in carcinoma. Analysis of 1,000 autopsied cases. *Cancer* 3:74–85, 1950
82. Selikoff IJ. Cancer risk of asbestos exposure. In: *Origins of Human Cancer,* ed. by HH Hiatt, JD Watson, and JA Winsten, Cold Spring Harbor, NY, Cold Spring Harbor Laboratory, 1799, p 1765
83. Beck B, Konetzke G, Ludwig V, Rothig W, Sturm W. Malignant pericardial mesotheliomas and asbestos exposure: A case report. *Am J Industr Med* 3:149–159, 1982
84. Churg A, Warnock ML, Bensch KG. Malignant mesothelioma arising after direct application of asbestos and fiber glass to the pericardium. *Am Rev Respir Dis* 118:419–424, 1978
85. Cohen JI. Neoplastic pericarditis. *Cardiovasc Clin* 7:257–269, 1976
86. Sytman AL, MacAlpin RN. Primary pericardial mesothelioma: Report of two cases and review of the literature. *Am Heart J* 81:760–769, 1971
87. Kobayashi Y, Takeda S, Yamamoto T, Goi S. Cytologic detection of malignant mesothelioma of the pericardium. *Acta Cytol (Baltimore)* 22:344–349, 1978
88. Spriggs AI, Jerome DW. Benign mesothelial proliferation with collagen formation in pericardial fluid. *Acta Cytol (Baltimore)* 23:428–430, 1979
89. Antman KH. Malignant mesothelioma. *N Engl J Med* 303:200–202, 1980
90. Mirvis S, Dutcher JP, Haney PJ, Whitley NO, Aisner J. CT of malignant pleural mesothelioma. *AJR* 140:665–670, 1983
91. Rabinowitz JG, Efremidi SC, Cohen B, et al. A comparative study of mesothelioma and asbestosis using computed tomography and conventional chest radiology. *Radiology* 144:453–460, 1982
92. Mendez G Jr, Isikof MB, Morillo G. Fatty tumors of the thorax demonstrated by CT. *Am J Roentgenol* 133:207–212, 1979
93. Scott RW, Garvin CF. Tumors of the heart and pericardium. *Am Heart J* 17:431–436, 1939
94. Harrer WV, Lewis PL. Metastatic tumors involving the heart and pericardium. *Pa Med* 74:57–60, 1971
95. DeLoach JF, Haynes JW. Secondary tumors of the heart and pericardium. *Arch Intern Med* 9:224–249, 1953
96. Hanfling SM. Metastatic cancer to the heart. *Circulation* 22:474–483, 1960
97. Malaret GF, Aliaga P. Metastatic disease to the heart. *Cancer* 22:457–466, 1967
98. Martini N, Freiman AH, Watson RC. Malignant pericardial effusion. *NY State J Med* 76:719–721, 1976

99. Syed S, Jung T. Cardiac tamponade caused by metastasising hemangioendothelial sarcoma of the liver. *Br Heart J* 40:697–699, 1978

100. Westfried M, Mandel D, Alderete MN, Groopman J, Minkowitz S. Sipple's syndrome with a malignant pheochromocytoma presenting as a pericardial effusion. *Cardiology* 63:305–311, 1978

101. Levitt LJ, Ault KA, Pinkus GS, Sloss LJ, McManus BM. Pericarditis and early cardiac tamponade as a primary manifestation of lymphosarcoma cell leukemia. *Am J Med* 67:619–623, 1979

102. Javier BV, Yount WJ, Hall TC, Crosby DJ. The clinical implications of cardiac mestastases from solid tumors. A clinical anslysis of 292 cases proved at autopsy. *Neoplasma* 14:561–573, 1967

103. Thurber DL, Edwards JE, Anchor RWP. Secondary malignant tumors of the pericardium. *Circulation* 26:228–241, 1962

104. Onuigro WIB. The spread of lung cancer to the heart, pericardium and great vessels. *Jpn Heart J* 15:234–240, 1974

105. Madianos M, Sokal JE. Cardiac involvement in lymphosarcoma and reticulum cell sarcoma. *Am Heart J* 65:322–326, 1963

106. Abrams HL, Adams DF, Grand HA. The radiology of tumors of the heart. *Rad Clin North Am* 9:299–326, 1971

107. Hipona FA, Paredes S. The radiology of pericardial disease. *Cardiovasc Clin* 7:91–124, 1976

108. Schiller NB, Botvinick EH. Right ventricular compression as a sign of cardiac tamponade. 56:774–779, 1977

109. Singh A, Usher M, Raphael L. Pericardial accumulation of Tc^{99} methylene diphosphate in a case of pericarditis. *J Nucl Med* 18:1141–1142, 1977

110. Schnittger I, Bowden RE, Abrams J, Popp RL. Echocardiography: Pericardial thickening and constrictive pericarditis. *Am J Cardiol* 42:388–395, 1978

111. O'Connell JB, Robinson JA, Henkin RE, Gunnar RM. Gallium-67 citrate scanning for noninvasive detection of inflammation in pericardial diseases. *Am J Cardiol* 46:879, 1980

112. Posner MR, Cohen GI, Skarin AT. Pericardial disease in patients with cancer. The differentiation of malignant from idiopathic and radiation induced pericarditis. *Am J Med* 71:407–413, 1981

113. Nakayama R, Yoneyama T, Takatani O, Kimura K. A study of metastatic tumors to the heart, pericardium and great vessels. Incidence of metastases to the heart, pericardium and great vessels. *Jpn Heart J* 7:227–234, 1966

114. Kline IW. Lymphatic pathways in the heart. *Arch Pathol* 88:638–644, 1969

115. Onuigro WIB. Cancer permeation: Process, problems and prospects—A review. *Cancer Res* 33:633–636, 1973

Chapter 11

Diaphragm

The diaphragm acts as a dome-shaped partition to separate the thoracic and abdominal cavities. Physiologically, the diaphragm is the chief muscle of inspiration. Anatomically, the diaphragm represents the interface, and, on occasion, the actual pathway for the spread of disease, between the abdomen and thorax. In this chapter, the normal cross-sectional appearance of the diaphragm will be reviewed. How this knowledge can be applied to the diagnosis of peridiaphragmatic pathology will be extensively illustrated.

GENERAL PRINCIPLES AND ANATOMY

Essential to the accurate interpretation of cross-sectional images through the base of the lungs and upper abdomen is identification of the hemidiaphragms (1). This is made possible by appreciation of the following principles.

The actual position of the hemidiaphragms generally must be inferred. This is because visualization of the normally thin line of the diaphragm itself is impossible when the diaphragm abuts structures of similar density, such as, for example, the liver and spleen. The hemidiaphragms can be visualized as separate structures only when their inner aspect is marginated by fat.

Despite this limitation, the position of the hemidiaphragms can be inferred from knowledge of characteristic anatomic relationships between the diaphragm and surrounding structures. Specifically, at all levels, the lungs and pleura lie adjacent and peripheral to the diaphragm, whereas the abdominal viscera, fat, and retroperitoneal spaces lie adjacent

and central to the hemidiaphragms. These principles are illustrated in Fig. 1.

Further analysis of the cross-sectional appearance of the diaphragm requires detailed knowledge of anatomy.

The diaphragm consists of a central tendon, with extensions to the right and left—the right and left leaflets (Fig. 2). Muscle fibers insert into the central tendon from all parts of the circumference of the inner aspect of the body wall (2). The pericardium is firmly attached to the upper surface of the central tendon.

Anatomically, the diaphragm consists of two parts. The costal portion arises from the posterior surfaces of the lower six costal cartilages, interdigitating with the slips of origin of the transversus abdominis muscle and inserting into the anterolateral border of the central tendon (3) (Fig. 2).

The posterior portion of the diaphragm is more properly referred to as the lumbar portion. It is composed, in part, of the two crura, which arise from the anterolateral surfaces of the bodies of the first three lumbar vertebra on the right and the first two lumbar vertebra on the left, respectively.

The remainder of the lumbar portion of the diaphragm arises from the medial and lateral arcuate ligaments. These ligaments represent thickenings of the thoracolumbar fascia overlying the anterior surfaces of the psoas and quadratus lumborum muscles. The medial arcuate ligament arises from the lateral margin of the L1 vertebral body and inserts on the transverse process of L1. The lateral arcuate ligament arises from the transverse process of the L1 vertebral body and inserts on the 12th rib. These structures are depicted schematically in Fig. 2.

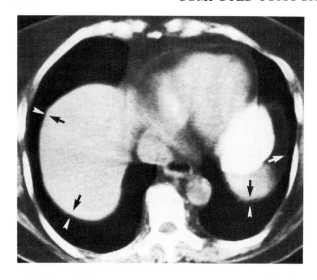

FIG. 1. Section through the domes of the diaphragm. The hemidiaphragms can be visualized as separate structures only when marginated centrally by fat *(white arrow)*. Visualization is lost when the diaphragms abut a structure of similar density (for example, the liver or spleen) *(black arrows)*. The position of the diaphragm can be inferred, however, from knowledge of characteristic anatomic relationships. At all levels, the lung and pleura lie adjacent and peripheral to the diaphragm *(white arrowheads)*; abdominal viscera, fat, and retroperitoneal structures lie adjacent and central to the hemidiaphragms.

Fibers arising from both the crura and arcuate ligaments arch forward to insert into the central tendon of the diaphragm and its extensions, the right and left leaflets. It is apparent from Fig. 2, as it is drawn, that there may be no clear line of demarcation between fibers arising from the crura and fibers arising from the arcuate ligaments. Furthermore, no clear line of demarcation separates the costal from the lumbar portions of the diaphragm.

The most cephalad section in which the crura can be identified is at the level of the esophageal hiatus (Figs. 3a and b, which are sections at, and 1 cm below, the esophageal hiatus, respectively). The same principles that applied in the evaluation of the diaphragm illustrated in Fig. 1 apply to these sections. Only those portions of the diaphragm marginated centrally by fat can be seen as separate structures: the right crus in its preaortic position coursing posterolaterally to the right, the left crus in its preaortic position coursing posterolaterally to the left, and the lateral and anterior portions of the left hemidiaphragm outlined centrally by intraperitoneal fat (Fig. 3). As pointed out by Meyers (4), the fat outlining the medial aspect of the right hemidiaphragm represents the most cephalad extension of the posterior pararenal space (Fig. 3a). In a recent review, fat within this space could be identified in approximately 80% of normal subjects (1). More inferiorly, the right adrenal gland can be recognized within the perirenal space (Fig. 3b). At this level, differentiation between perirenal fat and posterior pararenal fat can rarely be made.

On the left side, the anatomy appears less constant at the level of the esophageal hiatus. This is probably due to variability in the shape and position of the spleen. In Fig. 3a, the medial aspect of the left hemidiaphragm is outlined centrally by retroperitoneal fat within the posterior pararenal space. In Fig. 3b, a portion of the left adrenal gland and the upper pole of the left kidney can be seen, confirming that the fat adjacent to this portion of the diaphragm represents retroperitoneal fat. As on the right side, a clear distinction between fat in the left perirenal space and the left posterior pararenal space is not possible at this level. Differentiation between the retroperitoneal fat and peritoneal fat around the spleen is also difficult unless fluid is present in one or the other space.

The significance of identifying this fat as being retroperitoneal is of special consequence on the

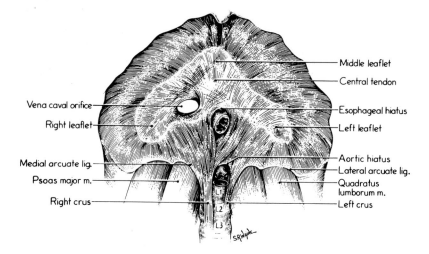

FIG. 2. Schematic diagram of the lumbar portion of the diaphragm, as viewed from below. This portion is composed of the crura, which arise from the anterolateral surfaces of the first three lumbar vertebra on the right and the first two lumbar vertebra on the left, respectively, and fibers that arise from the medial and lateral arcuate ligaments. These ligaments represent thickenings of the thoracolumbar fascia overlying the anterior surfaces of the psoas and quadratus muscles. Note that, as drawn, no clear line of demarcation separates the crura from the remainder of the posterior portions of the diaphragm.

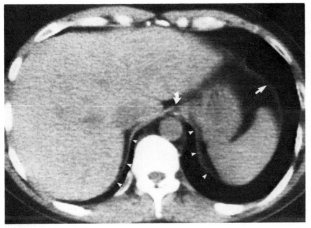
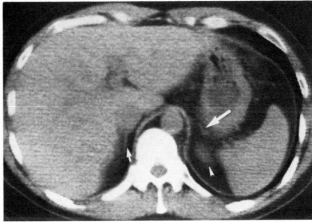

FIG. 3. a: Section at the level of the esophageal hiatus. A small gap can be identified separating the medial ends of the crura *(curved arrow)*. The medial portions of both hemidiaphragms can be identified as separate structures when outlined centrally by fat within the superior portions of the posterior pararenal spaces *(arrowheads)*. Anteriorly, the left hemidiaphragm is marginated centrally by intraperitoneal fat *(arrow)*. The inferior portions of the lower lobes lie adjacent and peripheral to the hemidiaphragms, which they help define. Medially, the lungs and pleura are in contact with the posterior mediastinum, on the left side in close proximity to the descending aorta. **b:** Section 1 cm below that shown in (a). Again, note that the crura merge with the remainder of the diaphragm laterally. The medial aspects of the hemidiaphragms are still outlined centrally by retroperitoneal fat. On the right side, the right adrenal gland can be seen *(small arrow)*; on the left side, the left adrenal gland *(large arrow)* and the upper pole of the kidney *(arrowhead)* can be visualized. In comparison with (a), differentiation between retroperitoneal and intraperitoneal fat on the left side is generally impossible.

right side because the most lateral extension of retroperitoneal fat along the posterior border of the right lobe of the liver serves as a marker identifying the right coronary ligament. Identification of the right coronary ligament is of particular value when attempting to differentiate intraperitoneal from pleural fluid.

As pointed out in Fig. 1, only those portions of the hemidiaphragms outlined centrally by fat will be identifiable as discrete lines (Figs. 3a and b). When the diaphragm abuts structures of similar density, such as the liver or spleen, the line of the diaphragm is lost. Intra-abdominal and retroperitoneal fat vary from patient to patient. In some cases, an unusual quantity of fat may be present anteriorly under the diaphragm. This appearance has been mistaken on liver–lung scintigraphy as subdiaphragmatic fluid (5). CT is efficacious in defining this apparent abnormality as a normal variant (see Fig. 4).

In a considerable percentage of cases, identification of the crura as distinct structures is not possible. This is illustrated in Fig. 3. Although the crura can be identified in their preaortic positions, laterally they merge with fibers from the medial arcuate ligaments.

Variations in the cross-sectional appearance of the crura have been defined (1,6). The crura can be divided into two classes: those in which there is a smooth transition between the crura and the re-

mainder of the lumbar portions of the diaphragms (that is, fibers arising from the medial arcuate ligaments) and those in which the transition is abrupt (Fig. 5).

Smooth transition.

This is by far the largest subgroup, present in approximately 90% of cases. This group can be further subdivided into three distinct subgroups.

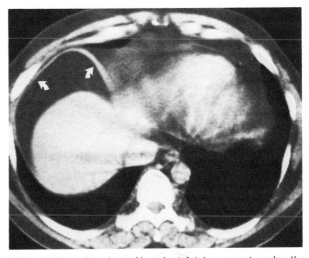

FIG. 4. Normal variant. Abundant fat is present under the anterior aspect of the right hemidiaphragm *(arrows)*. This appearance on routine radiographs and scintigrams has been mistaken for pathology in the right upper quadrant.

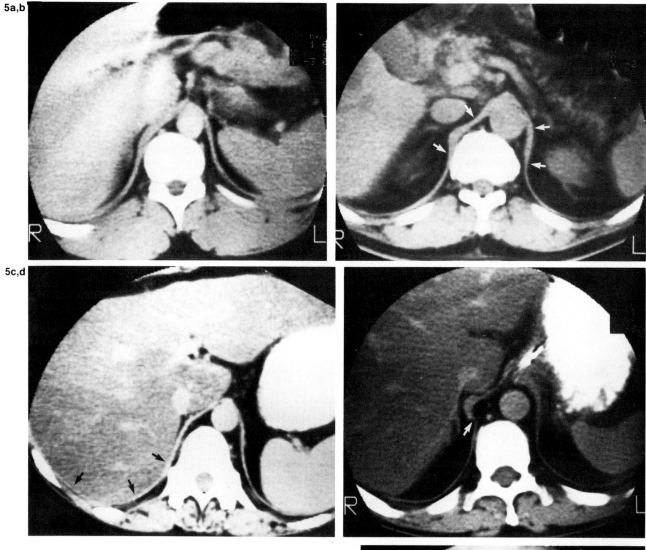

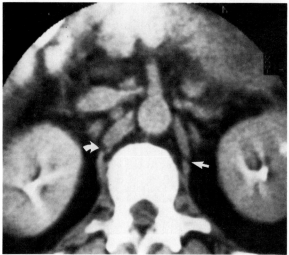

FIG. 5. Diaphragmatic crura: normal variants. **a.** Type 1A. The right crus is prominent. Laterally, the crura merge with the remainder of the posterior portions of the diaphragm. **b:** Type 1B. Accentuation of the appearance shown in (a). The crura are prominent; there is a smooth transition between the crura and the remainder of the posterior portion of the diaphragm. Despite this, the full extent of the crura can be identified bilaterally *(arrows)*. **c:** Type 1C. Atrophic crura. The crura are no thicker than any other portion of the diaphragm. The posterior spinal musculature is atrophic as well [compare with (a) and (b)]. In this case, the full extent of the right diaphragm can be identified because of diffuse fatty infiltration of the liver *(arrows)*. **d:** Type 2. There is an abrupt transition between the right crus and the remainder of the right diaphragm. **e:** Section through the lower portion of the diaphragm, at the level of the arcuate ligaments. There is clear separation between the crura anteriorly and the remainder of the diaphragm posteriorly *(arrows)*. The only reason to recognize these patterns is to avoid confusing normal variants with pathology.

The most common subgroup is illustrated in Fig. 5a. The right crus is prominent and thicker than the left one. Laterally, there is a smooth transition between the crura and the remainder of the lumbar portion of the hemidiaphragms. The exact point of transition cannot be identified with certainty.

The second subgroup represents an accentuation of the pattern illustrated in Fig. 5a. Both the right and the left crura are prominent, especially on the right side (Fig. 5b). Although the transition between the crura and the remainder of the posterior portions of the diaphragm is smooth, the crura themselves can be identified individually as separate structures.

The third subgroup is seen as frequently as is the type shown in Fig. 5b. In this subgroup, the crura are atrophic and are no thicker than any other portion of the diaphragm. In general this pattern can be seen in patients with generalized muscular atrophy from a variety of causes (compare the posterior spinal musculature shown in Fig. 5c with that shown in Figs. 5a and b).

Abrupt transition.

An abrupt transition can be seen between the crura and the remainder of the lumbar portions of the diaphragm. This is seen in approximately 10% of normal subjects, generally on the right side, as shown in Fig. 5d, and is especially frequent in the elderly.

On occasion, actual separation between the various components of the lumbar portions of the diaphragms can be seen. This separation is generally seen on sections through the lowest portions of the diaphragm, as shown in Fig. 5e.

The only significance of these variations is that they should be recognized as normal and not be mistaken for pathology. It cannot be overemphasized that identification of the crura *per se* has little diagnostic significance. It is the configuration and position of the full length of the hemidiaphragms that is of value.

The lungs and pleura always lie peripheral to the diaphragm when viewed in cross section (Figs. 1 and 3). This point is emphasized in Fig. 6, a schematic drawing of a sagittal section through the lateral arcuate ligament and upper portion of the quadratus muscle. The lung is invested with visceral pleura. Just below the most inferior portion of the lung there is a space–generally a potential space—referred to as the posterior pleural recess. This space is defined anteriorly and posteriorly by layers of parietal pleura. Fibers of the lumbar por-

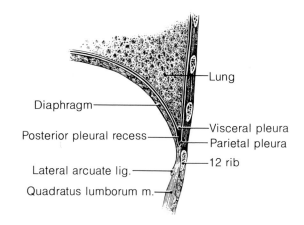

FIG. 6. Schematic diagram of a sagittal section through the lateral arcuate ligament. The lung is invested with visceral pleura. Below the inferior edge of the lung there is a potential space, which is the posterior pleural recess, which is defined anteriorly and posteriorly by layers of parietal pleura. The diaphragm always lies central to the lung and pleura when seen in cross section.

tion of the diaphragm extend below the posterior pleural recess, ending at the lateral arcuate ligament at the level of the 12th rib.

Identification of the posterior pleural recesses is critical when evaluating peridiaphragmatic fluid collections (7). This is because this space represents the most inferior, dependent recess of the pleural space; it is this space that will be filled first by free pleural fluid. As noted, the posterior pleural recess is usually a potential space. Occasionally it can be identified with CT in normal subjects. Figure 7a is an enlargement of a section through the inferiormost portion of the left lower lobe. The tip of the lobe is defined anteriorly by anterior visceral and parietal pleura, as well as by the left hemidiaphragm. Posteriorly, the lung is defined by posterior visceral and parietal pleura.

Figure 7b is an enlargement of a section 5 mm below that shown in Fig. 7a through the posterior pleural recess. At this level, below the left lower lobe, a thin space can be identified, bordered anteriorly by the anterior parietal pleura and left hemidiaphragm and posteriorly by the posterior parietal pleura.

These relationships between the various layers of the pleura and the hemidiaphragms is critical when evaluating the various types of peridiaphragmatic fluid collections. The intimate relationships between the pleural layers and the diaphragms—specifically, how far medially these relationships extend—are illustrated in Fig. 8 (a patient with asbestosis).

Inferiorly, the lumbar portion of the diaphragm

7a,b

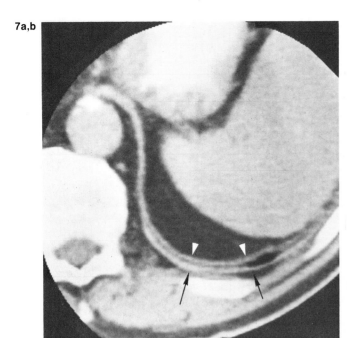
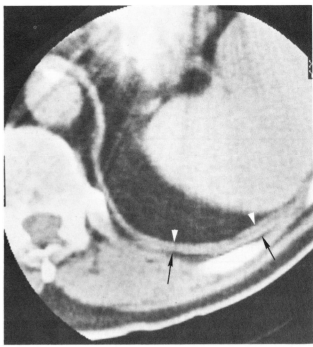

FIG. 7. a: Enlargement of a section through the left lung base. The lung is bordered anteriorly by the left hemidiaphragm and anterior visceral and parietal pleura *(arrowheads)*. Posteriorly, the lung is bordered by posterior visceral and parietal pleura *(arrows)*. **b:** Magnification of a section through the posterior pleural recess, 5 mm below (a). Visceral pleura is no longer present at this level. This space is bordered anteriorly by the left hemidiaphragm and anterior parietal pleura, which are indistinguishable *(arrowheads)*. Posteriorly, this space is defined by the posterior parietal pleura *(arrows)*.

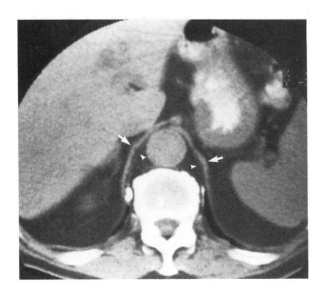

FIG. 8. Enlargement of a section 1 cm below the esophageal hiatus, at the level of the lung bases. There is focal calcification of the parietal pleura bilaterally due to asbestosis. The medial extent of the pleural reflections are seen *(arrowheads)* clearly separate from the posteromedial portions of the hemidiaphragms *(arrows)*. This shows the most medial extent of the inferior pleural recess. In this case, the medial portion of the inferior pleural recess is more cephalad than the posterior portions of this space (note that posteriorly there is a small portion of the lower lobes still visible).

extends to the arcuate ligament (Figs. 2 and 9a). As noted the arcuate ligaments represent thickenings of the thoracolumbar fascia overlying the anterior surfaces of the psoas major and quadratus lumborum muscles. In cross section, these muscles will lie just posterior and medial to the arcuate ligaments. A section obtained below the arcuate ligaments is shown in Fig. 9b. The only portions of the diaphragm that remain visible are the crura, which can be seen individually. The psoas and quadratus muscles can also be defined; they are no longer in contact with the hemidiaphragms. Figures 9a and b indicate the full extent of the inferior-posterior portions of the hemidiaphragms. These relationships are also easily defined with coronal reconstructions, as shown in Fig. 9c.

NORMAL VARIANTS
Retrocrural Air

Occasionally, air within the most medial and inferior portions of the lower lobes, in apparent isolation from the remainder of the lung, can be seen in cross section. This normal variant has been described by Silverman et al. (8), who have designated this as "retrocrural air". As shown in Fig. 10, this

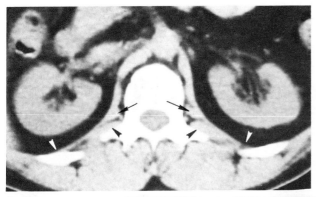

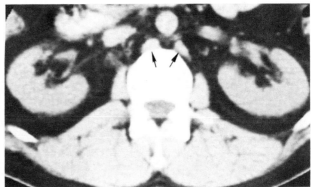

9a,b

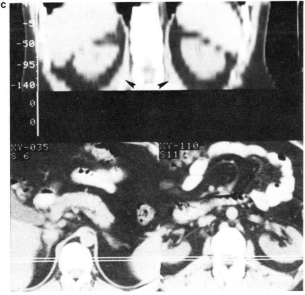

9c

FIG. 9. a: Enlargement of a section through the medial and lateral arcuate ligaments. These ligaments are anterior to the uppermost portions of the psoas *(arrows)* and quadratus *(black arrowheads)* muscles. The lateral arcuate ligaments insert into the 12th rib *(white arrowheads).* **b:** Magnification of a section below the arcuate ligaments. The psoas and quadratus muscles are no longer covered anteriorly by the diaphragm. The crura are all that remain of the diaphragm, and should not be mistaken for adenopathy *(arrows).* **c:** Coronal reconstruction through the medial arcuate ligaments and the psoas muscles in the same case shown in (a) and (b). The hemidiaphragms are seen as they trace a continuous curve beneath the medial inferior portions of both lower lobes. Inferiorly, at the level of the arcuate ligaments, the diaphragm covers the uppermost portions of the psoas muscles *(arrowheads).*

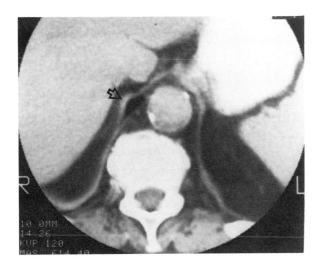

FIG. 10. Retrocrural air. Air within the medial and inferior portion of the right lower lobe can be identified; it is marginated anteriorly by the medial portion of the right hemidiaphragm *(arrow)* and posteriorly by visceral and parietal pleura.

represents air within lung posterior to the medial aspect of the right hemidiaphragm, marginated posteriorly by visceral and parietal pleura. This finding is present in approximately 1% of normal subjects. The only significance of this is that it is a normal variant not to be confused with true retrocrural (that is, retroperitoneal and/or posterior mediastinal) air.

Eventration

Eventrations of the diaphragm occur when the hemidiaphragms become exceedingly thin. In this case, protrusions of abdominal fat and/or omentum may occur, causing the diaphragm to have a mammillated appearance, especially on lateral radiographs (Fig. 11a). When viewing sequential images through the lower thorax and upper abdomen, care must be taken not to confuse focal protrusions of intraperitoneal fat with intrapulmonary masses

11a,b

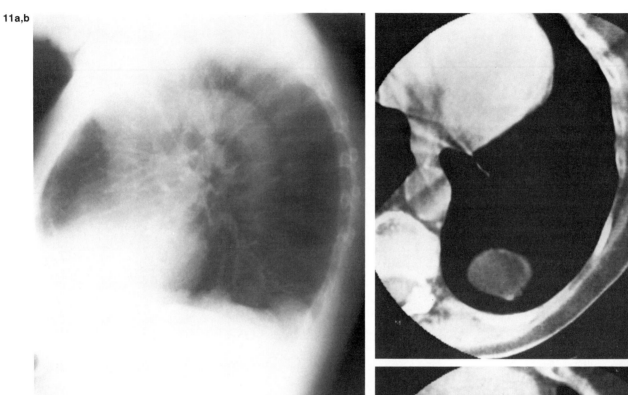

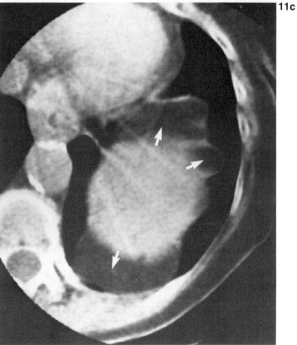

11c

FIG. 11. Eventration of the diaphragm. **a:** Lateral radiograph. **b:** Section through the uppermost portion of the left hemidiaphragm. Eventrated fat can be seen, which superficially mimics intraparenchymal pathology. **c:** Section 1 cm below that shown in (b). The diaphragmatic contour is irregular. Focal areas of eventrated abdominal fat can be identified *(arrows)*. The diaphragm is slightly serrated. Sections obtained between (b) and (c) confirmed continuity between the "mass" seen in (b) and the remainder of the diaphragm.

(Figs. 11b and c). Realization that this is a normal variant is contingent on recognizing fatty density within the "supposed" pulmonary mass and, further, tracing this abnormality in sequential sections to and through the level of the involved hemidiaphragm.

DIAPHRAGMATIC DEFECTS

The most common pathways that allow communication between the abdomen and thorax are the aortic and esophageal hiatuses. Less commonly, another potential pathway for spread of disease between the abdomen and thorax is focal defects in the hemidiaphragms. Posteriorly, the most common of these defects is caused by persistence of the embryonic pleuroperitoneal canal. Ninety percent of such defects are found on the left side (9). Herniation of abdominal structures through this defect may occur (Bochdalek hernia), and may simulate intrathoracic masses. Herniation is presumably facilitated by lower intrathoracic, as opposed to intra-abdominal, pressure. Interestingly, this pressure gradient is highest when patients are in a supine position, since in this position gravity causes the abdominal viscera to press on the undersurface of the diaphragms, forcing them up into the thorax.

As shown by Demartini and House (9), these defects are easily identified with CT. Usually, only fat herniates into the thorax; more rarely, abdominal organs, such as, for example, the kidney, will be displaced into the thorax (Figs. 12 and 13). CT is of obvious diagnostic value in such cases. When look-

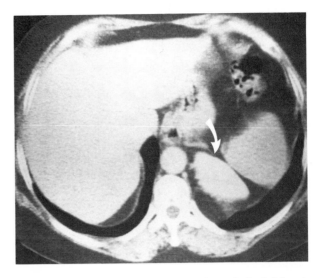

FIG. 13. Intrathoracic kidney. Section through the left hemidiaphragm. There is a diaphragmatic defect through which the left kidney has herniated from the retroperitoneum into the left hemithorax *(arrow)*.

ing at cross-sectional images through a Bochdalek hernia—especially when there is herniation of abdominal contents into the thorax—the images should be viewed through the defect in an anterior-to-posterior direction, since this is the general direction of herniation. Viewing these images in this manner makes evaluation conceptually more simple (Figs. 12 and 13).

Herniation of intra-abdominal fat and/or viscera may also occur in the anterior portions (costal portions) of the diaphragms, resulting in a paracardiac mass (so-called Morgagni hernia). CT is efficacious, first, in defining such masses as fatty and, second, in demonstrating continuity between this fat and abdominal fat (see Fig. 2, Chapter 3). The actual point of the diaphragmatic defect may be definable using parasagittal reconstructions.

PERIDIAPHRAGMATIC FLUID COLLECTIONS

Accurate localization of peridiaphragmatic fluid requires detailed knowledge of normal cross-sectional anatomy through the lung bases and upper abdomen. The key to accurate localization of peridiaphragmatic fluid is identification of the hemidiaphragms, because these represent the interface between the thorax and the abdomen. At all levels, the lungs and pleura lie adjacent and peripheral to the diaphragm; the abdominal viscera, fat, and intraperitoneal spaces lie adjacent and central to the diaphragm. Precise anatomic localization of the diaphragm depends on awareness of these anatomic relationships.

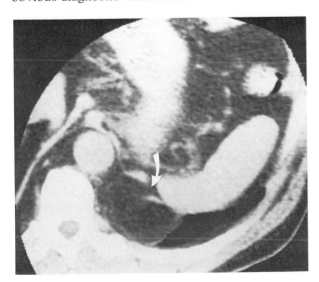

FIG. 12. Pleuroperitoneal canal. Enlargement of a section through the left hemidiaphragm in which a defect can be identified *(arrow)*. Retroperitoneal fat has herniated through this defect into the thoracic cavity.

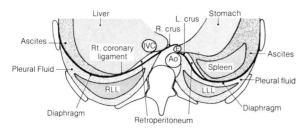

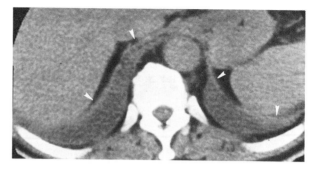

FIG. 14. Schematic drawing of the potential spaces in which peridiaphragmatic fluid may collect. Accurate identification of the diaphragm is critical. Fluid within the pleural space or lung lies peripheral to the hemidiaphragms; intraperitoneal or retroperitoneal fluid lies central to the hemidiaphragms. On the right side, intraperitoneal fluid is restricted medially at the level of the right coronary ligament. Ao, aorta; E, esophagus; IVS, inferior vena cava; LLL, left lower lobe; RLL, right lower lobe.

FIG. 15. Magnified section through the posterior pleural recesses, which are distended by bilateral subpulmonic effusions. The hemidiaphragms *(arrowheads)* can be identified bilaterally, outlined centrally by retroperitoneal and intraperitoneal fat.

Peridiaphragmatic fluid can be localized in one of four potential spaces: the pleural cavity, the lung, the peritoneum, or the retroperitoneum. This principle is illustrated in Fig. 14.

Pleural Fluid Collections

The most dependent portion of the pleural space is the posterior pleural recess (Figs. 6 and 7). This is generally a potential space beneath the lung base posteriorly, bordered anteriorly by anterior parietal pleura, as well as by the diaphragm, and bordered posteriorly by posterior parietal pleura.

Free pleural fluid initially accumulates within the posterior pleural recess, and, if restricted to this space, should be referred to as a subpulmonic effu-

sion. Initially, subpulmonic fluid was thought to be "atypical," but more recent work has confirmed that, in the absence of pleural adhesions, pleural fluid first accumulates normally in a subpulmonic location (10–12).

The appearance on CT of subpulmonic effusions is illustrated in Fig. 15. Fluid lies posterior to the hemidiaphragms, which are displaced anteriorly (13). Identification of the hemidiaphragms is facilitated in this case because the medial portions of the hemidiaphragms are well-defined centrally by retroperitoneal fat. The fluid conforms to the general configuration of the posterior pleural recesses. Note that pleural fluid extends quite far medially, coming in close contact on the right side with the descending aorta. This is in keeping with the general anatomic configuration of the pleural space, as

16a,b

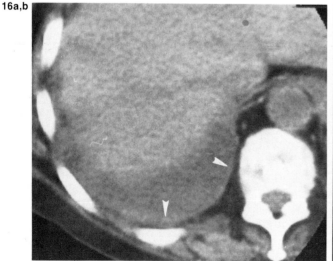

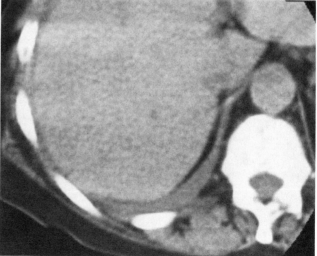

FIG. 16. a: Enlargement of a section on the right side shows a large pleural fluid collection. The interface between the fluid and the posterior aspect of the liver is indistinct. The posterior parietal pleura should not be confused with the right hemidiaphragm *(arrowheads)*. **b:** Magnification of a section 2 cm below that shown in (a), at the level of the right posterior pleural recess. Fluid lies posterior to the right hemidiaphragm.

shown in Figs. 6, 7, and 8, and is a principle useful in differentiating pleural from intra-abdominal fluid collections, especially on the right side.

The posterior pleural recesses are important anatomic landmarks because their characteristic configuration is easily identifiable, even in the presence of large quantities of pleural fluid.

As illustrated in Fig. 16, large pleural fluid collections abut the posterior surface of the liver. In these cases, superficially, the pleural fluid may appear to lie anterior to the right hemidiaphragm (Fig. 16a). With large pleural fluid collections on the right side, the interface between the liver and the pleural fluid may be poorly defined. Teplick et al. (14) have called attention to this hazy "interface sign" as being characteristic of pleural fluid collections. It is relatively easy to prove that this represents pleural fluid by obtaining sections through the posterior pleural recesses (Fig. 16b), because at this level fluid can clearly be identified as pleural due to the characteristic configuration of the pleural recesses.

In our experience, the easiest way to confirm the presence of pleural fluid is to scan through the posterior pleural recesses. This remains true even when fluid is present simultaneously within the pleural space and the abdomen (Fig. 17).

With supine cross-sectional imaging, variability in the appearance of pleural fluid at the lung base may be encountered; this probably reflects differences in the anatomy of the pulmonary ligaments. If there are incomplete attachments of these ligaments, the lower lobes are free to float on pleural fluid, provided the lung is not stiffened by disease and there are no adhesions between the lung and the adjacent pleura (Fig. 17; compare with Fig. 18).

Despite clarification of normal cross-sectional anatomy of the pleural spaces, certain cases remain difficult to evaluate. This is especially true when pleural fluid is sufficiently massive to cause inver-

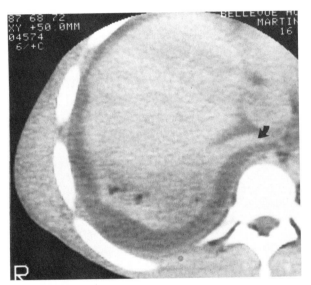

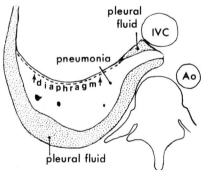

FIG. 18. Magnification of a section through the right lung base in a patient with right lower lobe volume loss and infiltrate and a right pleural effusion. There are a few, scattered areas of residual aeration within the lower lobe. Note that, despite volume loss and the presence of pleural fluid, the right lower lobe has retained its general configuration because of fixation by the pulmonary ligament *(arrow)* (compare with Fig. 4). Peripheral and anteromedial to the consolidated lower lobe is pleural fluid. Significantly, the density of the consolidated lung is intermediate between that of the liver anteriorly and that of the pleural fluid posteriorly. This helps to define the position of the right hemidiaphragm.

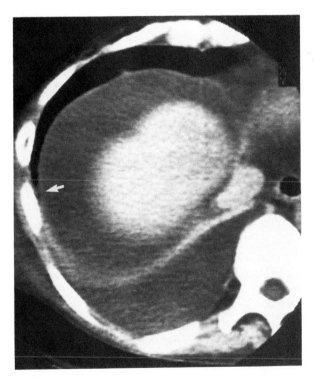

FIG. 17. Enlargement of a section through the right side near the dome of the liver in a patient with both ascites and pleural fluid. In this case, the line of the diaphragm can be seen distinctly. Note that the middle lobe interface with the chest wall laterally remains sharply defined, despite the presence of pleural fluid *(arrow)*.

sion of the hemidiaphragms, since pleural fluid may then simulate the appearance of intra-abdominal fluid (15). In these cases, parasagittal reconstruction may prove helpful (Fig. 19).

Pulmonary Consolidation

Superficially, pneumonia may appear to have fluid density, and hence may be mistaken for pleural or intra-abdominal fluid. In fact, consolidated lung almost never has a pure-fluid density—unlike ascites or pleural effusions. The density of consolidated lung represents an averaging of fluid and pulmonary parenchyma.

Localization is facilitated by the following. As is true with pleural fluid collections, consolidated lung always lies peripheral to the hemidiaphragms; in addition, consolidated lung usually conforms to the expected shape of the lower lobes. As with the pleural reflections, the medial portions of the lower lobes extend in close proximity to the descending

aorta and esophagus (Figs. 1 and 3a). Finally, residual areas of parenchymal aeration or air-bronchograms may be discernible to further aid in identification. These principles are illustrated in Fig. 20.

Infiltrate within the lower lobes may be present along with associated pleural effusion or even fluid within the abdomen. Careful attention to anatomic detail and the principles outlined above should allow proper identification of these variants (Fig. 21). It should be remembered that the configuration of the lower lobes will reflect, to some extent, the attachments of the inferior pulmonary ligaments (Fig. 18), and that identification of these is also helpful in differentiating pleural fluid from parenchymal consolidation. If doubt persists, scans obtained at a higher level should help confirm that the lower lobes are abnormal.

Intra-abdominal Fluid Collections

As illustrated in Fig. 14, intra-abdominal fluid may collect intraperitoneally or retroperitoneally,

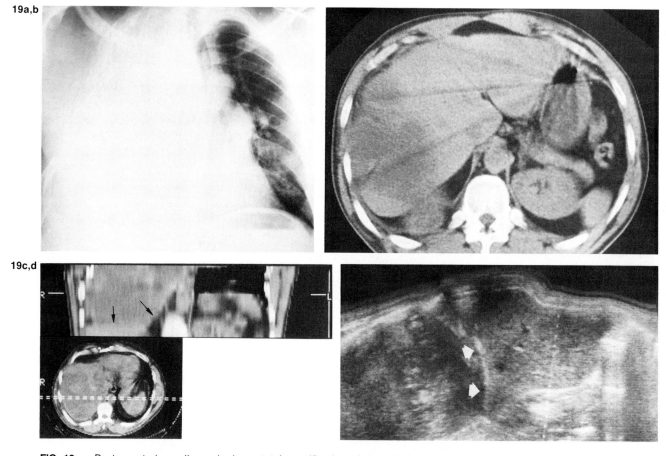

FIG. 19. a: Posteroanterior radiograph shows total opacification of the right hemithorax. This patient is status-post pneumonectomy. **b:** Section through the right lobe of the liver. There are ill-defined areas of decreased density in the lateral aspect of the liver. **c:** Coronal reconstruction through the midportion of the right lobe of the liver. There is a massive pleural fluid collection inverting the diaphragm *(arrows)*. The liver is displaced inferiorly. There is no evidence of subdiaphragmatic fluid. **d:** Longitudinal ultrasonic section through the right lobe of the liver. Inversion of the right diaphragm is apparent *(arrows)*.

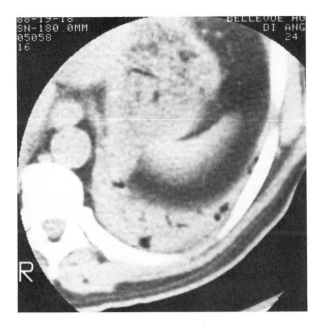

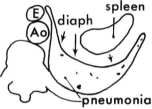

FIG. 20. Enlargement of a section through the base of the left lung. There is consolidation, as well as air-bronchograms, within the lower lobe. The consolidation conforms to the shape of the left lung base and lies peripheral to the left hemidiaphragm.

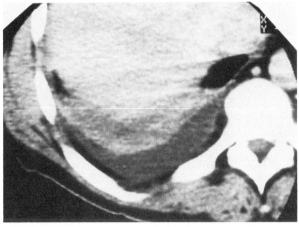

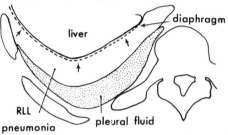

FIG. 21. Enlargement of a section through the right lung base in a patient with right lower lobe consolidation and a right pleural fluid collection. The density of the right lower lobe is intermediate between that of the "pure" fluid in the pleural space posteriorly and that of the liver anteriorly. There are no air-bronchograms present. The apparent air–fluid level medially is a common finding that represents residual aeration in the most medial portion of the posterior basal segment of the right lower lobe. This segment is frequently spared. The position of the right hemidiaphragm can be inferred accurately.

or both. Significantly, fluid collections in both spaces may abut the hemidiaphragms; in each case, the fluid will lie central to the diaphragm.

Retroperitoneal fluid will conform to the anatomic space and/or structures involved, e.g., posterior pararenal versus perirenal spaces. The psoas muscles are also retroperitoneal, and, as discussed above, are intimately related to the arcuate ligaments (16). Differentiation between retroperitoneal–psoas muscle fluid collections and pleural fluid collections is dependent on knowledge of normal anatomic relationships as shown in Fig. 22.

Generally, differentiation between retroperitoneal and intraperitoneal fluid is not difficult (17). Intraperitoneal fluid will collect in the peritoneal spaces and will therefore be restricted by the peritoneal reflections. On the right side, peritoneal fluid is restricted posteromedially by the right coronary ligament. The result is a characteristic medial tapering of intraperitoneal fluid, as shown in Fig. 23. It should be remembered, however, that superiorly,

ascites, when massive, may collect under the domes of the diaphragm on both the left and right sides (i.e., above the level of the coronary ligaments) (Figs. 17, 24, and 25).

On the left side, intra-abdominal (intraperitoneal fluid) is easy to identify because it will characteristically be central to the left hemidiaphragm, and, additionally, will surround the spleen (Fig. 25a; compare with Fig. 15). Even when fluid is present simultaneously within the left upper quadrant and the left pleural space, separation of these anatomic spaces is simple, provided an attempt is made to identify the inferior pleural recess (Fig. 26b; compare with Fig. 26a).

As already discussed, the medial aspect of the left hemidiaphragm is generally outlined by retroperitoneal fat in the upper portion of the left posterior pararenal space (Fig. 3). Unlike the right side, the configuration of this portion of the posterior pararenal space and its relationship to the diaphragm may be variable (Fig. 26c; compare with

22a

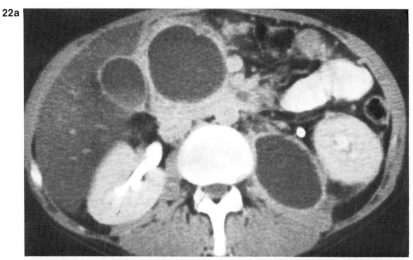

FIG. 22. Pancreatitis. a: Section through the head of the pancreas, showing a large well-defined fluid collection due to pancreatitis. Additionally, there is a large fluid collection in the left psoas muscle, which, at other levels (not shown), proved to be secondary to dissection of peripancreatic fluid into the psoas muscle. The overall density of the liver is markedly decreased due to fatty infiltration. b: Coronal reconstruction through the arcuate ligaments. There is a large pleural fluid collection superior to the inferior portion of the left hemidiaphragm *(arrows)*. Inferiorly, the psoas muscle is distended and largely replaced by a fluid collection. This image clearly demonstrates the relationships between the pleural space and diaphragm at the level of the arcuate ligaments.

22b

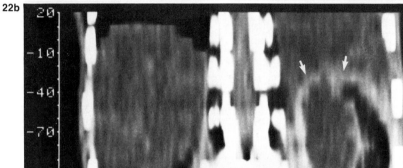

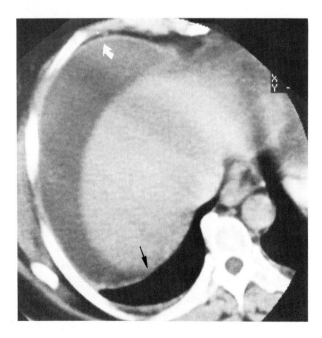

FIG. 23. Enlargement of a section through the right lung base in a patient with ascites. Medially, ascites tapers to a point, where it is restricted by the coronary ligaments *(arrow)*. Note that the intraperitoneal fluid lies central to the diaphragm, even anteriorly *(white arrow)*.

Fig. 25a). This variability should not cause confusion, since in both cases, intra-abdominal fluid can be localized central to the left hemidiaphragm.

Anterior subdiaphragmatic fluid collections also are characteristic in appearance. As shown by Halvorsen et al. (18), fluid may become confined to the anterior left subphrenic space. This space is defined on the right by the falciform ligament and on the left side by the left coronary ligament, which extends from the dorsal aspect of the liver posteriorly to the diaphragm (Fig. 27). The anterior subphrenic space extends superiorly to the dome of the diaphragm. Significantly, this fluid lies central to the anterior aspect of the left hemidiaphragm; additionally, fluid in this space will lie adjacent to the left lobe of the liver in a manner analogous to that of free intraperitoneal fluid, which surrounds the spleen posteriorly (Fig. 25; compare with Figs. 26a and c).

While CT is efficacious in defining the precise location of peridiaphragmatic fluid, in our experience, CT is of less value in differentiating among the various etiologies of peridiaphragmatic fluid. In the diagnosis of subphrenic abscesses, the most im-

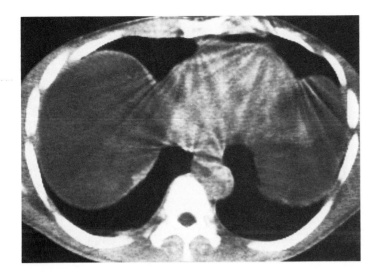

FIG. 24. Section through the domes of the diaphragm in a patient with massive ascites. The fluid lies central to the hemidiaphragms, which can almost be defined circumferentially. When massive, ascites can lie immediately beneath the hemidiaphragms. On the right side, there is no restriction of the intraperitoneal fluid, because this is a section above the level of the coronary ligaments.

portant role for CT is accurate localization of fluid. As has been shown by Alexander et al. (17), this is generally feasible, provided care is taken to define anatomy accurately. Subphrenic abscesses frequently form secondary to another focus of intra-abdominal disease. Communication between the subphrenic spaces and disease and/or fluid within the remainder of the abdomen may occur by way of small fistulous tracks. These may be difficult to define with CT, especially if they are serpiginous (19) (Fig. 25). The finding of fluid, especially loculated fluid, in the subphrenic spaces necessitates complete evaluation of the entire abdomen and pelvis.

THE DIAPHRAGM AS A PATHWAY FOR THE SPREAD OF DISEASE

The diaphragm usually serves to localize disease either in the thorax or abdomen. However, extension through the diaphragm can occur via several pathways. Direct contiguous spread most commonly occurs through the pre-existing normal channels of communication, that is, the aortic and esophageal hiatuses (20).

The esophageal hiatus is defined anatomically by the medial margins of the diaphragmatic crura. Generally, there is a small space between the crura through which the distal esophagus passes en route to the stomach. However, in a large percentage of cases, the medial margins of the crura are separated, as shown in Fig. 28. This separation provides a potential pathway between the abdomen and posterior mediastinum.

The most typical example of communication between the abdomen and thorax is herniation of in-

tra-abdominal fat and/or viscera through an incompetent phrenicoesophageal membrane that generally surrounds and fixates the esophagus to the diaphragm, i.e., a hiatal hernia (Fig. 29 and Fig. 3, Chapter 3). Just as characteristic is the spread of malignancy through this hiatus. Carcinomas of the fundus of the stomach will invade and track along the distal esophagus (Fig. 30). Esophageal varices also pass through the esophageal hiatus, and may be mistaken for periesophageal nodes or tumor (22). Difficulty in diagnosis is generally obviated by use of a bolus of intravenous contrast agent (Fig. 31).

Benign tumors may also pass from the thorax into the abdomen by way of the esophageal hiatus (23). An example of diffuse neurofibromatosis is illustrated in Fig. 32. Continuity between the posterior mediastinum and upper abdomen is apparent. In Fig. 32a, the right crus can be identified, marking this section at the level of the esophageal hiatus. More rarely, the esophageal hiatus serves as the pathway for the spread of pancreatic fluid collections (Fig. 33). The key to evaluating these fluid collections is analysis of contiguous sections from the lung bases to the upper abdomen.

The aortic hiatus is another important path for the spread of disease. As shown by Zerhouni et al. (21), malignant thoracic neoplasms, especially those involving the pleura, can extend into the retroperitoneum by this route. The propensity for spread of tumor through the aortic hiatus is related to two anatomic features. First, the phrenico-esophageal membrane affixes the esophagus to the crura in most individuals. This may preferentially direct tumor spread through the aortic hiatus. Second, the thoracic duct traverses the aortic hiatus providing a direct lymphatic pathway between the

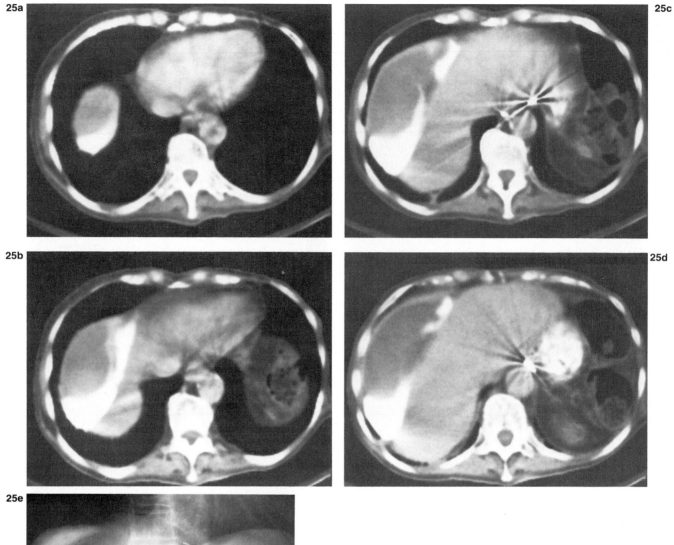

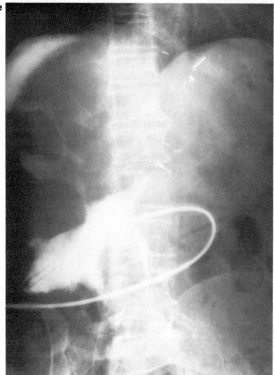

FIG. 25. Subdiaphragmatic abscess. **a–d:** Sequential sections from the dome of the diaphragm to the midportion of the liver. The abscess has been filled with contrast medium by an in-dwelling drainage catheter (see (e)). Notice that the abscess has a lenticular shape alongside the lateral margin of the liver; at each level, the fluid and contrast media lie central to the right hemidiaphragm. Above the coronary ligament, fluid and contrast agent lie directly beneath the right hemidiaphragm (see (a)). **e:** AP radiograph shows in-dwelling catheter in an abscess cavity in the midabdomen. A small, serpiginous fistula connects this cavity with the subdiaphragmatic collection. These fistulae may be difficult to detect in cross-sectional images. Any patient with a subdiaphragmatic fluid collection–abscess should have scans of the entire abdomen.

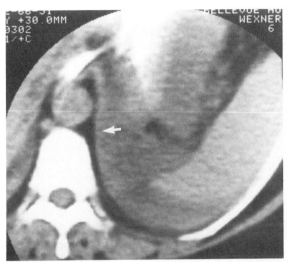
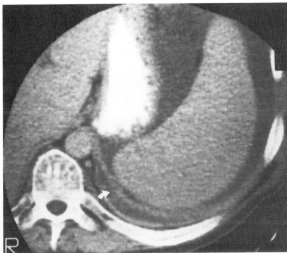

26a,b

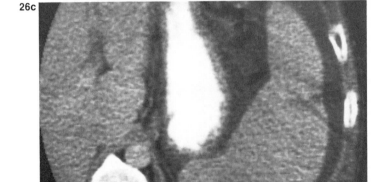

26c

FIG. 26. a: Magnified section through the upper abdomen shows intraperitoneal fluid surrounding the spleen. The fluid lies central to the left hemidiaphragm *(arrow)*. There is also a small quantity of fluid in the lesser sac, displacing the stomach medially. **b:** Magnified section through the left upper quadrant in a patient with a left pleural effusion and ascites. The effusion is easy to recognize, filling the left inferior pleural recess *(arrow)*. Intraperitoneal fluid lies central to the left hemidiaphragm, surrounding the spleen. **c:** Magnified section through the left upper quadrant in a patient with ascites. In this case, the superior aspect of the left posterior pararenal space can be identified *(arrow)*, separate from fluid within the peritoneum surrounding the spleen. The configuration of the superior aspect of the left posterior pararenal space is obviously variable.

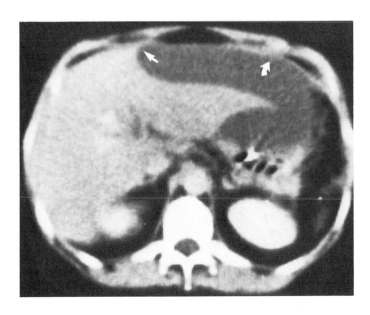

FIG. 27. Anterior left subphrenic space abscess. Section through the upper abdomen. A large fluid collection is present in the left anterior subphrenic space. This space is defined on the right side by the falciform ligament *(arrow)*, and centrally and to the left by the left coronary ligament, which extends from the dorsal aspect of the liver posteriorly. Note that this fluid collection lies central to the anterior aspect of the left hemidiaphragm *(curved arrow)*.

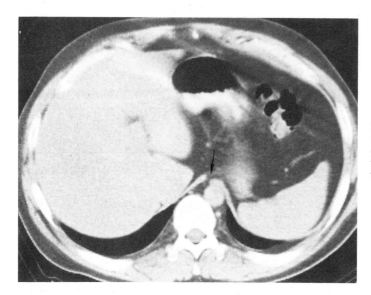

FIG. 28. Section through the esophageal hiatus, showing a small gap between the medial margins of the crura *(arrow)*. This gap represents a potential pathway for the spread of disease between the abdomen and the posterior mediastinum.

29a,b

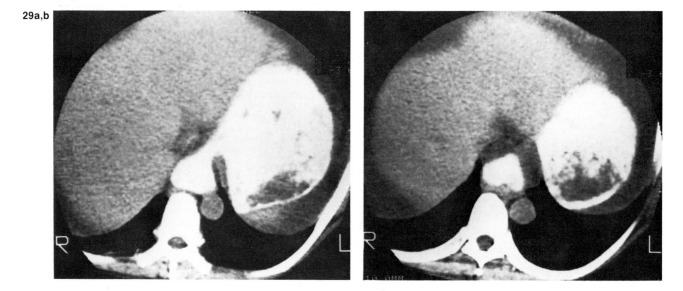

FIG. 29. Hiatal hernia. **a,b:** Sections through the esophageal hiatus and 1 cm cephalad, respectively. A large hiatal hernia can be seen.

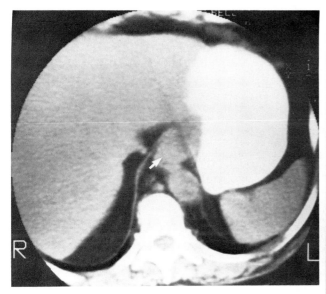

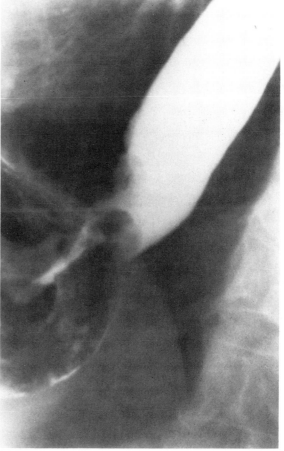

FIG. 30. Adenocarcinoma of the stomach extending into the distal esophagus. **a:** Section through the esophageal hiatus in a patient with gastric carcinoma arising in the fundus of the stomach. Tumor infiltrates and thickens the distal esophagus *(arrow)*. The right crus is displaced laterally. **b:** Coned-down view of the distal esophagus.

thorax and abdomen. These facts explain the frequent finding of retrocrural adenopathy as a clue to the simultaneous presence of intrathorax and abdominal malignancy. Less frequently, the aortic hiatus serves as the pathway for the spread of fluid between the thorax and abdomen (see Fig. 32, Chapter 3).

Other defects in the diaphragm occur and can be sites at which herniation of abdominal contents and/or fat may occur. These include Morgagni and Bochdalek hernias, and have been discussed in the section on normal variants (Figs. 12 and 13 and Fig. 2, Chapter 3).

Traumatic herniation following diaphragmatic rupture is another mechanism by which abdominal and thoracic pathology overlap. The appearance on CT of traumatic diaphragmatic rupture has been described by Heiberg et al. (24). This frequently occurs secondary to blunt trauma and may go undiagnosed for years. Diaphragmatic rupture following blunt trauma usually occurs on the left side (in up to 95% of patients). As pointed out by Heiberg et al., radiologic diagnosis of diaphragmatic rupture may be difficult; this entity is frequently misdiagnosed as an elevated hemidiaphragm, left lower lobe atelectasis, left pleural effusion, or left subphrenic fluid collections and/or abscess. CT can identify discontinuities in the course of the diaphragm, especially along the posterolateral aspect. An example is illustrated in Fig. 34.

While disease usually spreads between the abdomen and thorax by means of a diaphragmatic defect—either congenital or acquired—the diaphragm itself, on occasion, may actually serve as a pathway for disease. This is most typically encountered in patients with diffuse malignant pleural disease, especially mesotheliomas. In this setting, the diaphragm may become involved by tumor; the result

31a,b

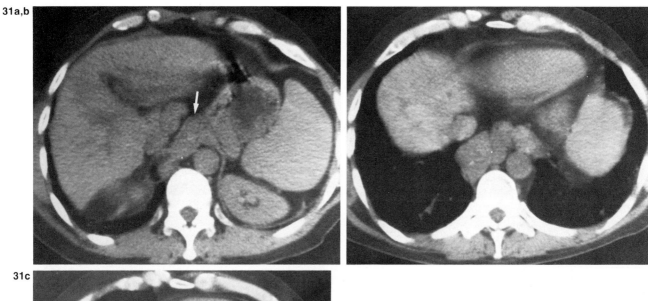

31c

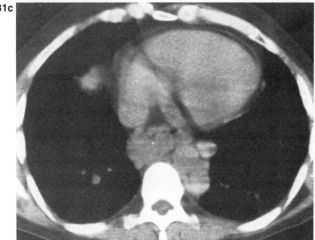

FIG. 31. Esophageal varices. **a–c:** Sequential images from below, then upward, in a patient with cirrhosis of the liver and esophageal varices. There is wide separation of the medial ends of the crura at the level of the esophageal hiatus [*arrows* in (a)]. Extra, nodular soft-tissue densities are present at the level of the esophageal hiatus, which can be tracked in subsequent sections into the posterior mediastinum. These nodular densities encompass the esophagus, making visualization of this structure difficult, and at the highest level illustrated (c), surround both the esophagus and descending aorta. This appearance may mimic other posterior mediastinal and/ or retroperitoneal masses. If the diagnosis is in doubt, the diagnosis can be confirmed with a bolus of intravenous contrast medium.

32a,b

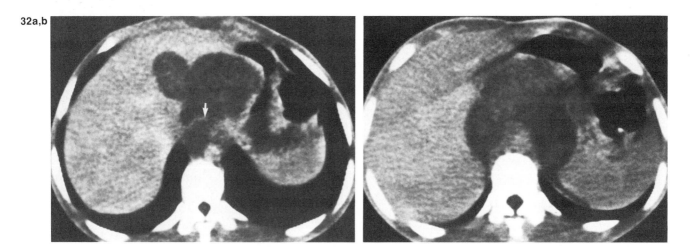

FIG. 32. Neurofibromatosis. **a,b:** Sections through the esophageal hiatus and upper abdomen, respectively. The entire posterior mediastinum is filled with a low-density mass, which, in fact, measures within the range of soft tissue. This mass of tissue extends into the abdomen via the esophageal hiatus (*arrow* points to medial aspect of the right crus). Biopsy proved neurofibromatosis.

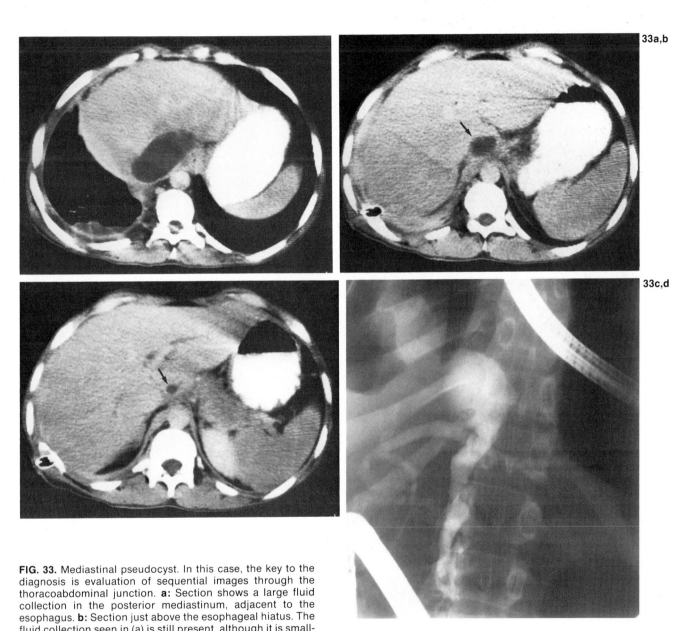

33a,b

33c,d

FIG. 33. Mediastinal pseudocyst. In this case, the key to the diagnosis is evaluation of sequential images through the thoracoabdominal junction. **a:** Section shows a large fluid collection in the posterior mediastinum, adjacent to the esophagus. **b:** Section just above the esophageal hiatus. The fluid collection seen in (a) is still present, although it is smaller lying anterior to the crura and lateral to the distal esophagus *(arrow).* **c:** Section at the level of the pancreas. A small fluid collection can be identified in the region of the head of the pancreas *(arrow).* In this case, fluid has tracked from the retroperitoneum through the esophageal hiatus to localize in the posterior mediastinum. Communication between these fluid collections could be established by reviewing sequential images (not all shown). **d:** Oblique view from an endoscopic retrograde, cholangiopancreatogram, confirming the diagnosis.

34a

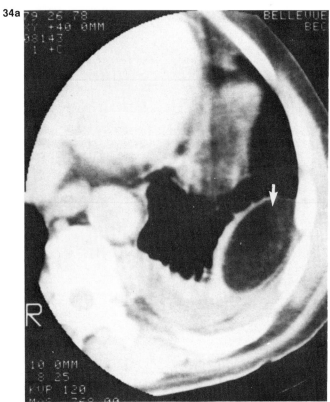

FIG. 34. Traumatic rupture of the left hemidiaphragm. **a–c:** Sequential images from above, then downward, in a patient who had blunt trauma some years previously. Intra-abdominal fat has protruded into the thorax (arrow in (a)), which can be traced in continuity to subdiaphragmatic fat (*arrow* in (b)). There are calcifications along the edge of the spleen (*double arrows* in (b) and (c)), as well as deformity along the lateral aspect of the spleen (c). These are due to an old subcapsular splenic hematoma (surgically confirmed).

34b,c

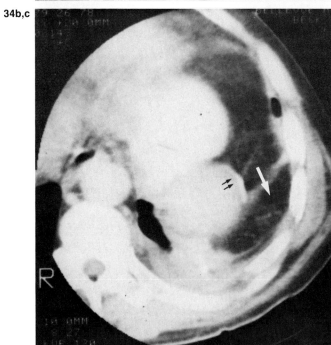

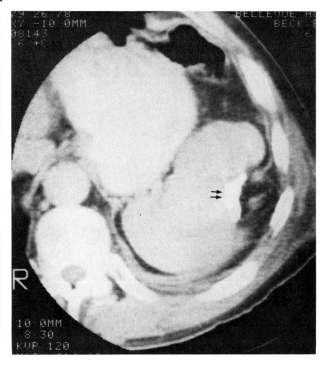

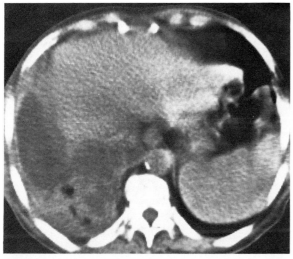

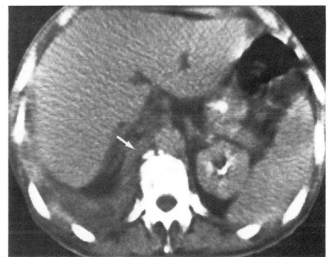

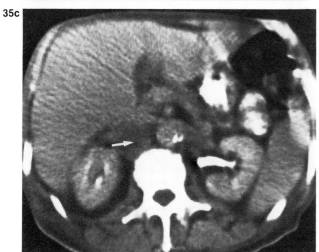

35c

FIG. 35. Mesothelioma. **a–c:** Sequential sections from above, then downward, through the right diaphragm in a patient with malignant mesothelioma. In addition to pleural fluid, the pleural surface and diaphragm are thickened and irregular. Note in (b) that the medial portions of the right hemidiaphragm and crus are markedly thickened, compared with the normal left side *(arrows)*. In (c), tumor has tracked along the entire length of the right crus to lie posterior to the vena cava *(arrow)*, medial to the right kidney. In this case, the diaphragm itself has acted as the pathway for spread of disease.

is that tumor tracks along the diaphragm to gain entry into the abdomen. This potential pathway is illustrated in Fig. 35.

Finally, tumors may arise within the diaphragm. This is exceptionally rare, and frequently presents diagnostic dilemmas. An example of a surgically confirmed hemangiopericytoma arising in the diaphragm is shown in Fig. 36. While the intimate relationship between the tumor and the diaphragm is obvious, the appearance should not be considered characteristic.

CONCLUSION

Various disease processes affect the diaphragm either directly or by contiguity. Delineation of disease is contingent on a thorough knowledge of the normal cross-sectional appearance of the diaphragm. Analysis is made difficult because of the overall oblique configuration of the diaphragm. In general, the exact position of the diaphragm can

only be inferred; it is visualized as an identifiable structure only when it is marginated by fat. Despite this limitation, the location of the diaphragm can be precisely defined, as illustrated throughout this chapter, by knowledge of the normal anatomic relationships between the diaphragm and surrounding structures.

Once the diaphragm has been localized, differentiation between intrathoracic and intra-abdominal disease, especially fluid collections, is facilitated. This is true even when fluid is present simultaneously in the chest and abdomen.

The diaphragm also can serve as a pathway for the spread of disease. This concept unifies evaluation of sections through the thoracoabdominal interface, and further reinforces the necessity for overall familiarity with the cross-sectional appearance of diseases within both the thorax and abdomen. As shown throughout this chapter, the notion that thoracic and abdominal disease are separate entities to be evaluated by independent specialists is unsatisfactory.

36a

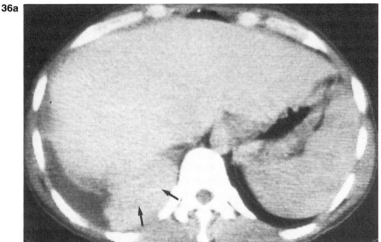

36b

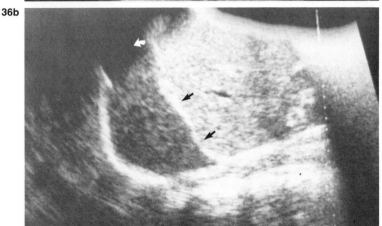

36c

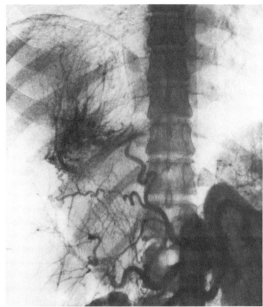

FIG. 36. Hemangiopericytoma (right diagram). **a:** Section through the inferior portion of the right pleural space. There is considerable pleural fluid, as well as a large oval soft-tissue mass, clearly peripheral to the hemidiaphragm *(arrows).* **b:** Longitudinal sonogram through the liver. The diaphragm is well-defined *(arrows).* Superior and adjacent to the diaphragm is an echogenic mass, above which pleural fluid can be identified *(white arrow).* **c:** Coned-down view from a celiac angiogram shows a markedly hypervascular mass being fed by a hypertrophied phrenic artery. Biopsy proven hemangiopericytoma arising in the right diaphragm. (Case courtesy of Dr. B. Nagesh Raghavendra, University Hospital, New York University Medical Center.)

REFERENCES

1. Naidich DP, Megibow AJ, Ross CR, Beranbaum ER, Siegelman SS. Computed tomography of the diaphragm: Normal anatomy and variants. *J Comput Assist Tomogr* 7:633–640, 1983

2. Romanes GJ, ed. *Cunninghams Textbook of Anatomy,* 12th edition. New York, Oxford University Press, 1981, pp 352–354

3. Williams PL, Warwick R, eds. *Gray's Anatomy,* 36th edition. Philadelphia; WB Saunders, 1980

4. Meyers MA. *Dynamic Radiology of the Abdomen: Normal and Pathologic Anatomy,* 2nd edition. New York, Springer-Verlag, 1982

5. Pozderac R, Borlaza G, Green RA. Radiographic exhibit: Subdiaphragmatic adiposity mimicking ascites by liver-lung scintigraphy. *Radiology* 132:154, 1979

6. Callen PW, Filly RA, Korobkin M. Computed tomographic evaluation of the diaphragmatic crura. *Radiology* 126: 413–416, 1978

7. Naidich DP, Megibow AJ, Hilton S, Hulnick DH, Siegelman SS. Computed tomography of the diaphragm: Peridiaphragmatic fluid localization. *J Comput Assist Tomogr* 7:641–649

8. Silverman PM, Godwin JD, Kobobkin M. Computed tomographic detection of retrocrural air. *AJR* 138:825–827, 1982

9. Demartini WJ, House AJS. Partial Bochdalek's herniation: Computerized tomographic evaluation. *Chest* 77:702–704, 1980

10. Mulvey RB. The effect of pleural fluid on the diaphragm. *Radiology* 84:1080–1085, 1965

11. Peterson JA. Recognition of infra-pulmonary pleural effusion. *Radiology* 74:34–41, 1960

12. Raasch BN, Carsky EW, Lane EJ, O'Callaghan JP, Heitzman ER. Pictorial essay. Pleural effusion: Explanation of some typical appearances. *AJR* 139:899–904, 1982

13. Dwyer A. The displaced crus: A sign for distinguishing between pleural fluid and ascites on computed tomography. *J Comput Assist Tomogr* 2:598–599, 1978

14. Teplick JG, Teplick SK, Goodman L, Haskin ME. The interface sign: A computed tomographic sign for distinguishing pleural and intraabdominal fluid. *Radiology* 144:359–362, 1982

15. Katzen BT, Choi WS, Friedman MH, Green IJ, Hindle WV, Zellis A. Pseudo mass of the liver due to pleural effusion and inversion of the diaphragm. *AJR* 131:1077–1078, 1978

16. Donovan PJ, Zerhouni EA, Siegelman SS. CT of the psoas compartment of the retroperitoneum. *Semin Roentgenol* 16:241–249, 1981

17. Alexander ES, Proto AU, Clark RA. CT differentiation of subphrenic abscess and pleura effusion. *AJR* 140:47–51, 1983

18. Halvorsen RA, Jones MA, Rice RP, Thompson WM. Anterior left subphrenic abscess: Characteristic plain film and CT appearance *AJR* 139:283–289, 1982

19. Aspestrand F. Demonstration of thoracic and abdominal

fistulas by computed tomography. *J Comput Assist Tomogr* 4:536–537, 1980

20. Thompson WM, Halvorsen RA, Williford ME, Foster WL, Korobkin M. Computed tomography of the gastroesophageal junction. *Radiographics* 2:179–193, 1982

21. Zerhouni EA, Scott W, Baker R, Wharam MD, Siegelman SS. Invasive thymomas: Diagnosis and evaluation by computed tomography. *J Comput Assist Tomogr* 6:92–100, 1982

22. Clark KE, Foley WD, Lawson TL, Berland LL, Middison FE. CT evaluation of esophageal and upper abdominal varices. *J Comput Assist Tomogr* 4:510–515, 1980

23. Ross CR, McCauley DI, Naidich DP. Clinical images: Intrathoracic neurofibroma of the vagus nerve associated with bronchial obstruction. *J Comput Assist Tomogr* 6:406–408, 1982

24. Heiberg E, Wolverson MK, Hurd RN, Jagannad-Larad B, Sundaram M. Case report: CT recognition of traumatic rupture of the diaphragm. *AJR* 135:369–372, 1980

Subject Index